# SANT'EGIDIO'S DREAM

# SANT'EGIDIO'S DREAM

How a Catholic People's Movement
Is Meeting the Challenge of AIDS
in Africa and Shaping
the Future of Global Health

**ROBERTO MOROZZO DELLA ROCCA**
**TRANSLATED FROM ITALIAN BY CAROLINE SWINTON**

Georgetown University Press / Washington, DC

© 2024 Georgetown University Press. All rights reserved. No part of this book may be reproduced or utilized in any form or by any means, electronic or mechanical, including photocopying and recording, or by any information storage and retrieval system, without permission in writing from the publisher.

The publisher is not responsible for third-party websites or their content. URL links were active at time of publication.

Cataloging-in-Publication data is on file with the Library of Congress.

ISBN 978-1-64712-429-8 (hardcover)
ISBN 978-1-64712-430-4 (paperback)
ISBN 978-1-64712-431-1 (ebook)

∞ This paper meets the requirements of ANSI/NISO Z39.48-1992 (Permanence of Paper).

25 24      9 8 7 6 5 4 3 2 First printing

Printed in the United States of America

Cover design by Trudi Gershenov
Interior design by Paul Hotvedt

# Contents

*Foreword by Jeffrey D. Sachs vii*

*List of Abbreviations xv*

1 The Lost Years 1

2 The Failure of Prevention 58

3 DREAM 116

4 Looking into the Future 183

5 Access for All 212

*Afterword by Paul Elie 261*

*Bibliography 271*

*Index 287*

*About the Author 297*

# Foreword
## Jeffrey D. Sachs

The COVID-19 pandemic claimed around eighteen million lives worldwide from 2020 to 2022, despite the fact that it could have been successfully contained even before the widespread use of vaccines, as was accomplished by several countries in the Asia-Pacific region during 2020–21. The successful suppression of the pandemic may seem to be a technical matter—how to mobilize testing, quarantining, and other public health and social measures needed to slash or stop transmission of the virus—but it is painfully evident that the deeper problems have been cultural and ethical. The fact that the United States, the world's wealthiest country, incurred around 1.4 million deaths by the end of 2022, despite having all of the advantages of wealth and early access to vaccines, is a sign of deep moral crisis.

The problem in the US has been that day after day neither the president nor Congress nor governors nor mayors could clearly define the crisis. Some treated it as a crisis of economic lockdowns, requiring first a reopening of the economy. Some thought of it as a crisis of freedom—the freedom to choose not to wear face masks. Some imagined it was a duty of older people to incur COVID-19 deaths so that younger people could be free to go about their business. Very few addressed the pandemic as a moral crisis: the right of every person to have the chance for life—indeed a dignified life.

Ironically, if it had been approached as a moral crisis, it would have been addressed much more readily. Leaders would have understood the moral significance of exploring why some countries but not others had succeeded in containing the virus. They would have been impelled by this moral perspective into a deeper inquiry: what could our country, our city, our community be doing better? They would have learned the practical arts of public health and thereby have saved both lives and the economy.

More than three years after the onset of the pandemic, the moral crisis still includes the marginalization of the poor and Africans' lack of access to adequate, massive, and sustainable vaccination campaigns in conjunction with improved health services more generally. Yet many rich countries, including the United States, have continued essentially to ignore the fate of the poorer nations, even as they largely ignore the well-being of their own poorer citizens.

Roberto Morozzo della Rocca has written a brilliant moral tale, with rigorous evidence and a deep knowledge of the history of AIDS in Africa. Like COVID-19, AIDS is a scourge that claims vast numbers of lives, currently around one million per year worldwide, down from three million at the peak in 2005. Africa has long been the epicenter of the global AIDS pandemic. Like COVID-19, the AIDS epidemic can be suppressed—many countries have succeeded—but generally has not yet been. As with COVID-19, the ongoing AIDS failure reflects a deep global moral blindness to understand what is most important: to save lives and to stop transmission completely. If AIDS had been understood to be a moral crisis, it too could have been solved much more resolutely and successfully. For well over a decade, we have had the key tools to end AIDS. We have simply not deployed them, obfuscating endlessly about that failure.

In both pandemics, the plain fact is that those in power are very casual about the loss of life, so casual that they turn their gaze from millions of readily preventable deaths per year while offering every kind of excuse, self-justification, platitude, empty denial, and often outright lies for why we are not making any real effort to save those lives. Far too many people who are not in power play along in ignorance, complicity, resignation, or utter indifference.

I have had deep policy engagement in both epidemics, so I've seen the problems up close. In the mid-1990s, when I was director of the Harvard Institute for International Development, I visited an advisory project in Lusaka, Zambia. When I arrived at the Zambian finance ministry, I was informed by a colleague that several of our

Zambian counterparts had recently died. I gasped. "What do you mean 'died'?" "They returned to their villages and died of AIDS." "Returned to their villages? Why didn't they go to doctors instead?" "Here they don't go to doctors but instead go to home villages to die." Thus began my professional lessons in life, death, disease, and the so-called global community.

It took me some time to understand the basics of the situation. AIDS was a known global crisis, a disaster of historic proportions. Surely, I supposed, the experts were on top of it, doing all that they could. Surely, the outpouring of speeches, handwringing, expressions of sympathy and solidarity, and declarations by scientists all added up to a massive global mobilization to fight the disease. How little did I know. I went to look up how much the world was spending on fighting AIDS. Lo and behold, I couldn't find the numbers. I tried the same with malaria, another deadly disease that was raging—indeed resurging—across Africa. Once again, I could not find the numbers for what I thought must surely be a huge global effort to contain an ancient and deadly scourge.

My colleagues and I slashed away at the dense statistical undercover to gradually uncover the truth. There was, in fact, no global effort, no mass mobilization, no war against the killer diseases. There was talk, pablum, and platitudes, and lots of deaths—millions per year. A new millennium was arriving, not with the "health for all" blithely promised by the world's health ministers back in 1978 but with three full-blown epidemics—AIDS, tuberculosis, and malaria—with almost no real effort to fight them.

I am a macroeconomist, so I could do the arithmetic of life and death. A typical poor country at the time—in the year 2000, for example—had an income of about $500 per person per year. That country might at best be able to devote 3 percent of its meager national income to health care, with the rest directed to education, water, sanitation, roads, rail, ports, power, public administration, and other budget lines. Three percent of $500 is just $15 per person per year directed toward health care—not enough to stay alive in "normal" circumstances, much less in the face of three large epidemics.

But here was another basic truth. The US at the time had a national income of $40,000 per person, and other rich countries had similar levels. The combined annual income of those countries, with around a total population of one billion, came to around $40 trillion. Insecticide-treated bed nets to prevent malaria cost $5 each. Around eight hundred million nets were needed over a period of four years, at a cost of $4 billion over four years. This was easily affordable by the rich countries. The required sum was just $1 per person per year for the rich countries.

The life-and-death arithmetic of AIDS was the same. On the surface, it seemed that the new antiretroviral medicines that were developed in the 1980s and 1990s were simply too expensive, with annual price tags of some $20,000 or higher per patient. Yet those prices were the sticker prices charged by companies that owned patents on those medicines. They were monopolistic prices. The actual production cost of the drugs was under $1,000 per year and by the early 2000s in the low hundreds of dollars per year.

Here was an easily understandable situation. Millions of poor people were dying of epidemic diseases that their own governments were too impoverished to fight. The costs of containing these epidemics, and thereby of saving millions of lives, was a pittance for the rich countries. Surely it would not be too much to ask that the rich act in solidarity with the poor, especially since the costs were so tiny and the stakes were so large.

Properly understood, this is a simple moral problem and not one that is at all hard to solve. A small inconvenience in the rich countries—around $1 per year of increased global health spending for every $1,000 of national income—could save millions of lives each year. And there would be added benefits. Ending disease epidemics would enable economic growth and development. Countries in need of aid today would achieve self-sufficient budgets in the future. And healthy societies would quarrel less, fight less, recruit fewer child soldiers, and resist having to migrate or flee as refugees. In the cold language of Anglo-American economics, the societal benefits of global disease control far outweigh the costs.

Yet this problem has proved to be very difficult for the rich world to solve. The G7 governments have failed the test. They got stuck on the issue of poverty. The African countries were too poor to stay alive, ergo the people in those countries, in some sense, were condemned to die. Aid would not work, they wrongly claimed; it would be stolen. Africans would not heed medical advice. Africans "could not tell the time" for adherence to their medicines. Africans would see traditional healers rather than dispensers of life-saving medicines. The antimalaria bed nets would be stolen, lost in warehouses, used as wedding veils, used as fishing nets. All of these despicable (indeed morally shocking) excuses were made, and some were even perhaps believed by those who made such casual and false claims. Morozzo della Rocca knows the story well and tells it brilliantly: the countless denials, deceits, lies, confusions, and claims justifying doing nothing, all standing in the way of a straightforward policy to collect modest funds from the rich to save many of the poor.

One Harvard ethicist explained the situation as follows, justifying triaging. Think of us on a lifeboat. There are too many on the boat. Some will make it; others will not. I responded that I was not impressed with his argument. We are not on a lifeboat—we are on an aircraft carrier. Nobody has to die.

I spent much of the period from 1999 to 2008 arguing for increased funding to save lives and enable the poorest countries to get on the first rung of development. From 2000 to 2001, I was fortunate to chair the WHO Commission on Macroeconomics and Health under the gifted WHO director general Gro Harlem Brundtland, one of the great statespersons of our time. From 2001 to 2007, I served as special adviser to UN Secretary-General Kofi Annan, who brilliantly led the adoption of the Global Fund to Fight AIDS, Tuberculosis and Malaria. I worked closely with Bono as he sealed the deal with George W. Bush to increase US contributions to fight AIDS. And from 2007 to 2015, I served as special adviser to UN Secretary-General Ban Ki-moon as he pushed the UN into the full-scale war on malaria with free distribution of bed nets and antimalarial medicines and then led the adoption of the Sustainable Development Goals and the Paris Climate Agreement.

Amazingly, the Community of Sant'Egidio's flagship program DREAM (today the abbreviation for Disease Relief through Excellent and Advanced Means; originally Drug Resource Enhancement against AIDS and Malnutrition) started without having access to the first official funding efforts. It is enough to look at the dates, since

DREAM program's structure and infrastructure was set up from 1998 to 2002 when the first antiretroviral therapies were distributed in Mozambique, as this book describes. Not surprisingly, given its provenance, the DREAM program was launched successfully by moral force, not official approval or funding.

The victories that came were therefore moral victories, won on the ground by courageous moral leaders. The Community of Sant'Egidio showed the path to success. The organization knew full well the great moral stakes involved and decisively responded to them. Guided by a commitment to human life and dignity, Sant'Egidio solved every practical problem to bring life-saving HIV treatment to the poorest communities in Africa. Its DREAM program set the standard for achievement, professionalism, creativity, and decency in the fight against AIDS. DREAM has inspired countless others in this remarkable mix of moral integrity and public health excellence. During the past decade, DREAM has helped to build strong scientific and human infrastructure in sub-Saharan Africa, enabling countries of the region to tackle a growing range of health challenges, including the COVID-19 pandemic, and thereby contributing to a sustainable path for global health worldwide.

The story of AIDS recounted by Morozzo della Rocca is one of lives lost, battles won, and unfinished challenges that lie ahead. The AIDS epidemic can be ended, as he precisely details, by ensuring that enough people infected today are put on successful treatment, the so-called 90-90-90 Initiative. This goal is practicable and readily within operational and financial reach, yet the world is even more distracted and disjointed than in 2000. Back then, the US signed on to help lead the fight against AIDS, TB, and malaria. Even with the success of the Global Fund and the broad global recognition that it has received, the US and other rich nations have still not stepped up to fund the 90-90-90 Initiative. As a result, the AIDS crisis continues, albeit at a moderate rate, when it could and should have been ended as a public health crisis.

Pope Francis, the world's greatest moral leader, has powerfully diagnosed our situation as "the globalization of indifference." The failure of rich countries to sufficiently help poor ones is indeed morally reprehensible. With COVID-19, we have experienced the failure of the rich countries even to save themselves.

Our challenge is above all a global moral renewal. With a moral renewal we will garner the courage, energies, and finances to implement the technical solutions. Roberto Morozzo della Rocca's important and insightful book offers not only a history of past struggles but also a global roadmap for success in the future.

Jeffrey D. Sachs is a professor at Columbia University and president of the UN Sustainable Development Solutions Network.

# Abbreviations

| | |
|---|---|
| AIDS | acquired immunodeficiency syndrome |
| ANC | African National Congress |
| ART | antiretroviral therapy |
| ARV | antiretroviral |
| AZT | azidothymidine |
| BMI | body mass index |
| CDC | Centers for Disease Control and Prevention |
| DAR | DREAM archives in Rome |
| DRC | Democratic Republic of the Congo |
| DOT | directly observed therapy |
| DREAM | Drug Resource Enhancement against AIDS and Malnutrition (first iteration) Disease Relief through Excellent and Advanced Means (second iteration) |
| FAO | Food and Agriculture Organization |
| FRELIMO | Liberation Front of Mozambique |
| HAART | highly active antiretroviral therapy |
| HIV | human immunodeficiency virus |
| ILO | International Labour Organization |
| ISAARV | Initiative sénégalaise d'accès aux antirétroviraux |
| MISAU | Mozambican Ministry of Health |
| MSF | Médecins Sans Frontières |
| NGO | nongovernmental organization |
| PEPFAR | President's Emergency Plan for AIDS Relief |
| PMTCT | prevention of mother-to-child transmission |
| RENAMO | Mozambican National Resistance |
| TB | tuberculosis |
| UN | United Nations |

| | |
|---|---|
| UNAIDS | Joint United Nations Programme on HIV and AIDS |
| UNDP | United Nations Development Programme |
| UNESCO | United Nations Educational, Scientific and Cultural Organization |
| UNFPA | United Nations Population Fund |
| UNGASS | United Nations General Assembly special session |
| UNHCR | Office of the United Nations High Commissioner for Refugees |
| UNICEF | United Nations Children's Fund |
| UNODC | United Nations Office on Drugs and Crime |
| WFP | World Food Programme |
| WHO | World Health Organization |

# 1

# The Lost Years

Acquired immunodeficiency syndrome (AIDS) was first defined as a disease in its own right on June 5, 1981, in the journal of the Centers for Disease Control and Prevention (CDC), the highest public health authority of the United States. To be precise, only its clinical manifestations were described because at the time its cause was unknown. The article was written by Dr. Michael Gottlieb, an immunologist at the University of California, Los Angeles School of Medicine, who first had the impression that this was a new pathology by observing the inability of the immune system of some homosexual patients to cope with a usually benign form of pneumonia.[1] The main outbreak of the epidemic in the United States occurred in the gay communities in San Francisco and Los Angeles, but other specific contexts came to light almost immediately afterward: Haitian immigrants, hemophiliacs, and heroin addicts. There was still no official name for the disease, although some people called it GRID (gay-related immune deficiency). The acronym AIDS was coined in July 1982, although nobody was yet able to explain the origin and mechanisms of the pathology. The AIDS virus was identified and then certified as the cause of the disease in 1983–84 and generated the well-known dispute regarding the claim for the scientific discovery between the French professor Luc Montagnier and the American professor Robert Gallo. The virus itself was given the name "human immunodeficiency virus" (HIV) in 1986 by an international committee of experts.

In the years following, HIV/AIDS became a significant public health concern in the West. In the United States, the federal government, headed by President Ronald Reagan, was slow to address the disease or even to acknowledge it. In response members of the gay community, seeing the government as indifferent to (or contemptuous of) gay people, organized campaigns to raise public awareness, spur government funding of research and treatment, and combat discrimination against seropositive people and people with AIDS. In the beginning, though, there were not a vast number of cases. In 1984 four thousand people were estimated to have AIDS throughout the world, six hundred in San Francisco alone.[2] The figures in North America and Western Europe, including both new cases of infection and deaths, went initially from thousands of confirmed seropositive people to one and a half million in the 1990s.

Whether these figures are high or low, what was terrifying is the fact that the disease could not be treated. Fighting to live requires hope: it was not so much the clinically devastating and physically painful forms of full-blown AIDS that were frightening as the inevitability of the final outcome, which was in a sense anticipated by the stigma and by the loneliness that surrounded sick people. It was not the "loneliness of the dying" in modern civilization, made famous by Norbert Elias.[3] Rather, it was a moral and social censorship that made it very difficult to experience what, in the past, was defined as *ars moriendi*—the art of dying.[4] Through widespread (often superficial) coverage in the mass media, AIDS was characterized as "the gay plague" or the plague of modern times. People who knew they were HIV-positive saw no hope of survival, even though they were dying from full-blown AIDS about ten years after being infected. The virus's long period of incubation ends with the breakdown of the immune system and the outburst of various types of diseases that the body's defense system is no longer able to keep at bay. AIDS did not spare anyone. Famous personalities such as Freddie Mercury, Rock Hudson, Arthur Ashe, and Rudolf Nureyev succumbed, demonstrating the implacable character of the virus. Unlike other modern epidemics, such as tuberculosis and smallpox, AIDS was 100 percent deadly. This threat was exacerbated by the fact that HIV-positive people do not present symptoms, they have no organic lesions, they look healthy, and they can unknowingly spread the virus without their sex partners being aware of it. The invisible way HIV spreads through apparently healthy carriers is disheartening. The course of HIV/AIDS is very different from that of other diseases, such as smallpox in the past and Ebola today, where infection is immediately followed by the manifestation of the pathology, if not rapid death.

At first AIDS was considered a catastrophe affecting people in specific social groups— homosexuals, drug addicts, and hemophiliacs— but as soon as the percentage of those infected through heterosexual relationships increased, it became an object of fear among the general public. The Western health care systems started fighting AIDS in many different ways: health education regarding the disease and its forms of transmission, screening of the categories of people at risk, prevention based on the use of condoms, syringes distributed free of charge, checks on blood transfusions. Scientific experimentation in particular was extremely well funded. Although the research on AIDS did not identify a vaccine, it produced drugs, called antiretrovirals, that since 1996 have made it possible for HIV-positive people not only to survive but also to have a good quality of life, despite not actually being cured. The name "antiretroviral" comes from the fact that the virus known as HIV belongs to a group of so-called retroviruses. The antiretroviral drugs counter the replication of HIV in human cells—that is, in the lymphocytes that are essential for the immune system and that are otherwise taken over by HIV. These drugs are only effective as a combination; if taken individually, their efficacy is very short-lived because the virus mutates very easily and quickly produces variants that are resistant to the drugs. The treatment therefore consists of a cocktail of three antiretroviral drugs, the so-called triple antiretroviral therapy, also known as HAART (highly active antiretroviral therapy). The specific drugs that make up the cocktail can vary depending on how well the patient tolerates them and on the development of resistance. Thanks to the antiretroviral drugs, AIDS is no longer a death sentence.

After 1996 the alarm over AIDS in the Western public health care systems subsided almost as abruptly as it had surged just a few years earlier, but AIDS was still a priority concern. From an acute fatal disease, it had turned into a chronic one that was compatible with a normal life, on the condition that the patient scrupulously adhered to the therapy prescribed. Taking the antiretroviral drugs quickly reduces the viral load in the body fluids so the patient is almost no longer infectious at all.[5] The therapy is thus also an effective way to prevent the epidemic from spreading. In fact, the epidemic is reduced to the same extent as access to the therapy increases. Every year on December 1, World AIDS Day is celebrated in order to keep people aware of the disease and make sure it is not forgotten, especially by young people, who did not experience the emergency phase of the pandemic before 1996, resulting from reckless sexual behavior. For one day a year in which AIDS is dutifully remembered, the other 364 days go by with just a few words mentioned about it. This is a sign on one hand of lightheartedness and distraction but also of a battle that is basically considered won.

The discerning reader will have already noticed that what has been described up until now is the history of AIDS in the mind of the Western individual. The year 1996 is only the turning point in the Western story of AIDS, which is only a part of the whole picture. The first historical studies on AIDS, at the end of the 1980s, hardly talked about the rest of the world at all.[6] There was no perception that AIDS could be a greater threat for countries with limited resources than for the rich countries. There was also the question of collecting data. In sub-Saharan Africa, with the exception of Uganda, there were virtually no sentinel sites.[7] Neither were there any HIV tests for ascertaining whether a person was HIV-positive. People were dying from AIDS without having been diagnosed, so they just thought they were dying of dysentery, tuberculosis, pneumonia, cancer, or other pathologies. They did not have the slightest idea that that these were opportunistic infections caused by AIDS. This situation led the World Health Organization (WHO) to present a somewhat unconvincing estimate in 1989 of only twenty-three thousand cases of AIDS in all of Africa. At this time, AIDs was actually prevalent in approximately 10 percent of the populations of about a dozen African countries, and in Uganda, Zambia, and Zimbabwe the percentage was even higher.

The West had the scientific ability to identify AIDS and then to create the pharmacological arms to block the epidemic and save the infected people. However, because of the origin and development, prevalence and incidence, and morbidity and mortality of AIDS, it is mainly a question that concerns Africa and countries with limited resources, which used to be known as the third world. Needless to say, neither Africa nor these developing countries are to blame for AIDS. It is, however, a fact that in 1996, a watershed year from a therapeutic point of view, 22.6 million people in the world had HIV, 64 percent of whom lived in sub-Saharan Africa, whereas less than 5 percent lived in the West.[8] It is also a fact that in the same year, 74 percent of the 8.4 million full-blown cases of AIDS in the world were in sub-Saharan Africa. AIDS is therefore primarily an African story. Westerners tended to ignore its global epicenter until 1996, when they somehow managed to contain the epidemic in their countries and then realized that in other countries HIV was anything but under control. They had been absorbed by their own hardships and indulging in their ethnocentrism. The peripheral areas, however, as far as AIDS was concerned, were involved to a far greater extent than this alleged center that had been determined by the West. Besides, there is a marked difference between AIDS and other epidemics in the history of man (the plague, cholera, smallpox, etc.), which is that AIDS is not a catastrophe limited to a certain geographical area or a period in time but rather is a long-lasting and global event. AIDS is the bitter fruit and a pathology of globalization.

There are several interconnected theories regarding the origins of the pandemic. The most commonly accepted hypothesis is that HIV spread as a result of the end of the isolation of the thick equatorial forests in Central Africa: southeastern Cameroon, the Republic of the Congo, and the Democratic Republic of the Congo (DRC; originally the Belgian Congo and called Zaire from 1965 to 1997). This is where the transmission of the original virus from animals to man allegedly happened. The progenitor of HIV, or rather the viral matter that later evolved through various mutations into the different HIV strains that are known today, is said to have passed to one of the few humans living in that nearly impenetrable place. This apparently happened at the beginning of the twentieth century, according to the hypotheses accredited by molecular phylogenetic studies.[9] The host animal from which the progenitor of HIV probably jumped to the human species may well have been a chimpanzee, identified as such by scientists after years of exhausting studies of various nonhuman primates. In Africa many types of nonhuman primates also had viruses that were the forefathers of HIV, and the researchers called them SIV (simian immunodeficiency virus) because of the similarity with the abbreviation of the human immunodeficiency virus that was believed to be its more or less close relative.

However, these nonhuman primates were not threatened by the pathogen that they had probably harbored for thousands if not millions of years. The predecessor of HIV was dangerously active in chimpanzees, though, which was a sign that they had been infected not too long before, maybe a few hundred years ago. The passage of the immunodeficiency virus from chimpanzees to humans may have happened after the chimpanzees were captured, while they were being slaughtered, after they had been found dead, or at any other moment during which men with even only minimal or unnoticed wounds and cuts touched raw, bloody meat, causing contact with infected blood and biological fluids.

It is more than likely that the virus adapted to the human carriers and gradually reached the closest urban centers, first settling in the stations along the river and then in the emporiums and towns, up to the two colonial capitals that faced each other along the Congo River: Brazzaville, which belonged to France, and Léopoldville, which belonged to Belgium and was named Kinshasa after colonialism. Colonialism probably encouraged the migration and spread of the virus due to the increase in trade and improved communication routes. HIV was found in human blood samples collected in Léopoldville and Kinshasa in 1959 and fortuitously preserved, despite political upheavals and civil wars.[10] If in this area during those years the disease was already claiming its first victims, it was not identified, as it had not been identified in the previous decades in the cases in which it had manifested. In both the French Congo and the Belgian Congo, the life expectancy of the local population was low, death was treated as a matter of fact, medicine was a luxury available to only the affluent few, and little attention was paid to the fate of ordinary people. If a doctor confirmed the cause of death, which rarely occurred, what was recorded was one of the opportunistic infections or forms of cancer that typically follow HIV immunodeficiency during full-blown AIDS. Then there is the fact that because life in Central Africa was so precarious, when HIV-positive people died from a great variety of causes before they even had full-blown AIDS, nobody noticed anything unusual about it. People there had always died from unknown infections and fevers. In any case there was never such a large number of suspicious deaths that they had to be investigated, which might have stimulated the identification of a new disease.

In the meantime, year after year, among the increasing number of infected people, HIV replicated, and continuous mutation was taking place. It was becoming increasingly aggressive and deadly. If the pathogen circulated in man at the beginning of the twentieth century, it had first moved slowly and invisibly as an infection with low morbidity, until some specific conditions had given it a boost. At this point one should remember that Léopoldville was developing into a crowded city with multitude forms of trade, a hub for the coming and going of goods and of travelers by every means of transport, including airplanes. On the other hand, one could also mention a modern aspect of Africa in the 1910s, which was the use of the hypodermic syringe for mass health campaigns. There were obviously no disposable syringes, and the needles and syringes were never sterilized between one injection and the next. At best they were rinsed. Campaigns to fight sleeping sickness and venereal diseases were carried out with hundreds of thousands of injections that used the same limited number of syringes.[11] And this continued for decades.

How did the disease get from Léopoldville in 1959 to San Francisco and Los Angeles in 1981? The early spread of AIDS among Haitians living in the United States is an indication that it came from New York City and Miami, not from California. The route may have been as follows. The Belgian Congo became independent in 1960, but it had no doctors, teachers, or managers of any kind because the Belgians had not trained anyone before they left.[12] The United Nations thought it would be a good idea to send to the new country temporary staff from Haiti, where there was no lack of doctors and teachers, despite François "Papa Doc" Duvalier's dictatorship. It looked like an ideal solution, since Haitians were Blacks of African origin whose mother tongue was French, the same language that colonialism had given the Belgian Congo. Whether this unusual experiment in cooperation was successful or not, halfway through the 1960s the Congolese people were already occupying the positions left by the Belgians, and one by one the Haitians started going back to the Caribbean. As someone observed, the Haitians arrived in the DRC as single men, but they had no intention of living in solitude.[13] The rest is easy to imagine. According to laboratory research carried out on samples of that period, the most lethal HIV strain, the one of the subsequent pandemic, probably reached Haiti around 1966. Some men, just back from their experience in the DRC, are said to have soon moved to the United States, often New York or Miami. Moreover, there was a flourishing blood trade on the Caribbean island at the end of the 1960s. The plasma was collected from thousands of habitual donors with particular industrial mechanical processes that mixed the blood, so one infected donor would contaminate the whole product that was obtained. The plasma was exported to the United States at the rate of sixty to seventy thousand liters a year, a practice that was stopped in 1972 for political reasons.[14]

The facts and timing match. HIV would certainly have reached the United States even without the Haitians but probably later on. The first Californians who died of AIDS had been infected at the beginning of the 1970s and were carriers, without knowing it, for about ten years. It is not illogical to think that the fact that they were infected has something to do with the emigration to North America of Haitians who had worked in DRC. Miami is an hour-and-a-half flight from Port-au-Prince, and this is where the infection was first noticed among the Haitians and then duly reported to the CDC. It was the same immunodeficiency syndrome that Michael Gottlieb had observed among gays in California.[15] Recent studies on blood samples reveal the presence of HIV in New York as early as 1970, and in this case too "the genetic evidence supports the theory that the virus came from the Caribbean, perhaps Haiti."[16] If the virus was not already in San Francisco, it would soon be active there. HIV may have spread fast because of the export of infected blood products from Haiti to the United States, and there was also the other highly vulnerable group of people, according to the initial clinical observations of the disease—hemophiliacs.

In conclusion, the Haitians who went to the DRC may have been the main transoceanic carriers of HIV, from the DRC to Haiti and then to Miami and New York and possibly elsewhere in the United States. They were direct carriers, with their bodies, or indirect carriers, through the bags containing their blood. They had absolutely no idea of the danger that they represented when they came back from Africa, considering that several years would pass before their HIV would become full-blown AIDS, which was in any case an unknown pathology at the time. This chain of transmission of HIV, which is passed on above all through the blood, in sexual intercourse, and in blood transfusions, appears from authoritative studies to be plausible,[17] so the link between AIDS and intercontinental globalization from its very early manifestations is extremely strong.

The above observations reflect recent studies. However, from the middle of the 1980s, researchers (or, more precisely, their epidemiological studies) had pointed the finger at Africa and its nonhuman primates and started to detect the presence, in some species, of viruses that were more or less similar to HIV. This meant that the origin of HIV was not only the subject of academic discussions among Western scientists but also of controversies between the Global North and Global South.

African intellectuals and politicians, out of patriotism and their ideologies, contested the thesis that HIV had come from their continent.[18] They considered the thesis defamatory and racist. On the other hand, there was no shortage of Western authors who, despite confirming the African genesis of HIV, blamed European colonialism for spreading it, since colonialism is what allegedly caused the cultural and environmental changes that freed the virus from its original context, made it aggressive and deadly, and spread it.[19] It was probably the exploitation of the land and the colonial powers' trade-expansion strategies, as well as the syringes used time and again by the colonial public health systems for preventive and therapeutic campaigns and mass vaccinations, that were responsible for AIDS.[20] Considering Africa as the origin of the virus, this interpretation held Westerners responsible for spreading AIDS. The African élite could have made this their own interpretation. The people's self-respect would have been protected: another historical evil in Africa would have been attributed to colonialism. However, the narrative was already going a different way.

Since the 1980s there was a tendency in the sub-Saharan countries to deny the existence of the epidemic. Whether or not the political leaders, intellectuals, élites, and doctors of every field and level were irritated by the Western assertions that HIV may have originated in Africa or by the consequential controversy about alleged African sexual promiscuity, they did exclude the possibility that there could be a serious AIDS epidemic because they considered it to be a decadent Westerners' foreign disease. African governments accepted advice and funds in order to carry out propaganda to prevent AIDS. Nonetheless, there was a widespread belief that if HIV was really spreading in Africa, it had come from outside the continent, perhaps imported by homosexuals on safari. The stigma that characterized the way the disease was experienced socially in the West, at least in its first fifteen years, and that promised to be even more cruel in Africa (as indeed it is), frightened the authorities of the sub-Saharan countries, who did not want to acknowledge an epidemic whose fate was played out in sex and blood. Nonetheless, denial, skepticism, and disbelief are in contrast with what happened and is happening in the continent. All in all, with prevalence rates that vary from area to area, HIV is definitely present, even if one does not want to see it.

Apart from the HIV-positive blood samples of 1959 found in Léopoldville, cases of AIDS were retrospectively reported in the late 1970s in Tanzania, Uganda, and again in the former Belgian Congo, which had been renamed Zaire.[21] In the 1980s the first African countries that saw vast numbers of cases of HIV-positive people and therefore experienced subsequent massacres were in the middle of the continent: Uganda, Zaire, Zambia, Rwanda, Burundi, the Central African Republic, and Zimbabwe (but also Ivory Coast, which is in West Africa). In the 1990s the epidemic spread rapidly toward eastern and southern Africa, and South Africa soon had the highest number of infected people in the world—millions of people—which is even more shocking considering the size of its population was nothing like the planet's demographic giants. In 1990, while South Africa was setting up an epidemic surveillance network, the percentage of seropositive adults was 0.73 percent; around ten years later it had increased incredibly to 20 percent. However, at the turn of the century, countries near South Africa had the world's highest adult HIV/AIDS rates: Botswana 38.8 percent, Zimbabwe 33.7 percent, Swaziland 33.4 percent, and Lesotho 31.0 percent.[22] The situation was slightly different in West Africa, where French is spoken in most of the countries.

AIDS was less devastating there because its morbidity was limited by a less aggressive strain (the so-called HIV-2[23]) and by a measure of economic and social stability as well as by practices encouraged by religious customs, such as circumcision.

There are many causes for the vast spread of HIV/AIDS in sub-Saharan Africa, and they vary from area to area. In short, the prevalence of HIV/AIDS in Africa can be linked to ongoing war, migration, the national health care systems' organizational and technical issues, chronic lack of education, and ancestral and deep-rooted social customs such as polygamy and levirate marriages. However, it can also be linked to even more particular African characteristics, such as the often more superstitious than scientific approach to reality. The harsh stigma that for decades destroyed HIV-infected Africans made them people to avoid literally like the plague because of their transgressions—because they were guilty, cursed. So, relatively few acknowledged that they were seropositive to the day they died, let alone took precautions to avoid infecting other people.

Much has been said about the supposed sexual promiscuity of Black Africans, which it is said also contributed to spread the virus. Regarding this point, it is important to make a difference between prejudice and reality. Polygamy is sometimes taken for sexual promiscuity. Moreover, phenomena such as transactional sex—that is, sex in exchange for food or protection, not necessarily with more than one partner in the same period—depends on the objective poverty and fragility of the women. On the other hand, in Africa, like elsewhere, there is the ideology of virility. It is undeniable that Africa has very unbalanced gender relationships to the detriment of the woman, who is dominated by the man and not really protected at all. The massive migrations of male labor, in particular to southern African mining townships, do not imply sexual promiscuity a priori but rather a sex market, there one uncontrolled and consisting almost completely of single men who contracted HIV and spread it when they got back home. Philippe Denis, a scholar of southern Africa, offers plausible observations:

> The research on sexual behaviour carried out at the beginning of
> the 1990s in several African countries with a high rate of seropositive

people did not provide significantly different results from those obtained in Western countries or in African countries with a low rate of seropositive people. . . . Variations observed in the prevalence of seropositive people are due more to factors regarding the transmission [of the virus], like the lack of circumcision or the prevalence of sexually transmitted diseases than to the frequency of high-risk behaviour. Sexuality certainly plays a role in the transmission of AIDS but in a more complex way than previously believed. It is not necessary to postulate intense sexual activity in order to explain the rapid transmission of the virus among people living in towns and in the suburbs. It is the general instability that makes sexual behaviour dangerous, an instability that has grown, even for decades, due to urbanization, migrant labour, poverty.[24]

Let us now take a small step forward in order to deal with the decisive issue on AIDS in sub-Saharan Africa, the one regarding the therapeutic possibilities. At the beginning of the twenty-first century, AIDS had been treated in the West for four years. The therapies had proved to be valid and reliable, despite the fear of resistances and the evolution of the virus. Nonetheless, similar treatments for AIDS in Africa remained purely hypothetical. The point of view of the international development agencies and donors was that "in sub-Saharan Africa, AIDS treatment was thought of as largely unfeasible to implement, to finance, and to sustain at any level of responsibility or success (i.e. impractical to 'roll out' or 'scale up,' as it were)."[25] Treating AIDS in Africa was taboo, and whoever violated this taboo was considered idiotic. There were an increasing number of documents, guidelines, warnings, and standpoints all saying that the right conditions did not exist for treating AIDS in countries with limited resources, the way it is treated in the first world.

The figures in 2000 were terrifying. The number of people infected by HIV increased throughout the world to 36.1 million. In North America and Western Europe there were fewer than 1.5 million seropositive people. Two thirds of the total number (25.3 million) were in sub-Saharan Africa, even though it contained only one tenth of the world's population. The prevalence rate in African adults was 8.8 percent, in North American adults it was 0.6 percent, and in

Western Europeans it was 0.24 percent.[26] Eight countries in the world had prevalence rates in the adult population of over 20 percent, and they were all in in the south and east of the African continent: South Africa, Botswana, Lesotho, Swaziland, Namibia, Zimbabwe, Zambia, and Kenya, where in the 1990s the epidemic had progressed exponentially.

HIV-positive people in rich countries had been able to use antiretroviral drugs since 1996, and they no longer died from AIDS if their treatment was started before their immune system was too badly compromised. This has already been said: AIDS, which kills fast, has become a sustainable chronic disease. HIV-positive Africans, on the other hand, were left to their fate: four-fifths (2.4 million) of the 3 million people who died of AIDS were from poor sub-Saharan countries. Moreover, 17 million of the 21.8 million people who died of AIDS at the beginning of the pandemic were African. In addition, 3.8 million of the 5.3 million newly infected people lived in sub-Saharan Africa. Ninety percent of all children with HIV were infected in sub-Saharan Africa, generally through mother-to-child transmission. These children were destined not to live long—in fact, 40 percent of them died within their first year of life. Many others, even healthy children, became orphans because AIDS killed their parents: 95 percent of all AIDS orphans live in Africa.

A very relevant fact, although poorly highlighted at the time, is that HAART lowers a person's viral load—the amount of viral particles circulating in body fluids—to the extent that their levels become so low that they are undetectable. The virus does not disappear, but the possibility of transmission is reduced practically to zero, and it is no longer present in the plasma and other body fluids, which are the vehicles for infection. The person is no longer infectious. This also explains how it is possible that in the year 2000 there were 75,000 newly infected people in the Western world and in countries below the Sahara, as mentioned, there were 3.8 million. Where the treatment is available, the level of infectivity is reduced until it disappears. On the other hand, the international discussion on AIDS in Africa concentrated on prevention alone and denied treatment. In the West the treatment was provided alongside prevention and was itself a form of prevention. The same can be said for public spending. For example, in its 1993 health budget, the United States allocated $4.9 billion for AIDS, only 12.6 percent of which was for prevention.[27] Conversely, throughout the 1990s, in countries with limited resources, including the African countries, funds were allocated for prevention alone. This basically meant stating how dangerous HIV was, teaching people to fear it, providing information regarding its transmission, distributing condoms, and abandoning infected people to the inevitable prospect of their death.

The red herring that was useful to distract from the inaction of the global aid community regarding AIDS in Africa was the hope of a vaccine that would solve the problem. This was what those in favor of prevention alone were really thinking: since there would soon be a vaccine, there was no point in setting up therapeutic regimens. The identification of a vaccine seemed to be just round the corner. According to a famous statement made by Margaret Heckler, the US secretary of health and human services in 1984, "a vaccine [will be] ready for testing in approximately two years."[28] The research was never completed, though, and forty years after the first cases of AIDS in the West there is still no vaccine. In around 2000 several researchers announced the imminent identification of a vaccine, but nothing ever came of it. A vaccine would make it possible to overcome the obstacles that are presented in order to deny the treatment of AIDS in Africa, from the high cost of the drugs to the shortcomings of the public health care systems—but there was and is still no vaccine.

In 2000 Roy Anderson, an epidemiologist from the University of Oxford, wrote, "Drugs can reduce [the length of time that somebody is infectious] to some extent, by bringing people's viral load down to the point where they will not pass on the disease. But effective therapies are currently expensive and . . . are unlikely to become cheap enough for routine use there [in developing countries] for some time."[29] Anderson knew that treating meant preventing; nonetheless, he was not against people who denied treatment to Africans who had AIDS in order to concentrate on prevention that was totally unrelated to any hypothesis of treatment. It was mainly the economic factors that disconcerted him. If this could happen to an epidemiologist who was aware of how the disease spread through a country, it was even more likely that those who did not know much about these dynamics would deny people with AIDS in Africa the hope of ever becoming healthy again. These decision-makers were, for example, politicians who were afraid of the risks involved in taking action, health care managers concentrating on their budgets, bookkeeping-style economists, theoretical researchers of human science, doctors who were not specialized in viruses and epidemics, and so on. How was it possible, though, to accept that the therapy was unavailable in South Africa, Botswana, Lesotho, Swaziland, Namibia, Zimbabwe, Zambia, and Kenya, where the prevalence of AIDS was between 20 percent and 40 percent of the adult population and where the life expectancy was plummeting to forty years after just having reached sixty? In Uganda and in Mozambique, despite lower prevalence rates, life expectancy was already under forty years because it had been low in the first place. AIDS is a multiplier of poverty. It mainly kills people of productive age. Large numbers of teachers, doctors, nurses, technicians, farmers, miners, drivers, and builders died, and African societies lost their invaluable professional figures, crucial for the development of their future.[30] The young people were affected most. Consequently, the macroeconomic indicators showed that every sub-Saharan country was in trouble. In 2000 in the West, which was well supplied with antiretroviral drugs, 0.4 percent of the adult population was seropositive, compared to the above-mentioned average in Africa of 8.8 percent, with peaks of nearly 40 percent in the southern regions. Without drugs, prevention was ineffective, and it was easy for the epidemic to snowball.

## THE UNAIDS POLICY

From the beginning of the 1990s, the global leader in the fight against AIDS was the WHO, the United Nations agency responsible for public health. The Joint United Nations Programme on HIV and AIDS (UNAIDS) was set up in 1995 to work within the network of UN agencies and was given the task of coordinating the fight against HIV/AIDS. Scandinavia and France in particular wanted UNAIDS because in their opinion the WHO, whose president at the time was Hiroshi Nakajima from Japan, was insufficiently committed to the fight against AIDS and paid even less attention to the epidemic's social implications. The promoters and directors of UNAIDS aimed to tell a different story from that of the WHO, as though a modern minister of social affairs was contradicting an old-fashioned minister of health. They insisted that AIDS was far more than a medical issue and that in order to deal with the epidemic a multifaceted approach was necessary. The UNAIDS buzzword was "multisectorial," which dominated international development jargon for about ten years. It was no coincidence that the poor countries repeated it obsessively in the projects they presented to international donors in order to obtain funds. What did it mean, though? UNAIDS argued that before being epidemiological, the approach to the HIV pandemic had to be social, political, pedagogical, and demographic.[31] The medical aspect was considered marginal. The skills of the UN agencies that did not work in the field of health care therefore became very useful. For example, the United Nations Population Fund (UNFPA) agreed with UNAIDS that HIV spread because of poverty, armed conflict, "gender inequality in sexual and social relations," and problems regarding "sexual and reproductive health," and it deplored that "yet, research into the social causes, context and consequences of the epidemic is still often heavily influenced by the health perspective."[32] AIDS was therefore taken out of the purely medical context. UNAIDS was set up in order to direct the work of its various cosponsoring UN agencies in a social sense (a euphemism so as not to say that UNAIDS, at least in its own field of competence, considered them subordinate).[33] In 2006 the epidemiologist Anne Buvé, of the Institute of Tropical Medicine in Antwerp, wrote,

> Several social, economic and cultural characteristics of African societies contribute to aggravate the vulnerability of their populations with respect to HIV, and in particular the women's inferiority status, poverty, rapid urbanization and modernization, and above all war and armed conflict. . . . The only way out [of the HIV/AIDS epidemic] consists in bearing in mind the general contextual factors that contribute to the spread of HIV and to take them into consideration by developing programmes to control the epidemic. This reasoning led to the dissolution of the WHO Global Programme on AIDS and the creation of UNAIDS, a joint programme of the

United Nations that brought together 9 international agencies in a multi-sectorial approach to fight the AIDS epidemic.[34]

UNAIDS was created in the context of an ideological battle that had lasted since the 1980s and that continued for a long time. The WHO continued to state that AIDS was a medical issue and would have preferred to deal with AIDS itself. Other UN agencies that were also interested in dealing with it said it was more of a social question than one regarding public health. On one hand, HIV/AIDS was perceived as a pandemic that was to be dealt with by doctors, public health specialists, and local and international health care organizations with preventive health care activities and as far as deemed possible with treatment for infected people. On the other, HIV/AIDS was considered a societal issue for which "responses have to take account of cultural context, sexual practice, reality and denial, the status of woman and education of girls,"[35] an approach that was basically prevention from a social point of view. UNAIDS's criticism was that the WHO culture offered technical short-term solutions—simply medical solutions—that were destined to be ineffective because they did not address the multiple factors that caused HIV to spread.

The reason for setting up UNAIDS was valid enough. AIDS, above all in poor countries, was definitely a social issue regarding poverty, development, education, human rights, war, and migration. It was unrealistic to prevent and treat it without taking this into account. Nonetheless, while broadening the discussion, UNAIDS marginalized the medical approach. In this way it tended to avoid the patient's main need, which is to be treated and to survive. Treatment is given immediately; cultural changes take generations. Diseases are treated there and then; mentalities evolve like geological epochs. The UN's response to the pandemic ended up being essentially political: *leadership at all levels* and *political advocacy* were the UNAIDS leitmotifs, where "at all levels" meant from the heads of state to the people, all the way to the individual people with AIDS. This is what the executive director of UNAIDS, Peter Piot, said, after a visit to Uganda in 2000: "I met with women who are preparing their children to be orphans, organizing everything from memory books to sustainable arrangements for micro-credit. These women are truly leaders."[36] Maybe those mothers would have preferred to stay alive thanks to the antiretroviral drugs, which in 2000 were already available in developed countries, so their children would not become orphans at risk, rather than be recorded as "truly leaders" in UN records.

All the agencies within the framework of the UN system are traditionally rivals in regard to resources, skills, and prerogatives. UNAIDS spent its first years affirming its coordination of the UN agencies regarding AIDS. UNICEF naturally did not appreciate receiving instructions on breastfeeding in poor societies, the WHO did not like feeling observed when drawing up health care guidelines, and the World Bank did not like being controlled when allocating its funds, nor did UNHCR like being told how to organize refugee camps, and so on. UNAIDS publications indicate political clashes among various agencies in the UN, which took up a great deal of energy. As far as external action was concerned, UNAIDS did not have many resources, and in any case it did not appear to intend carrying out operations on the field. It was conceived as a political advocacy and lobbying device, which in order to sponsor the cause it stood for collected data on the pandemic, wrote annual reports, and hired experts and consultants. Moreover, in every country under its patronage, it created national committees to fight AIDS, including the local representatives of the various UN agencies. One particular feature of UNAIDS was its sort of ongoing statistical studies, since it owed much of its acclaim to the graphs and tables that were continuously generated. Another peculiarity of UNAIDS was its criticism of the bureaucratic systems, almost as though it claimed it was not guilty of what is considered the original UN sin.

UNAIDS was directed by the above-mentioned Peter Piot, who, by virtue of this position, which he held from 1995 to 2008, was one of the most influential decision-makers in the worldwide fight against AIDS at an institutional level. Piot, a Flemish microbiologist, had characteristics such as ability, instinct, and a politician's sense of opportunity.[37] He was informal, at ease in the politically correct Anglo-American world, jealous of his supervision of the AIDS planet, and had spent many years in the higher levels of the UN, where he was an undersecretary for Boutros Boutros-Ghali, Kofi Annan, and Ban Ki-moon. In his first years as the director of UNAIDS, Piot only provided support for countries with limited resources in terms of prevention of AIDS, since he considered it unfeasible to provide therapy.[38] The results of the pilot projects for therapies with antiretroviral drugs promoted by UNAIDS discouraged adopting the triple therapy in Africa.[39] UNAIDS basically suffered from a superiority-inferiority complex with respect to the WHO, an agency with infinitely greater traditions, skills, funds, and staff. UNAIDS felt that the WHO, to whose alleged incapacity it owed its creation, was a detrimental entity, to be put under surveillance, despite the fact that Piot himself, after a few years as executive director of UNAIDS, started cultivating his aspiration to become the director of the WHO.[40] This is the most prestigious position in the world for people involved in public health care. Moreover, within the health care sector, the senior positions of the UN system (and of similar organizations such as the Global Fund and PEPFAR[41]) are relatively interchangeable: we can find the same names of senior executives in different years at the top of UNAIDS, the WHO, UNICEF, the World Bank, and so on, not to mention in the senior management of the UN itself.

The approach developed by UNAIDS was supposed to inspire all the UN agencies and consequently determine the decisions of each country, all the more so if they needed international assistance, as was the case for every single sub-Saharan country. The African countries certainly did not dare criticize the guidelines that came from New York or Geneva (the latter being the headquarters of UNAIDS and the WHO), on pain of incurring financial retaliation and cuts in aid. So, from 1996 to 2002, when AIDS exploded in Africa, all Piot and the senior management of the agencies involved talked about with respect to the fight against the epidemic, especially for the sub-Saharan countries, was prevention.[42] Treating the disease, on the other hand, was denied. Since the "magic bullet," whether it be the AIDS vaccine that had been announced several times but never made or the drug to kill the virus for people who were already infected, did not exist, and since the antiretroviral drugs were excluded a priori, the idea was to solve the problem through a "social immune system": "AIDS can only be curbed through a sustained social mobilization that systematically reduces vulnerability. . . . Reducing vulnerability to AIDS and its impact is about creating a social vaccine or, better still, a social immune system that continually learns, builds and rebuilds itself in protecting against the impact of AIDS."[43]

In the Western world, as already mentioned, providing therapy also meant preventing infection because the viral load in patients who were treated was undetectable and they were no longer contagious. This observation was not considered valid for HIV-positive Africans, who were denied the therapy that Western patients were given. Even if Africans with AIDS were treated, they were still considered plague spreaders. In a chilling epidemiological perspective, what was important was to bring down the number of new infections, not to save lives, without realizing that treating would also mean preventing the spread of infection.

## 1996–2002: PREVENTION VERSUS TREATMENT

How was it possible to get to the point of considering prevention alone, in the nonpharmacological sense, as legitimate for Africa? What strategic decisions did the international institutions responsible for fighting AIDS adopt? In July 1996 the XI International AIDS Conference in Vancouver announced the great results achieved with a combination of three antiretroviral drugs, which drastically reduced the viral load and developed very infrequent resistances, unlike the single and double antiretroviral therapies that HIV always managed to counter successfully. The Vancouver conference's motto was "One World, One Hope"—famous last words. It was immediately clear that the triple therapy was not going to be for everyone. Also apparent was that the divide between the rich and the poor was accepted. In 2007 three senior officials of UNAIDS, the WHO, and the Global Fund wrote the following, partially in order to justify themselves: "Delivery of complex treatment regimens needed advanced health systems, and the cost exceeded by several orders of magnitude the average overall health budgets of most developing countries. These apparently insurmountable obstacles allowed the worldwide community to ignore the inequity between rich and poor countries with regard to treatment access."[44] After the Vancouver conference, all that most of the international community's public health experts offered the countries of sub-Saharan Africa was "surveillance, education, information,"[45] which continued for over five years, often within a framework of a general political and social mobilization.[46] Basically nothing clinical or therapeutic was provided, so seropositive people were all destined to die. In other words, "the international consensus recommended prevention in the countries of the Global South, rather than treating AIDS; none of the international institutions were prepared to finance therapeutic treatments."[47] What counted were the economic reasons (treatments that were considered too expensive for the small health care budgets of the countries in the Global South, prices of the antiretroviral drugs that were high everywhere, an imbalance between the cost of the treatment per inhabitant and the GDP per inhabitant, so a patient would have cost far more than what little they produced for the country) and the medical reasons (presumed incapacity of the weak public health systems to take on complex treatments, the presumed inability of Africans to adhere to the treatments, and fear that the treatments taken badly would lead to resistances and serious virological consequences).

One of the few people who took "One World, One Hope" seriously was French president Jacques Chirac, who said in Ivory Coast on December 7, 1997,

> We do not have the right to accept that there are by now two ways to fight AIDS: treating patients in developed countries, and just preventing infection in the South of the world. . . . Watching without reacting to the onset of a two-speed epidemic would be shocking, unacceptable and contrary to one of the most elementary principles of solidarity. . . . We have to do everything possible to extend the benefits of the new therapeutic treatments to the poor populations in Africa and in the rest of the world, the populations that are the most harrowed by the disease.[48]

This appeal provoked a wave of contrary reactions. Michael W. Adler of University College London Medical School slammed France's idea in the *Lancet*:

> While the annual per capita health budget in most African countries is less than US$10, triple antiretroviral therapy against AIDS in the

developed world costs $12,000–14,000 per patient per year. Calculations based upon a lower per patient cost of $7,000, and treating all 1.4 million African AIDS cases, would cost US$10 billion per year for drugs alone, more than 30 times the amount currently spent annually by international donors for AIDS programs in the entire developing world. Basic infrastructural requirements would have to be met [for] antiretrovirals [to be] made widely available, ranging from HIV screening and counseling to the provision of clean water with which to consume the required 20–30 tablets per day. High program costs will challenge long-term sustainability. Universal access to care and treatment for HIV infection and AIDS is not a reality in the developed world, let alone feasible in developing countries. Given the competing health care priorities in developing countries, the high costs of antiretroviral agents, poor infrastructure, and inability to sustain such a program, the French initiative is ill-advised and foolish public health practice.[49]

The international development agencies unanimously confirmed that it was economically and technically impossible to provide antiretroviral treatments to the poor countries. A chorus of donor countries proceeded to say that treatment was unsustainable "given the costs and the parlous nature of most developing countries' health services."[50] In a UNAIDS–WHO report of June 1998, this is presented as obvious and beyond doubt: "Such [antiretroviral] therapies are expensive, hard to administer, and require regular medical monitoring."[51] In particular, no developed country had any intention to take on people to treat for their whole lives and bind the contributors with no time limits.

After Vancouver it was clear that if AIDS were treated, it was no longer necessarily a death sentence. So, UNAIDS devised a drug-access initiative on an experimental basis, which aimed to treat around four thousand HIV-positive people in Ivory Coast, Uganda, Chile, and Vietnam with antiretroviral drugs. The initiative started in 1998 and was presented as a research survey in order to understand what to do in the Global South. Nonetheless, it looked as though it had been devised in order to confirm that antiretroviral drugs could not be used in Africa. In Ivory Coast the government funded the cost of the treatment, but the forecasts of the expenses were wrong, and the antiretroviral drugs were not supplied continuously. In addition, the treatments were basically ineffective, especially the double therapies that were adopted at the beginning, instead of the triple therapies, which are the only ones that can counter HIV. The outcome of the pilot program was disappointing. It was even worse in Uganda. In this case, the patients were asked to pay the full cost of their treatments. The drugs were procured from the multinational pharmaceutical companies, following agreements mediated by UNAIDS at a discount of 40 percent—that is, $7,200 per person for a year. Many patients ran out of money and abandoned the treatment, consequently developing resistances to the first-line antiretroviral drugs, which prevented them from resuming the treatment had they been able to. They resigned themselves to dying. This phenomenon is said to have affected three-quarters of these patients.[52] At the beginning of their treatment, 80 percent of the Ugandan patients had a CD4 count of less than 200 per milliliter of blood, a very low number for these lymphocyte cells that act as soldiers for the immune system.[53] Their immune system had therefore been seriously compromised. Moreover, 34 percent of the patients were at the final stage of the disease. A cohort of patients who were difficult to treat had been selected, with a high number of terminal cases, and not surprisingly fifteen months later only 54 percent of the patients were still alive and under treatment. The initiative was started in Chile and Vietnam in 2000. In Chile, a country with Western characteristics, the results were positive. In Vietnam the focus was on mother-to-child prevention of HIV by administering one antiretroviral drug, Nevirapine, which was erroneously believed to be particularly effective as a single-dose therapy in countries with limited resources.[54] Even though the desperate African patients' capability to adhere to the therapy turned out, surprisingly enough, to be the same as, if not superior to, that observed in the patients in the West, UNAIDS claimed to have proof that at that time it was too difficult to treat AIDS in Africa. It would be hard to imagine a more clumsily organized drug-access initiative. In any case, UNAIDS drew evidence from this initiative in order to exclude not only a decisive therapeutic scale-up in the countries tested but also to disapprove of excessive investments made in the therapeutic field rather than in the development of "prevention technologies."[55]

Again in 1998 a clinical experiment using the antiretroviral therapy started in Senegal, and this one was a great success. The Dakar government had asked UNAIDS to include Senegal in the drug-access initiative, but the request was refused. Acting out of pride, the government decided to launch a pilot program using the triple therapy and to do it alone. This surprising decision taken by the country, whose president at the time was Abdou Diouf, was due in particular to the doctor and scientist Ibrahim Ndoye, who was in charge of Senegal's national AIDS program. Ndoye disagreed with the UNAIDS's skepticism regarding the antiretroviral therapies in Africa. He knew that patients treated with antiretroviral drugs are no longer contagious or at least the percentage of infection is very low. While UNAIDS, with its drug-access initiative, started its therapeutic trials in Ivory Coast and Uganda, Senegal decided to treat AIDS patients on its own and distanced itself from the passive attitude of the other African countries.

Without financial aid from abroad,[56] Senegal started treating patients with the triple therapy. A top-down financial plan was implemented and also a system providing treatment partially or totally free of charge, depending on the patients' income, elements that in Ivory Coast and in Uganda, respectively, were missing from the clinical experiments promoted by UNAIDS. The Initiative sénégalaise d'accès aux antirétroviraux (ISAARV) concentrated on quality rather than quantity, hoping that the expected drop in the price of the antiretroviral drugs would make it possible to increase the number of patients in therapy. In order to be cautious from an economic point of view, they started with just fifty patients, who were treated according to the best Western therapeutic standards. The numbers gradually increased. The patients started the program when they were not too badly compromised from an immunological and virological point of view, in order to optimize the efficacy of the triple therapy; they were asked to contribute to the cost of their therapy in proportion to their income, to a minimal extent; they were scrupulously looked after by medical teams in order to support their adherence to the regimen; they were regularly monitored for toxicity and resistances; and they were included in reciprocal support groups where they could get encouragement and benefit from solidarity.

ISAARV shows that treating AIDS in Africa is feasible and that the antiretroviral therapies are no less effective there than in the developed countries in the Global North. At the end of one or two years, the viral load of most of these patients was undetectable, their immune system had partially recovered, and they were fit enough to work.[57] It is not that ISAARV was perfect. The figures were low, the health care services were supported by the qualified reference center in Dakar and some patients died because they started the treatment with low CD4 levels—that is, too late. Nonetheless, ISAARV was a medical first for Africa.

It was not surprising that the Senegalese initiative, which strongly challenged the development cooperation agencies and the current line of thought, was not talked about at the time. It started to be mentioned in scientific discussions when, around 2002, the international approach regarding low-income countries changed from prevention to treatment. In the meantime, Senegal had had its pilot project revised by the most important French experts on AIDS (the ANRS—Agence nationale de recherches sur le sida), who together with the researchers from Dakar had published its flattering results. At the same time, the CDC had scientifically assessed the drug-access initiative's results in Uganda, and the ANRS and the CDC had assessed its results together in Ivory Coast. The atypical case of Senegal was recognized as best practice.

But let us continue to talk about the years in which low-income countries were denied treatment. While little was said about Senegal, the lamentable results of the UNAIDS drug-access initiative in Ivory Coast and Uganda confirmed the views of the majority, those in favor of prevention. In June 1999 the World Bank stated that "AIDS is completely preventable," so "preventing HIV infection must remain as the highest priority for all countries." It drew up a report in which it hypothesized intervening in an average African country (indicated with a made-up name, Muzumbaka) in a multisectorial way and came to the conclusion that the antiretroviral drugs were "simply not affordable": "The cost of the ARV [antiretroviral] drug regimens is prohibitive for Muzumbuka as for most countries in Africa, especially when drugs for palliative care to treat opportunistic infections and reduce suffering are not available. The ARV drugs are expensive, and they require patients to follow a complicated, strict daily regime of medication, with frequent contact with health care providers. Muzumbuka does not have the health infrastructure to administer these drugs successfully nor to perform the complex tests needed for follow-up."[58]

The European Union too, in its guidelines written at the end of 1999 on projects for fighting AIDS in countries with limited resources, placed "prevention and essential care" as the priorities and insisted on "sexual health" and "women's rights and empowerment." As for the triple antiretroviral therapies, the European health care executives pointed out their exorbitant cost and the spending capacity of developing countries. They also expressed doubts about how practical these therapies were, because they were so complicated in terms of administering the drugs, medical monitoring, and the overly complex support required from the laboratories. It was better to resort to "basic care" and strengthen the health care services. The HAART regimen was considered "presently not affordable nor sustainable for developing countries," especially because Africans' expected poor adherence to the triple therapy would create resistances to the cheaper first-line drugs, necessitating more expensive drugs.[59]

In June 2000, confirming the above, the annual UNAIDS report did not ignore the antiretroviral drugs, but it excluded them for countries with limited resources. The report presented three care-and-support packages—one essential, one intermediate, and one advanced—to be applied according to the level of development of each country. Antiretroviral therapies were only included in the third package, for countries with plenty of human, infrastructural, and financial resources: "Where the ability to mobilize resources is extremely limited (such as in most of rural sub-Saharan Africa) or somewhat limited (as in northern Thailand), the package will necessarily be more limited than where resource availability is relatively unrestricted."[60] The essential package, for Africa, included psychosocial support, the opportunity to be tested for HIV, palliative treatment only for some opportunistic infections caused by AIDS ("pneumonia, oral thrush, vaginal candidiasis and pulmonary tuberculosis"), infection prophylaxis with cotrimoxazole (better known by its trade name Bactrim), and support for local community activities in order to reduce the social impact of HIV. Nothing that would affect the course of HIV/AIDS and promise survival.

From July 9 to 14, 2000, there was the Durban International AIDS Conference. It was a turning point. The most prominent participants, with their biting speeches and passionate demonstrations, were the South African activists of Treatment Action Campaign, the best-organized and most numerous activists in the continent, led by the charismatic Zackie Achmat. The activists, demonstrating in front of thousands of journalists, were calling for the introduction of antiretroviral drugs in Africa and specifically in their country, which had the highest number of HIV-positive people in the world (4.2 million out of fewer than 40 million inhabitants, with a prevalence rate in the adult population of 20 percent). With less than 1 percent of the world's population, South Africa had 13 percent of all the HIV-positive people in the world. The governments, international development agencies, and donor countries were harshly criticized for their strategy of prevention alone. Brazil was praised for fighting for the production and distribution of generic antiretroviral drugs and for having halved the number of people who were dying from AIDS. The scandal of Africa's health care apartheid broke out in the media. The world's public opinion was confronted with reports on the double standard for AIDS, which was killing people in Africa but appeared to have been neutralized in the Global North. After ten years of scientific research and, in 1996, validation of the triple therapy, Durban represented for Africa what the vast emotional mobilization of public opinion had represented in the fight against HIV/AIDS for the West. The international opinion became that in the West AIDS was no longer considered a catastrophe but a routine health care issue, whereas elsewhere its effects were devastating. During the Durban conference, *Le Monde diplomatique* wrote, "Before being a danger, AIDS is first of all a disease. The absence of any prospect of therapy does not encourage people who are sick to find out whether they are seropositive and then have to accept the consequences. . . . Insisting exclusively on prevention, which marginalizes the efforts made for access to treatment, accelerates the spread of the epidemic. The *tout-prévention* policy is in fact in itself what has made it fail."[61]

In Durban, Piot also raised his voice in favor of universal access to antiretroviral treatments. Had he been converted? Or was this just temporary alignment with the supermotivated activists sitting next to him? One month earlier he had released the UNAIDS report presenting that essential package, by which Africa was denied both antiretroviral drugs and ordinary treatments for the opportunistic infections caused by AIDS. In fact, Piot's seeing eye to eye with Achmat lasted just for the duration of the conference, until he got on the plane that took him back to his office in Geneva. Here he again started spreading his political approach to AIDS: "The only way the epidemic can be reversed is through a total social mobilization. Leadership from above needs to meet the creativity, energy, and leadership from below, joining together in a coordinated program of sustained social action.... We are facing the most devastating epidemic humanity has ever known. Our response must therefore be equally unprecedented: the most concerted, sustained, coordinated, full-scale assault on a disease the world has ever known."[62]

The effects of the Durban conference were not immediately felt, although the approach of prevention with as little health care as possible prevailed. The development cooperation agencies, whatever the orientation of their directors, remained hostile to sending antiretroviral drugs to poor countries. In its update at the end of January 2000, UNAIDS confirmed that it was opposed to the antiretroviral therapy in Africa. Its directors were afraid of being overtaken in the fight against AIDS by those who at the time were planning what was going to become the Global Fund, a sort of Marshall Plan with vast resources for fighting AIDS in Africa. They therefore decided to make a substantial request to the rich countries, $3 billion. However, none of this amount was destined to treat people with full-blown AIDS. Half was for prevention in the usual so-called multisectorial way. The other half was for palliative remedies and treatments for opportunistic infections for a necessarily limited number of patients, considering the funds that were planned. And all this was with the understanding that the funds would only be available if the sub-Saharan countries were able to provide adequate health care facilities and had sufficient competent medical staff. The message that came across was that without a health care system that worked properly, without human skills, without "strategic thinking, planning and management," not even the $3 billion would make a difference: "Money can only be used wisely if people are available to use it wisely." A discouraging passage in the text says that if one was to promote the antiretroviral therapies in Africa, which was in any case an alien proposition for the authors, since they made the request for $3 billion sound as though it were already incredibly daring, this would mean adding "several billion dollars annually to the bill."[63]

In South Africa, it was difficult to put into practice what was understood during the Durban conference. President Thabo Mbeki had acquired a different view of AIDS, which interpreted the disease as a cruel consequence of the poverty and malnutrition that the West had pushed Africa into and argued that there was no relationship between HIV and full-blown AIDS. Mbeki defined the antiretroviral drugs as an initiative that aimed to poison Africans because they were extremely toxic. From a political point of view, this pseudo-medical position was very powerful: it exalted African nationalism in a country marked by the recent struggle between Blacks and whites. The South African government of the African National Congress (ANC), the glorious movement/party of the victory over apartheid, fell in line with Mbeki, although Nelson Mandela had a different opinion of the disease.[64]

Nine months passed after the Durban conference, and nothing new happened until April 26, 2001. At a summit of African leaders in Abuja in Nigeria, Kofi Annan announced the creation of the Global Fund, which would collect funds to be used to fight AIDS, malaria, and tuberculosis.[65] Annan hoped that the fund would make the appropriate therapies accessible for everyone with AIDS all over the world and overcome the double standard for rich countries and poor countries. The aim of this new organization was to annually collect a war chest of $10 billion, a figure that those fighting HIV had never dreamed possible. A few months earlier UNAIDS, with great caution, although merely hypothetically, had started to talk about spending $3 billion for Africa. However, it had never aimed for such a high figure as $10 billion per year because it was skeptical about the feasibility of mass therapies and the improvement in the health care systems in countries with limited resources. Prevention, even when massively emphasized, was ultimately a low-cost activity, with limited expenses, not permanent like the treatment. The cost of condoms, for example, was negligible, even though they had been bought by the millions, as UNAIDS liked to point out. In 1999 just over $300 million in international aid was available for 24.5 million HIV-positive Africans—that is, $12 per person. UNAIDS was not totally to blame for this absurd amount because where were the international leaders?

The Global Fund announced by Annan was created under the auspices of the United Nations, but as an organization it was outside the UN, so it would not be "devoured by a voracious UN bureaucracy," as the *Economist* wrote.[66] It was basically set up as a container and multilateral guarantor for large public and private donors. The definition of the Global Fund owes much to the suggestions of the Harvard *enfant prodige* Jeffrey Sachs, a brilliant economist who considered eradicating the main endemic diseases in poor countries an imperative condition for their development, starting with AIDS, tuberculosis, and malaria. Sachs's main principle was that investments in the health care sector in developing countries not only saved lives but also produced enormous progress from an economic point of view. According to Sachs, health and economic success go together.[67] Sachs was president of the WHO's Commission on Macroeconomics and Health and was one of the advisers that Annan listened to most. It was Gro Harlem Brundtland, the former prime minister of Norway, who wanted to involve the world of finance in the health of poor countries and who invited Sachs to work for the WHO.

The idea of an international financial organization that would fight the endemic pathologies in countries with limited resources had emerged in the WHO at the end of 1999 under the provisional name of Massive Attack on Diseases of Poverty, without its aims and potential having yet been clearly identified. So, Sachs described this moment:

> Essentially, this pandemic was running its complete natural course without any intervention from the rich world. The surprising thing, and the thing that's not so easy to figure out, is that there's lots

of talk going on. There's speeches; there's hand-wringing; there's pronouncements; there's summits. So you imagine with all that noise that there's actually some action. You have to parse through all of the fog that's intentionally thrown up to find out there is nothing there. There is no treatment. There is no health promotion. There's almost nothing. That's what I discovered at the end of the 1990s to be the case. Officialdom doesn't exactly hold up a sign that says, "We're doing nothing." And they're not so happy when anyone else holds up a sign, either.[68]

Sachs took part in the Durban conference and insisted on the idea of a global fund of several billion dollars to fight AIDS because, as he said provocatively, the World Bank and international donors were not doing their work. In January 2001 in the *Lancet*, Sachs talked about allocating $7.5 billion to immediately fight against AIDS within the framework of what was soon to become the Global Fund. This money was understood to be grants and not loans, considering the poverty of the countries involved. This was the opposite of what the World Bank, the main provider of funds for fighting AIDS, was doing.[69] Sachs had a vision, he was thinking big, and he was not shy about asking for funds. Durban had shocked him. Apart from the discussions on costs, convenience, and sustainability, Sachs pointed out that the medicines did not reach the poor countries and that people were dying: "The notion that parents should be sent to their graves for lack of $500 a year in drugs strikes me as a mind-boggling miscalculation from an economic development point of view as well as being immoral."[70] Sachs therefore proposed introducing the therapies in resource-limited countries, which up to that point had denied them. This was why the Global Fund was so necessary. In the Consensus Statement on Antiretroviral Treatment for AIDS in Poor Countries, dated April 4, 2001, a prelude to Kofi Annan's announcement in Abuja on April 26, Sachs brought together 133 Harvard academics who wanted to set up an experimental scientific program in developing countries to treat one million AIDS patients with the triple antiretroviral therapy within three years, at an estimated cost of $1,123 a year per patient. Five hundred dollars of this was to be gradually spent for the drugs in total, while waiting for further reductions in price, and the rest was to support adherence, to cover clinical and laboratory costs, and for scientific research on what was being done to identify best practices and guidelines.[71] Once a program like that was set up,[72] there had to be a more ambitious goal—to make the same treatment available to three million people with AIDS over a period of five years. The statement, known as the Harvard statement, did not underestimate the difficulties: inadequate health care facilities, possible resistances to the drugs, and less funds for prevention. However, it did underline the urgency of becoming operative. It was necessary to invest in and build infrastructures, the patients' adherence had to be guaranteed in order to avoid resistances, and the global budget for the fight against AIDS from the rich countries had to be increased in order to provide money for prevention.

Sachs was very confident about the scientific approach: "There has been a tremendous amount of amateurism and seat-of-the-pants operations by donor agencies. Somehow proper science just doesn't get into the story."[73] The appeal for knowledge did not save the Harvard economist from being criticized by those who argued that prevention saved more lives than the drugs and who therefore wanted to avoid the diversion of funds from prevention to the antiretroviral therapies. He was attacked by the Bill and Melinda Gates Foundation, the Rockefeller Foundation, and the United Nations Foundation. Even some people from the Harvard Medical School disagreed with him.[74] Sachs discussed the resistance in a February 2020 television interview:

> Of course there was resistance. Immediately there was pushback. Oh, the pendulum is swinging too far from prevention to treatment, some foundations said. I was shocked, because how can you say the pendulum swung? Not one person yet was on treatment from actual donor dollars. The rich world had not treated one person on a donor project up until the middle of 2001. This was the reality—millions dying, drugs available, proven successes, and nobody being treated by the rich countries. It's the most shocking reality.[75]

The World Bank challenged the idea that it was possible to find so much money to fight AIDS.[76] UNAIDS was also in a political frenzy because Sachs had observed that its "global efforts have been ineffective in preventing the further spread of the disease" and had also proposed joint and equal direction of the future Global Fund by the WHO and UNAIDS, which would downgrade the latter's alleged leadership. The Harvard statement contained truths that were unpleasant for UNAIDS to hear:

> Over the past 2 decades, the international response to HIV/AIDS in poor countries has emphasized HIV prevention, primarily due to the high cost of treatment and the limited resources available to developing countries. Despite this emphasis, the available scientific tools for prevention, in the absence of effective vaccines, remain inadequate to stop the spread of the disease. The very mention of AIDS treatment has often been avoided by donor agencies in wealthy countries, for fear that raised expectations would increase the financial and operational demands upon them, and detract from prevention efforts. The disparity in access to effective treatment between wealthy countries and developing countries is neither scientifically nor ethically justified at this time.[77]

Sachs did not ask for the work on prevention to be reduced—he pointed out the limit of prevention being considered separate from treatment. On the basis of what had been widely observed in the West, he believed that the therapeutic treatment was in itself prevention. The Harvard statement, after saying "the immediate humanitarian rationale for treatment" was to save millions of lives, went on to state,

> Treatment is necessary to optimize prevention efforts. When treatment is not available, less incentive exists for an individual to take an HIV test, since HIV-positive status not only is associated with social stigmatization but also is tantamount to a death sentence. It is only when HIV testing is coupled with treatment that people have an incentive to be tested, thus enabling a rational response to AIDS: primary prevention for those who are HIV-uninfected, and antiretroviral treatment for those who are HIV-infected. Effective antiretroviral treatment of HIV-positive people also lowers the viral load within

infected individuals, which in turn has a major effect in reducing the likelihood that they will transmit HIV infection to others. Ultimately, then, appropriate treatment of infected individuals may become a major tool in AIDS prevention.

The answers that Sachs gave those who disagreed with him were not theoretical. When talking about the infrastructural problems, he said that part of the funds available would have to go to strengthen the health care facilities. He did not underestimate the issues concerning the adherence of the patients to the treatment and recommended they be accompanied by people, paid if necessary, who would check that they were taking their medicine properly and minimize the development of resistances, according to the model previously tested for tuberculosis (the so-called directly observed therapy, or DOT). This Harvard economist was convinced that prevention would always fail if not accompanied by therapeutic treatment: "I'm utterly convinced that people will not get tested, will not consider themselves infected, if this is not put in a medical context."[78]

Unlike so many documents from UN agencies and international foundations, the statement that Sachs promoted did not consist of just a list of obstacles but also proposed solutions. For the poor countries it advocated nothing less than what was being done in the West, albeit in an operational context that took into account a series of local variables. The statement did not talk about a multisectorial approach, not even using that somewhat vague term. Rather, it started with the simple affirmation that there is a HAART regime:

> In wealthy countries, there has been dramatic success in the fight against HIV/AIDS, success that has been largely achieved through the use of antiretroviral therapy. Those with access to this treatment have enjoyed tremendous gains in survival and quality of life. Yet despite this success, antiretroviral therapy remains largely inaccessible in the world's poorest countries, where interventions have focused almost exclusively on prevention. With soaring death rates from HIV/AIDS in low-income countries, both the prevention of transmission of the virus and the treatment of those already infected must be global public health priorities.[79]

At the time, Sachs and his Harvard colleagues were clearly in the minority with their approach. Nonetheless, Annan, who was African, agreed with this approach, naturally with all the diplomatic caution that his position required, and he proved it in Abuja. The Global Fund to Fight AIDS, Tuberculosis and Malaria was to deal with the prevention and treatment of the three major infectious diseases. Its headquarters were to be in Geneva, next to the WHO and UNAIDS, but it was to be independent of the UN system, although its employees would be formally considered WHO staff. The funds arrived, which made it possible to draw up a spending budget in 2007 of $10 billion.

Soon after that, on June 25–27, 2001, the first UNGASS (United Nations General Assembly special session) on AIDS took place and was organized by UNAIDS. For the occasion, Bernhard Schwartländer, the UNAIDS chief epidemiologist, limited the extent of the economic and health care proposals put forward by Sachs. According to Schwartländer and his epidemiologist colleagues from the UN in Geneva and from other institutions, in an article published in *Science*, $9.2 billion would be made available in 2005 for fighting AIDS throughout the world. More than half this amount, according to them, was to be used for prevention (10 percent of the total to purchase six billion condoms) and the rest for care and support, within which HAART would count for 27 percent of the total (a little less than $2.5 billion). The antiretroviral therapies were included, but the funds to be allocated for them were just a quarter of the total. The summary of the article confirms that the triple therapy was not the main issue:

> Government and civil society representatives meet for a Special Session of the General Assembly of the United Nations (UNGASS) 25 to 27 June 2001 to consider an expanded response to HIV/AIDS. This policy forum estimates that by 2005, that response will require about US$9 billion annually, with half of these resources needed in sub-Saharan Africa. About US$4.8 billion is required for prevention including interventions focusing on youth, workplace programs, mother-to-child transmission and condom distribution. US$4.4 billion is needed for palliative care, treatment and prophylaxis of opportunistic infections, support for orphans, and antiretroviral

therapy. One-third to one-half of these resources can come from domestic sources, both public and private, with the remainder needed from international sources.[80]

The final UNGASS appeal, prepared beforehand by UNAIDS, did not mention therapeutic treatments. Much was said about prevention, accompanying and supporting patients, treating opportunistic infections, and palliative remedies for terminal patients. Only the pressure of the so-called Rio Group (a block of eleven Latin American countries including Brazil) led to the addition of treatment (actual therapy) to the usual general recommendations of care and support in the final declaration of commitment on HIV/AIDS, whose main statement was, yet again, "Prevention must be the mainstay of our response." This was what most of the donor countries wanted, since they were not prepared to spend money on treatment. According to Eamonn Murphy, who represented the Australian goverment at the time: "From a donor's perspective, quality, capacity for delivery, patient adherence and cost issues were essentially questions without answers. How were these drugs going to be delivered and to whom were they going to be accessible? Are they just going to go to the wealthy in the cities? Plus, for a donor, the question always is, how to make commitments that are sustainable?"[81] This was a step back from the spirit of Durban and Annan's proposal. It was also a move backward with respect to the solemn promises set out in 2000 in the Millennium Development Goals. Identified by the United Nations after exhausting global negotiations, these were eight targets to reach by 2015 for human development worldwide. One goal, the sixth, called for universal access to HIV/AIDS treatment within ten years.

At the same time that UNGASS committed to fighting AIDS, UNFPA, supervised by UNAIDS, produced its *Strategic Options for HIV/AIDS Advocacy in Africa*, which stated, "Since no cure exists, preventing infection and controlling the spread of the virus constitute the prime line of defence against HIV/AIDS."[82] As far as the antiretroviral drugs were concerned, they were once again described as a treatment but not a cure that would heal people, even though there had been a drop in prices, which up to then had made them inaccessible to many Africans. It continued:

Other obstacles to widespread distribution remain: weak health infrastructures and the shortage of skilled medical personnel to prescribe the drugs and monitor their impact are likely to minimize the impact of these promising developments. In the short term, therefore, treatment options in Africa are likely to be limited largely to palliative treatment and the treatment of opportunistic infections, such as tuberculosis. In the poorer countries and among poorer PLWHA [people living with HIV/AIDS], access to even these forms of treatment is limited.[83]

As far as the rest was concerned, *Strategic Options* described the various phases and methods of prevention, correlated with an idea of democracy that was under construction. If this prevention had taken place within a context of an open society, of civic education, and of participation, it would have encouraged the desired individual change in behavior.

UNFPA was still suffering from its failure to lower fertility rates in Africa after the 1994 Cairo Conference on Population and feared a similar lack of success in the prevention of HIV/AIDS. It was therefore determined to "address deep-rooted social and psychological factors that determine sexual attitudes and behaviours."[84] This, it said, "requires that dynamic and creative relations to social science are established," considering that "research into the social causes, context and consequences of the epidemic is still often heavily influenced by the health perspective."[85]

Stephen Lewis, a UN special envoy for Africa, has talked about his attempt at the end of 2001 to convince the World Bank to fund treatment programs for AIDS. In this prestigious institution in Washington, Lewis counted on good relationships with the senior management. Nonetheless, he recalled that he was told, "You see, Stephen, it's difficult. Let's face the painful truth: the people with AIDS are going to die. The money would probably be better used for prevention. It's all a matter of trade-offs." Lewis responded, "You speak to me of trade-offs? You have drugs to keep people alive, and you're going to let them die because of a trade-off? Why don't you find more money and do both treatment and prevention, and screw the trade-off?" The people he was talking to were adamant. Lewis went on: "I mention it now because for the longest time, this pernicious frame of mind ruled the dialectical roost. Somehow the people living with AIDS were expendable, in vast numbers, while people in power persuaded themselves that it was better to practice prevention."[86]

However, the climate outside the big, cold development agencies was changing. Even though the talk about the therapies was inconclusive, it encouraged the WHO in 2002 to publish the first guidelines for treating AIDS in resource-limited settings. These specified simplified, minimalistic regimens far below the standards of excellence found in the Western world, but they established an essential therapeutic regulatory framework for the international modus operandi. The antiretroviral treatment of AIDS in the Southern Hemisphere was now legitimate. The guidelines mentioned the aim defined by the WHO's 3 by 5 Initiative, which was to have three million people treated with HAART in the poor countries by 2005. This was the proposal that Jeffrey Sachs had made a year before. The WHO was harshly criticized by those who advocated prevention as the first-line response to the epidemic and who claimed that funds allocated for the therapies represented an unnecessary expense.[87] However, it is also true that in the spring of 2002, the World Bank, which up to just before then had been firmly against spending on treatments, made an agreement with the WHO in order to finance not only prevention but also treatments. Its president, James Wolfensohn, managed to overcome the deep-rooted aversion of his board of directors to any AIDS therapy proposed for countries with limited resources.[88] Wolfensohn interpreted his high position not only from technological and financial points of view but also from a moral one: he was convinced of the need to save the lives of people with AIDS regardless of the cost-effectiveness criteria venerated by his organization. The World Bank's senior management maintained that treatment was less convenient than prevention without understanding the preventive value of the therapy itself, which was indeed far more cost-effective than prevention alone. However, in the meantime it had to reluctantly comply with and in some way indulge its president. This is a relevant fact because the World Bank (the UN's safe), together with the Global Fund (then being set up) and George W. Bush's PEPFAR (which was in its early days), represented the greatest possibility of financing the fight against AIDS in poor countries.

In Barcelona in July 2002, at the biannual International AIDS Conference, which followed the one in Durban, Joep Lange, the president of the International AIDS Society, stated the following about bringing the antiretroviral drugs to millions of people with AIDS in countries with limited resources: "It is actually quite simple. . . . Do not be fooled: People make simple things complex to condone their inertia, and the inertia of those who are living off this epidemic. Or maybe not inertia, but simple lack of imagination. We need to be creative." He added, "If we can get cold Coca-Cola and beer to every remote corner of Africa, it should not be impossible to do the same with drugs."[89]

In the meantime, there was the conversion of Bill Clinton, which was no less impressive than that of Wolfensohn. As US president, Clinton had defended the patents and earnings of the multinational pharmaceutical companies producing the antiretroviral drugs, without hesitating to take drastic measures against countries that produced generic antiretroviral drugs at low prices. This policy seriously hindered the treatment of people with AIDS in countries with limited resources. When Clinton was once again a private citizen, he created the foundation with his name on it and committed himself to the greatest global tragedy of the time, AIDS. What he wrote in the *New York Times* on December 1, 2002, confirmed his political acumen:

> Historians will look back on our time and see that our civilization spends many millions of dollars educating people about the scourge of H.I.V. and AIDS, which has already taken 25 million lives and could infect 100 million people over the next eight years. But what they will find not so civilized is our failure to treat 95 percent of people with the disease. Given that medicine can turn AIDS from a death sentence into a chronic illness and reduce mother-to-child transmission, our withholding of treatment will appear to future historians as medieval, like bloodletting. . . . Confronted with these awful facts, we can offer the historians of the future our excuses: too many countries are still in denial about the scope of the problem

and what has to be done about it; many countries lack the nationwide health infrastructure to treat such a disease; most countries don't have enough health-care personnel to run a complicated treatment program; the necessary drugs are expensive and unavailable to people in the poorest, hardest-hit countries. But those facts only serve to outline the extent of the problem. They do not justify our failure to recognize the moral and practical imperatives to mount a full-throttle treatment program in conjunction with ongoing education and prevention efforts.[90]

There was, however, still no action. Neither the Global Fund with its financial sponsorship nor the WHO with its 3 by 5 Initiative managed to even get off the starting blocks. UNAIDS, the WHO, and the major donating countries were invited to The Hague by the Dutch government in October 2002 to discuss access to treatment in developing countries, but "much of the discussion still focused on why treatment scale-up was not possible—or dangerous—rather than on how to overcome the obstacles."[91] The participants continued to refuse to invest in treatment for a pathology that would in the future become chronic. "Lifelong" is a word that nobody wants to hear. The Global Fund launched its first funds, for 154 projects, but only a few of them were for treatments with antiretroviral drugs, and when these treatments were included, they were not for the triple therapy but as single doses for mother-to-child prevention. This was a shortcut with little or no effect, as will be explained further on: in the developed world, the triple therapy for pregnant mothers almost completely eliminated the transmission of HIV to newborns.

The Global Fund received applications for four hundred projects from developing countries, most of them along the lines of prevention, with no mention of the triple therapy. This was the approach that had prevailed until then at an international level, and it had been enthusiastically absorbed at a national level. The Global Fund's board complained of "insufficient focus on disease treatment rather than prevention or other aspects of care."[92] The head of auditing of the projects, Michel Kazatchkine, reported to the board in an open plenary session that "developing countries were 'shy' about applying for ARV Tx [therapy], and believed that applications would be rejected if there were significant treatment components."[93] In the meantime, a study summarizing the antiretroviral treatments administered to Ivorians and Ugandans within the context of the UNAIDS drug-access initiative and to Senegalese patients within the context of ISAARV showed that African patients reacted to the treatment exactly as Western patients did: "Virologic and immunologic outcomes, adverse events, and estimated survival are similar among patients in African DAIs and ART-treated patients in Europe and the USA."[94] The news was not in the outcome of the study but in that it was felt necessary to demonstrate these facts. Perhaps someone thought that the anatomy of Africans was different or that the effect of the drugs depended on latitudes and climates.

Clearly the WHO still needed time to finalize the 3 by 5 Initiative. Finally, in December 2003, two and a half years after it had first been mentioned publicly, the program became operative. The Global Fund received a boost for a financial commitment that was less dispersive, after having distributed money like rain on the most diverse projects. So, Africans with AIDS started rushing for the therapy. The experts who had advocated "prevention first" were disappointed. The UNAIDS Board welcomed the 3 by 5 Initiative in June 2004, but it also expressed the fear that the increasing focus on treatment would make prevention seem less important. It is underlined that "prevention must remain a cornerstone of a comprehensive response, not only to prevent new infections but also to reduce stigma and discrimination."[95] Shortly afterward, Michel Caraël, a UNAIDS manager in charge of the prevention sector, appeared to see more negative than positive effects in the treatment: "The new context of possible access to the treatment, which is still very far away in most of the African countries, could revitalize the prevention programmes but also re-medicalise prevention and curb the dynamism of the civil society associations, as it clearly appeared in the high income countries where there has been a large number of new infections."[96]

Once again the intention was to ignore the lesson learned about AIDS patients treated in the West: the treatment was in itself prevention, thanks to the reduction of the viral load to almost zero. Neither did these people understand that when patients on HAART made an astonishing recovery, this allowed the whole African society to look at

AIDS in a different way. The stigma diminished, not because of the advertising campaigns but because everyone could see that the patients had been born again, so people there started doing the test to find out whether they were positive or not. The best advertising came from the fast and stable improvement of the patients' vital parameters and from the quality of life of all the patients on HAART, even those whose condition had been severe when they started the treatment. Without being able to receive treatment, nobody was interested in doing the test: it would have been like going to court voluntarily to be sentenced to death. Up to then, in order to encourage people to do the test, there had only been an offer of counseling in which the health officers could basically give two answers: If they are negative, then they have an incentive to stay that way. If infected, the message is "positive living," where that term means simply eating well, not getting tired, having a balanced life, not getting drunk, and not taking drugs.[97] In theory UNFPA and UNAIDS were right: the antiretroviral drugs did not actually cure people. They were a treatment rather than a cure. However, they were really worth much more than a treatment because it was as if people were actually being cured. They became healthy again, they had physical energy, they were happy to be alive, they experienced a good quality of life, and they no longer could pass on the disease.

In any case, the WHO had taken the brakes off, the delay was over, and the path was open. Treatment was being given, despite the skepticism of many people in the so-called family of the United Nations, where rivalry and envy sometimes even led people to want others to fail. Even in the WHO there were factions that criticized the new therapeutic approach. Since they were not able to disapprove of the attempt to save lives, their complaints were more in terms of form than of substance, especially with respect to the 3 by 5 Initiative, claiming that it was wrong to commit to such specific aims and timing. By proposing to treat three million people with antiretroviral drugs in countries with limited resources by 2005, the WHO would contradict its first rule of economic predictions: "give 'em a number or a date, but not both."[98] These were absurd considerations. The WHO had started moving, and this annoyed the people in New York and Geneva who preferred bureaucratic sclerosis, brainstorming, verbal marathons, and solemn and politically correct proclamations.

## ANTITHERAPY OBSTINACY

From 1996 to 2002 the international development cooperation agencies were not alone in saying that it was impossible to treat AIDS in Africa. Scientific journals, prestigious media, scholars, and scientists were all of the same opinion. The yearly publications of the *Lancet* reveal the situation clearly. In November 1997 Robert Hogg, a Canadian demographer of the British Columbia Centre for Excellence in HIV/AIDS, published a study with his colleagues on the costs of the triple therapy for the hypothetical treatment of 25 percent of the AIDS patients in each country in sub-Saharan Africa. It quantified the percentages of expenditure in relation to their GDP. This limited treatment was estimated as corresponding to 84.4 percent of Malawi's GDP, 66.8 percent of Mozambique's, 61 percent of Uganda's, 51.2 percent of Tanzania's, and so on, down to 26.2 percent of the DRC's GDP and 25.5 percent of Togo's. This is a timid contribution to the feasibility, in underdeveloped countries, of the "known survival benefit associated with the triple-combination therapy."[99] This prestigious medical journal published a categorical contradiction by a professor from Heidelberg, Olaf Müller, et alia. It was a summary of current opinions:

> We do not agree with Hogg and colleagues' proposal that such combination therapies be made widely available in Africa. In countries of sub-Saharan Africa, where less than $10 per capita per year is spent on health, large-scale antiretroviral drug treatment is an unrealistic option because of the prohibitive high costs. The limited availability and quality of health services in most of these countries, where patients often do not even have regular access to simple antibiotic or antimalarial treatment, calls for great caution with respect to the introduction of complex therapies. Only experts from specialized centers equipped with the necessary laboratory facilities

to measure HIV-1 viral load or CD4 lymphocyte counts would be able to manage antiretroviral regimens. The large-scale introduction of antiretroviral therapy within the regular health services of sub-Saharan Africa would not ensure the safety of and the compliance with these complicated combination regimens. This would lead to severe side-effects in patients and to rapid development of drug resistance in the community. . . . Instead of promoting expensive and potentially dangerous antiretroviral drug therapies, policy makers should invest limited resources into improving the infrastructure of the existing health services to enable them to cope with the increasing number of cases of tuberculosis, pneumonia, and other opportunistic infections.[100]

During the Durban conference, the *Lancet* published an equally clear opposition to the triple antiretroviral therapy in poor countries:

Highly active antiretroviral therapy is not affordable on a large scale in less-developed countries either privately or by government, nor is it a technology that most poor people could adhere to or that existing health systems in poor countries are equipped to support. Even if the drugs were cheap, this type of therapy would probably not be cost-effective as implemented for most patients compared with treatment of opportunistic infections because of problems with non-compliance and erratic supplies of drugs. Weak compliance can generate the spread of drug-resistant strains of HIV, to the detriment of future AIDS patients.[101]

A year later, still as a reaction to an initial event, the above-mentioned UNGASS session devoted to fighting AIDS, an editorial in the *Lancet* criticized the declaration of commitment on HIV/AIDS because it mentioned treatment. Before providing drugs, it said, it was necessary to strengthen the national health care systems, which were unable to distribute antiretroviral drugs:

Yet the reality of Africa is that there is no working primary healthcare infrastructure for large parts of the continent. . . . Is provision of antiretroviral agents an answer to the health problems many

Africans face? Certainly, it is part of the answer. But far more crucial are the elements of a sustainable primary health-care system. These are given only passing acknowledgement in the UN declaration and in the speeches that surrounded it. Such fundamental services are not an eye-catching platform for politicians and policy-makers. Yet they remain desperately needed—for without them, any effort to distribute medicines will fail.[102]

Another relevant person during this period was Luc Montagnier, who was still in dispute with Robert Gallo about who had discovered HIV. Montagnier seemed to appreciate some of the South African president Mbeki's ideas and went to Johannesburg to be a member of the commission on AIDS that the president had set up. Montagnier tended to be skeptical about the effects of the drugs for AIDS, and it was easy for him to agree with the mainstream opinion of those in favor of prevention, which was that the triple antiretroviral therapies were not indicated for Africa.[103] The French virologist did not accept the denialist theories of American biologist Peter Duesberg that Mbeki was interested in—that would be to deny his own scientific undertakings—but he was getting the idea that an energized immune system could get rid of HIV in a natural way.[104] This led him to say that antioxidants, an appropriate diet, fighting opportunistic infections, and genital hygiene were enough to cure people of AIDS. Despite his bizarre theories about the miracles of papaya, Montagnier continued to be given credit by the scientific community. In 2008 he received the Nobel Prize for medicine, before his theories about oxidative stress and his stand against vaccines led him to be considered a scientist who had gone astray.

In turn, Alan Whiteside, a prolific and established South African AIDS scholar working for UNAIDS, considered the HIV epidemic to be "a development crisis, which deepens poverty and increases inequality at every level." However, precisely by virtue of this analysis, he ruled out treatment by exasperating its negative aspects:

> The treatment regimens are complex. A patient has to take a number of drugs during the day, at set times, some on a full stomach, some on an empty one. If these regimens are not adhered to then

the prospects for successful treatment are not good. Linked to the inability to take the drugs regularly is the issue of resistance. HIV mutates rapidly and can become resistant to drugs, hence inconsistent or incorrect use of the drugs will speed this up. Another problem is that the drugs are toxic. Due to drug toxicity side effects may occur, such as anemia, liver disease, kidney stones, diabetes, and heart disease. In addition, there is the question of what drugs should be given in which combination and when. Research suggested that the best option is to start treatment when the CD4 cell count drops below 350/mcl of blood. There are also issues of cost and the associated tests incurred. Another is the issue of sustainability. It is noted that HIV is a "long wave" disaster, thus continued treatment regimens are needed. Finally, there is a real danger that treating symptoms does not get to the cause. In view of this, prevention must remain a priority. Moreover, the need to respond to the consequences of the epidemic: the millions of orphans, the families pushed into destitution, and the elderly caring for scores of grandchildren.[105]

In September 2001 Whiteside published an economic analysis of AIDS in Africa in the *British Medical Bulletin* that clearly said that "without effective treatment of HIV infection, people will die of AIDS" but that the therapy was unworkable: "It is too expensive, requires a fairly sophisticated delivery system, and people need to know they are infected in order to access it."[106] Another UNAIDS adviser, the English academic Tony Barnett, published in 2002 the ponderous study *AIDS in the Twenty-First Century*, in which he stated the following:

> Even if the drugs are available, they could not and cannot be ladled out like aspirin. These are complex treatment regimens. . . . HIV/AIDS leads back to the poverty. These drugs are less effective if patients do not have appropriate lifestyles and a good diet, and if the treatment is not monitored. Such conditions are untenable in poor countries. . . . In other words, ARTs [antiretroviral therapies], even at much lower prices, are not "the answer." They are part of an answer, which must include head-on confrontation with the conditions that contribute to the epidemic in the first place. Those conditions

are poverty-related risk.... The poor world's best response is to recognize the role of appropriate treatment in prevention and mitigation.[107]

In May 2002, while the Global Fund with its money and the WHO with its 3 by 5 Initiative were planning on spreading antiretroviral drugs in Africa, the *Lancet* published articles that aimed to confirm that prevention was absolutely more advantageous than treatment. These articles insisted on cost-effectiveness—that is, the economic advantage in relation to the results. Andrew Creese and some other academics from Northern Europe denied that antiretroviral drugs were appropriate in Africa, arguing that investing in condoms, controlling transfusions, treating infections, counseling and testing, and single doses of Nevirapine for women in labor were much more profitable.[108] Elliot Marseille from the University of California and other experts of health policy claimed that the cost-effectiveness of prevention was twenty-eight times greater than that of treatment: "Data on the cost-effectiveness of HIV prevention in sub-Saharan Africa and on highly active antiretroviral therapy (HAART) indicate that prevention is at least 28 times more cost-effective than HAART. We aim to show that funding HAART at the expense of prevention means greater loss of life. To maximize health benefits, the next major increments of HIV funding in sub-Saharan Africa should be devoted mainly to prevention and to some non-HAART treatment and care."[109]

This time it was too much. Cost-effectiveness is considered very important in the Anglo-American world, but it should not be used to insult humanitarian consciousness. It was already known that millions of Africans had died of AIDS and a different variant was spreading. Readers of the *Lancet* from England and from South Africa protested:

> Treatment and prevention are inextricably linked, offering treatment strengthens prevention measures, and prevention is less effective without treatment. Cost-effectiveness alone is a misguided way to justify one over the other. Social and economic benefits are vast: children saved from being orphaned, and longer life means people can contribute to society. Cost-effectiveness analyses represent a narrow viewpoint from which relevant stakeholders are entirely

excluded. Such analyses have never been an exclusive prescription for health-care choices in the developed world. . . . How are doctors in Africa to tell their patients they cannot treat them because it is not cost-effective?[110]

A gay activist in New York observed, "Data need to be put into a larger socioeconomic context before they are used to guide public policy on HIV/AIDS. For instance, what is the cost of not treating HIV infection in the countries of sub-Saharan African, where tens of millions of people with HIV/AIDS now reside? What will be the effect on: the stability of business, communities, families; countries' gross economic products; degree of poverty; educational opportunities; food, security, and other indicators?"[111]

Peter Piot also intervened, together with representatives of the World Bank and of the WHO. They described the idea of prevention and treatment being in competition with each other as a "simplistic and out-dated proposition," when both need to be increased because HIV was by then putting populations, societies, economies, and whole countries at risk. Now that the cost of the antiretroviral drugs had come down, it was possible to treat as well as prevent AIDS. Hospitals would be less crowded with AIDS patients who had opportunistic infections, so they would save on resources, and in general public health systems would be better off.[112]

The two above-mentioned controversial studies, one by Creese et alia and one by Marseille et alia, were noticed by Senegalese and French scholars who were responsible for assessing the ISAARV, the first African public health program for treating AIDS:

> Two studies on the cost-benefit ratio of different intervention strategies suggest allocating the new funds available mainly to prevention and treatment, with the exclusion of long-term multiple (antiretroviral) therapies. These analyses are based on fragmented data that underestimate the benefits of organized programs for access to antiretroviral drugs and ignore the request by HIV+ people and the individual and collective importance of keeping them in good health. In the Global North, there was no demand to legitimize the treatment from an economic point of view compared to the cost of

prevention before making the antiretroviral treatment available to whoever needed it. On the other hand, making multiple antiretroviral therapies available in "poor" countries is permanently threatened by "appeals to reason" based on arguments presented as "scientific." Many studies, against imposing the "burden of proof" on HIV+ people living in countries in the South, have proposed ending this biased debate and consider it over by now: prevention and medical therapy are undeniably complementary, whatever the circumstances. The real economic questions concern the reduction of the cost of the therapies and finding the necessary funds.[113]

The discussion was ended in July by an unusual editorial in the *Lancet*. It talked about the almost thirty million HIV-positive Africans who died in 2001, the dramatic fifteen-year reduction in the life expectancy (from sixty-two to forty-seven) in the sub-Saharan countries, and the fact that millions of children died or became orphans. The editorial continued, in its empirical Anglo-American manner, to combine the health and economic factors:

> There are no simple solutions to the global HIV/AIDS epidemic and its economic consequences, but unless action is taken soon there will be no workforce to develop Africa. . . . A shift in thinking about the disease is necessary. . . . HIV should be considered an infectious disease like any other, with testing and treatment being the norm, rather than the exception. Kevin de Cock and colleagues argue for such a strategy in Africa. . . . They suggest that public health approaches to the African AIDS pandemic are more appropriate than the human rights approaches that have prevailed as the model in the developing world. . . . Such a refutation of the exceptionalist approach to AIDS would require commitment from political leaders at the highest level.[114]

This represented a radical change in perspective. Nonetheless, prevention continued to be proposed as an alternative to treatment. Catastrophic forecasts of the spread of AIDS (e.g., the US National Intelligence Council believed that in a few years China, India, Russia, Nigeria, and Ethiopia would have had between fifty and seventy-five million cases) always called for prevention instead of treatment. With a critical jolt, in October 2002 the *Economist* commented on similar epidemic forecasts: "Prevention is said to be better than cure. It is, however, often hard to get people to act on this sensible advice."[115] The projections were wrong, but they were not surprising. Apocalyptic data offered to the media was not uncommon in the political history of AIDS. It served to shock, to give a sense of insecurity and of emergency, and therefore to obtain funds or to affirm directives like prevention with no treatment. In the following years, while it was becoming increasingly clear that treatment and prevention complemented and supported each other—that treatment was not a parallel activity to prevention but was the best form of prevention—there were still nostalgic comments that prevention should have been given the priority over treatment.

## NOTES

1. Gottlieb, "Pneumocystis Pneumonia," 250–52.
2. Levy, "Isolation of Lymphocytopathic Retroviruses."
3. Elias, Über die Einsamkeit der Sterbenden. All translations are my own.
4. Martini, "Vivere e morire di AIDS oggi," 5–15, 7.
5. The viral load (also called viraemia) is the number of copies of a virus in a person's blood. In the case of the HIV infection, it corresponds to the number of copies of the acquired immunodeficiency virus present in a millimeter of venous blood.
6. Grmek, *Histoire du sida.*
7. Sentinel sites are the health care sites included in a surveillance system for diseases. These systems are used when high-quality health data are necessary but unavailable through passive surveillance. Some sentinel health care centers are therefore selected in order to record and then report the cases of certain diseases and other associated variables. The sentinel system is particularly useful in countries that have weak national health care systems and where passive surveillance only provides unreliable data.
8. Palombi, "Dove l'AIDS è un flagello incontenibile," 121–30.
9. Worobey et al., "Direct Evidence of Extensive Diversity," 661–64.
10. Zhu et al., "African HIV-1 Sequence," 594–97.
11. Pépin, "Origins of AIDS," 473–75. See also Pépin's book of the same name.
12. See Kuyu, *Les Haïtiens au Congo.*
13. Quammen, *Spillover,* 484.

14. *New York Times*, January 28, 1972.

15. Pitchenik et al., "Opportunistic Infections and Kaposi's Syndrome."

16. Maggie Fox, "New Study Shows HIV Epidemic Started Spreading in New York in 1970," NBC News, October 26, 2016, https://www.nbcnews.com/health/health-news/new-study-shows-hiv-epidemic-started-spreading-new-york-1970-n673371.

17. Pépin, *Origins of AIDS*.

18. See the extensive literature on Western prejudice and African denial, such as Chirimuuta and Chirimuuta, *AIDS, Africa, and Racism*; Bibeau, "L'Afrique, terre imaginaire du sida"; Mbali, "AIDS Discourses"; Khonde, "L'histoire du sida au Congo"; and Mulwo, Tomaselli, and Francis, "HIV/AIDS and Discourses of Denial."

19. Setel, Lewis, and Lyons, *Histories of Sexually Transmitted Diseases*.

20. On these facts and their interpretation with reference to AIDS, see Quammen, *Spillover*, 412–19, 429–31.

21. See Khonde, "L'histoire du sida au Congo," and Buvé, "L'épidémie de VIH en Afrique subsaharienne."

22. Data referring to 2001 from UNAIDS, *Report on the Global HIV/AIDS Epidemic: July 2002*.

23. The definition of HIV-2 is valid for differentiating it from HIV-1, which in these pages is simply indicated as HIV.

24. Denis, "Pour une histoire sociale du sida," 17–40, 36.

25. Steenberg Olsen, "Structures of Stigma," 7.

26. For these data, see UNAIDS and WHO, *AIDS Epidemic Update*.

27. *Le Monde*, October 10, 1992.

28. Statement reported in Esparza, "Global Effort to Develop a Preventive HIV Vaccine."

29. "A Turning-Point for AIDS?," *Economist*, July 13, 2000.

30. Annan, *Address to African Summit*. The topic recurs in the economic literature on HIV/AIDS.

31. This approach derives from the WHO program that had been in charge of the fight against HIV/AIDS since 1987, the Global Programme on AIDS (GPA), which in turn was the transformation of a similar program that had existed since 1986. Some of the GPA's directors worked in the subsequent UN agency against AIDS (the Joint United Nations Programme on HIV and AIDS, or UNAIDS), including Peter Piot (later the first executive director of UNAIDS). See Knight, *UNAIDS*.

32. UNFPA and UNAIDS, *Report of the Planning Meeting on Strategic Options*.

33. Including the first agencies and those added over time, UNAIDS has altogether eleven cosponsoring agencies: UNHCR (Office of the United Nations High Commissioner for Refugees), UNICEF (United Nations Children's Fund), the WFP (World Food Programme), UNDP (United Nations Development Programme), UNFPA (United Nations Population Fund), the ILO (International

Labour Organization), UNESCO (United Nations Educational, Scientific and Cultural Organization), the WHO (World Health Organization), the World Bank, UNODC (United Nations Office on Drugs and Crime), and UN Women (United Nations Entity for Gender Equality and the Empowerment of Women).

34. Buvé, *L'épidémie de VIH en Afrique subsaharienne*, 89–90.
35. Knight, *UNAIDS*, 24.
36. Knight, 118.
37. Peter Piot (1949) started his career at the Institute of Tropical Medicine in Antwerp. After field research and academic teaching experiences in Belgium, Zaire, and Kenya, at the beginning of the 1990s he started working for the WHO and became an expert in public health policies. From 1995 to 2008 he was the executive director of UNAIDS and an undersecretary of the United Nations. Since 2010 he has been the director of the London School of Hygiene and Tropical Medicine. This is how he introduces himself in his memoir, published in 2012: "At times I was an outbreak detective in the heart of Africa, a scientist studying antimicrobical resistance in bacteria or the genetic diversity of HIV, a desperate clinician caring for patients when there was no antiretroviral treatment, a researcher and public health practitioner designing prevention and treatment programs, a UN official leading a complex multilateral organization in eighty countries and spearheading UN reform, a patient diplomat negotiating political resolutions and price reductions of antiretroviral drugs, a stubborn campaigner reaching out to the powerful of this world and bringing AIDS awareness to unexpected places, a frustrated fighter of bureaucracy, an activist from the beginning . . . and so often all of the above simultaneously" (Piot, *No Time to Lose*, x). Two aspects of his book put Piot in the spotlight because he had been in charge of UNAIDS and had taken part in the identification of the Ebola virus. An investigation into his involvement in the discovery of the Ebola virus in 1976, sometimes attributed to him, came in 2016 from the medical journalist Helen Branswell (see her "History Credits This Man"). However, see his memoir too. A scientific illustration of these circumstances shows that Joel G. Breman and Karl M. Johnson of the CDC played key roles (see Breman et al., "Discovery and Description of Ebola Zaire Virus"). Apparently it all began with a Belgian doctor in Zaire in 1976, who sent a thermos to the Institute of Tropical Medicine in Antwerp containing blood samples taken from a nun who was very sick from an unknown pathology. Piot was a twenty-seven-year-old trainee at the institute's laboratory and was involved in investigating the samples, under the guidance of Prof. Stefaan Pattyn. A virus believed to be of the Marburg strain was isolated, without the certainty that it was something new. Since Marburg-type viruses are highly lethal, only a few laboratories in the world, with the maximum level of biosecurity, were authorized to deal with them, and Antwerp was not among them. The blood samples were sent to the British military laboratories at Porton Down; a sample was then sent to the CDC. The CDC allegedly determined that it was a new virus and fulfilled the criteria for a discovery of this kind. It was still necessary

to establish how lethal the virus was and its actual effects. A scientific expedition to Zaire in 1976, organized and guided by the CDC, included researchers from Belgium, whose colonial dominion of the country had ended a few sixteen years before. Piot was in this group. The expedition gave the virus the name of a local river, the Ebola.

38. Piot's *No Time to Lose* was published in 2012, when the international policy on AIDS for countries with limited resources required the triple antiretroviral therapy. In it Piot claims he originally wanted to save AIDS patients in poor countries, and specifically in Africa, through treatment after the discovery in 1996 of the effectiveness of the triple antiretroviral therapy: "We had no choice but to do everything possible to bring antiretroviral treatment where the needs were greatest: in the first place, Africa" (Piot, 299). This commitment is repeated several times in his book (Piot, 239, 309, 314–15). At the same time, he criticizes the therapeutic skepticism of the institutions, experts, large agencies, and donor countries as well as African governments. Nonetheless, the book also lists the obstacles to the triple therapy in Africa, which by the end of the 1990s Piot considered to be, realistically speaking, insurmountable. These obstacles involved the feasibility of carrying out HIV tests, the lack of health care services and laboratories, the availability of drugs at accessible prices, the adherence of patients to their therapy, uniform therapeutic regimens to avoid the development of resistances, and taking on the long-term responsibility of vast numbers of chronic patients (see in particular Piot, 300–301). This was precisely what was alleged by the institutions, experts, large agencies, and donor countries in order to deny therapy in countries with limited resources, especially in Africa. Not even at the end of 2000 did the increasing requests for funds to fight AIDS from UNAIDS include any for the triple antiretroviral therapy in countries with limited resources. See UNAIDS and WHO, *AIDS Epidemic Update: December 2000* (a document signed by both UNAIDS and the WHO, although the experts indicated in the text all appear to be from UNAIDS). Assuming that UNAIDS did want to take the antiretroviral therapy to Africa, it did not distinguish itself by disagreeing with the rest of the mainstream international antitherapy approach to Africa, which, moreover, it had institutionally inspired and supervised. At the time, Piot appeared to have decided to be involved in essentially just one endeavor: negotiations with the large pharmaceutical industry to bring down the costs of the antiretroviral drugs.

39. Infra in this chapter regarding the *UNAIDS Drug Access Initiative*.

40. Lewis, *Race against Time*, 140.

41. On the Global Fund, see infra in this chapter PEPFAR: President's Emergency Plan for AIDS Relief.

42. Only toward 2002 did Piot appear to go along with the international trend that was increasingly in favor of extending the therapeutic approach to Africa too. Years later, when necessary, he still attributed the success of the fight against AIDS more to prevention than to the therapy, as though the therapy was not in

itself prevention. See, for example, his speech at the Tsinghua University of Peking on September 17, 2008, https://www.unaids.org/sites/default/files/media_asset/20080917_sp_pp_tsinghuauni_en_3.pdf. In it, the reduction of the incidence of new cases of HIV/AIDS is attributed to prevention initiatives (e.g., "Young people in . . . African and Caribbean countries are waiting longer to become sexually active, having fewer sexual partners, and using condoms more"), and the success of the fight against AIDS is first related to "political leadership and activism—political action," second to "funding," third to "HIV prevention and treatment" programs, and fourth to "science," as long as it was not only biomedical but also social and inexpensive.

43. Peter Piot's speech at the Second Africa Development Forum, Addis Ababa, December 3–7, 2000, reported in Knight, *UNAIDS*, 118.

44. Schwartländer, Grubb, and Perriëns, "10-Year Struggle," 541–46.

45. Katzenstein, Laga, and Moatti, "Evaluation of HIV/AIDS Drug Access Initiatives," 1.

46. Dozon, "Des appropriations sociales et culturelles du sida," 679–88.

47. Ndoye et al., "Présentation de l'initiative sénégalaise," 5.

48. "Discours de M. Jacques Chirac, Président de la République, sur la lutte contre le Sida en Afrique, l'aide au développement, la solidarité internationale pour la prévention et la mise en oeuvre de traitements coûteux, Abidjan le 7 décembre 1997," https://www.vie-publique.fr/discours/207830-discours-de-m-jacques-chirac-president-de-la-republique-sur-la-lutte.

49. Adler, "Antiretrovirals for Developing World," 232.

50. Knight, *UNAIDS*, 68.

51. UNAIDS and WHO, *Report on the Global HIV/AIDS Epidemic: June 1998*, 46.

52. For the setting of the drug-access initiative in Ivory Coast and Uganda, see "A Turning-Point for AIDS," *Economist*, July 13, 2000; Schwartländer, Grubb, and Perriëns, "10-Year Struggle," 541–42; Vidal and Moatti, *L'accès aux traitements du VIH/sida*; Uganda Ministry of Health, UNAIDS, and CDC, *Preliminary Report*; and Weidle et al., "Pilot Antiretroviral Drug Therapy Programme," 34–40.

53. The CD4s are the lymphocyte cells that make up the immune system, and they are used and destroyed by HIV in order for it to reproduce itself. In people with HIV, the CD4 count is drastically reduced, with the consequent deterioration of the immune system and the onset of ever-changing opportunistic infections to the point of full-blown AIDS and then death. If the antiretroviral therapy is started when a seropositive person has enough CD4s and their immune system is therefore only partially compromised, the therapeutic outcome can be successful. Otherwise, the outcome is unlikely to be very good.

54. On this, see infra in chapter 5.

55. Knight, *UNAIDS*, 87.

56. It was only since 2000 that funds from abroad were granted, starting with the European Union.

57. On ISAARV, see the voluminous Desclaux, *L'Initiative sénégalaise.*
58. Africa Region, World Bank, *Intensifying Action against HIV/AIDS*, 60.
59. European Commission, *HIV/AIDS and Population Related Operations*, which is dated November 12, 1999.
60. UNAIDS, *Report on the Global HIV/AIDS Epidemic: June 2000*, 97.
61. Philippe Rivière, "Sida, fin de l'indifférence," *Le Monde diplomatique*, July 7, 2000.
62. UNAIDS, *Global Strategy Framework on HIV/AIDS*, preface.
63. UNAIDS and WHO, *AIDS Epidemic Update: December 2000.*
64. Mbeki's denial could be interpreted as a jolt of African pride after the ANC itself became aware of the epidemic. See Butler, "South Africa's HIV/AIDS Policy," 591–614: "If only formally, the ANC came to power with a very impressive strategy to fight AIDS. A South African National Conventional on AIDS (NACOSA), first held in 1992, brought together the ANC, its ally the United Democratic Front and the Minister of Health of the National Party's government to finally, in 1994, agree on an overall national plan for AIDS, based on credible predictions: 'HIV/AIDS is emerging as a major public health problem, with over 2,000 reported cases at the end of 1993, and 500,000 people infected with HIV.' By 2000, the plan noted, 'there will be between four and seven million HIV-positive cases, with about 60 percent of total deaths due to AIDS, if HIV prevention and control measures remain unaddressed.... Credible predictions indicate that by year 2005, between 18 and 24 percent of the adult population will be infected with HIV, that the cumulative death toll will be 2.3 million, and that there will be about 1.5 million AIDS orphans.'"
65. United Nations, "Secretary-General Proposes Global Fund."
66. "Gambling with Lives," *Economist*, May 31, 2001.
67. "We have to get serious about public health in the poor countries if we are to be serious about economic development." This is Sachs's conclusion to his 2001 lecture at the Office of Health Economics in London, "The Link of Public Health and Economic Development."
68. "The Age of AIDS: Interview Jeffrey Sachs," *Frontline*, May 30, 2006, https://www.pbs.org/wgbh/pages/frontline/aids/interviews/sachs.html.
69. Attaran and Sachs, "International Donor Support," 57–61.
70. As quoted in Vogel, "Dollar and Cents," 2422.
71. "Consensus Statement on Antiretroviral Treatment."
72. The Harvard statement calls the Global Fund "the New Global Initiative," "the Global Program," and "the HIV/AIDS Prevention and Treatment Trust Fund," but it is exactly the same fund.
73. Vogel, "Dollar and Cents," 2422.
74. Cohen, "Call for Drugs."
75. "Age of AIDS."
76. The Harvard statement contained passages like "At approximately $1,100

per patient per year, the total cost of treatment for 1 to 3 million HIV-infected individuals in Africa within 3 to 5 years would be easily managed by the world's wealthiest countries. Even at the 5-year mark, the annual expenditure of about $3.3 billion would represent only about 0.01 percent of the aggregate GNP of these countries—or about 1¢ of each $100 of income in these economies."

77. "Consensus Statement on Antiretroviral Treatment."

78. As in Vogel, "Dollar and Cents."

79. "Consensus Statement on Antiretroviral Treatment."

80. Schwartländer et al., "Resource Needs for HIV/AIDS," 2434–36. Strangely enough, this article, which appeared at the end of June 2001, was considered by UNAIDS to be inspiration for the economic demands expressed by Kofi Annan when he announced the Global Fund in Abuja on April 26, 2001. See Knight, *UNAIDS*, 129. Piot, in *No Time to Lose*, states that the article by Schwartländer and his colleagues intended to "provide treatment to a majority of patients" (290). The figures seem to say otherwise, unless in this case only a very limited number of terminal AIDS patients were considered eligible for HAART.

81. Knight, *UNAIDS*, 134.

82. UNFPA and UNAIDS, "Report of the Planning Meeting on Strategic Options," 8.

83. UNFPA and UNAIDS, 9.

84. UNFPA and UNAIDS, 9.

85. UNFPA and UNAIDS, 11.

86. Lewis, *Race against Time*, 157–58.

87. An indicative episode: the US National Institutes of Health had funded the WHO for the drafting of the first guidelines for treating AIDS in resource-limited settings but later disagreed with the proposed approach so vigorously that the WHO returned the funds.

88. Wolfensohn led the World Bank from 1995 to 2005. He was a banker, economist, and jurist and cultivated the idea of worldwide development based on a humane approach.

89. This is what Lange said on July 12, 2002, at the closing ceremony of the 14th International Conference on AIDS in Barcelona. See Zackie Achmat, "Treatment Access as a Human Right," TheBodyPro, October 1, 2002.

90. William J. Clinton, "AIDS Is Not a Death Sentence," *New York Times*, December 1, 2002.

91. Schwartländer, Grubb, and Perriëns, "10-Year Struggle," 544.

92. Ramsey, "Global Fund Makes Payments," 1581–82.

93. Press release after the Global Fund board of directors meeting of April 22–24, 2002, by the activist Paul Davis of the Health GAP Coalition and the AIDS Coalition to Unleash Power (ACT UP).

94. DAIs: drug-access initiatives. ART-treated patients are those taking the triple antiretroviral therapy. Katzenstein, Laga, and Moatti, "Evaluation of HIV/

AIDS Drug Access Initiatives." It added, "These pilot programs also suggest that once financial barriers to access to drugs have been overcome, adherence to HAART can be as high among HIV-infected patients in Africa as that generally observed in industrialized countries."

95. Knight, *UNAIDS*, 172.

96. Caraël, "Face à la mondialisation du sida," 43–61, 59.

97. Tony Barnett and Alan Whiteside, *AIDS in the Twenty-First Century: Disease and Globalization* 333, 338.

98. "Treating AIDS, 3 by 5," *Economist*, March 30, 2006.

99. Hogg et al., "Triple-Combination Antiretroviral Therapy," 1406.

100. Müller et al., "Antiretroviral Therapy in Sub-Saharan Africa," 68. In fact, what Hogg proposed was an academic reflection on the feasibility of the triple therapy in underdeveloped countries, without taking a clear stand. Moreover, in his following article (Hogg et al., "One World, One Hope), the Canadian scholar calculated the cost of antiretroviral treatments for every infected individual in every country in relation to the overall population. In southern and eastern Africa, with so many HIV-positive people, each inhabitant would have had to pay six or seven times the American per capita cost. He then concluded, "Our results demonstrate that the cost of making combination antiretroviral therapy available worldwide would be exceedingly high, especially in countries with limited financial resources."

101. Ainsworth and Teokul, "Breaking the Silence," 58–59. Ainsworth worked for the World Bank.

102. "Global Health Fund," 1.

103. Gehler, *Un continent se meurt*, 173.

104. Peter Duesberg is one of the best-known scholars who denied the viral origin of AIDS—that is, the correlation between HIV and AIDS. See Duesberg, *Inventing the AIDS Virus*.

105. Whiteside, "Drugs," 3.

106. Whiteside, "Demography and Economics," 73–88.

107. Barnett and Whiteside, *AIDS in the Twenty-First Century*, 340, 342.

108. Creese et al., "Cost-effectiveness of HIV/AIDS Interventions," 1635–42.

109. Elliot Marseille, Paul B. Hofmann, and James G. Kahn, "HIV Prevention before HAART," 1851–56.

110. E. Goemaere, N. Ford, and S. R. Benatar, "HIV/AIDS Prevention and Treatment," 86.

111. Gregg Gonsalves, "HIV/AIDS Prevention and Treatment," 87.

112. Letter from P. Piot, D. Zewdie, and T. Türmen, *Lancet* 360, 9326 (July 6, 2002).

113. Ndoye et al., "Perspectives," 248.

114. "Editorial: The Economics of HIV in Africa."

115. "The Next Wave," *Economist*, October 17, 2002.

# 2

# The Failure of Prevention

Let us have a look at the arguments in favor of prevention as opposed to treatment. Some are fairly reasonable, some less so, and some are purely cynical.

First of all, there is the unsustainable cost of the antiretroviral drugs, to be considered in a worldwide context in which the greatest spread of HIV/AIDS was precisely in the countries with the least resources. In 2001 the *New England Journal of Medicine* estimated that a year of triple antiretroviral therapy carried out in the United States, using the most scrupulous and advanced clinical and diagnostic means available, cost between $13,000 and $23,000.[1] The average amount spent on health care per person in underdeveloped countries in 2001 was $13. This difference appeared to justify the inaccessibility of the treatment for the majority of people with AIDS throughout the world.

In 1998 the annual per capita income in South Africa was $3,336, in Cameroon $789, and even less in Kenya, Senegal, the DRC, Uganda, Tanzania, and Mozambique, all the way down to $148 in Burundi and $123 in Ethiopia, not to mention countries such as Liberia and Somalia engulfed in war, which completely disrupted their economic activities.[2] The average per capita annual income in sub-Saharan Africa was $621. Well, in Africa in 1996, the cost of a year's antiretroviral drugs produced in the West was on average $20,000; in 1998 it was brought down to $7,200, and in 2000 it was $1,200. At the turn of the century, the Accelerating Access Initiative, in which UNAIDS acted as an intermediary between countries with limited resources and pharmaceutical companies in order to bring down the prices, took into consideration a range between $950 and $1,850, depending on the specific antiretroviral cocktail.[3] In 2001 there was another drop in prices, to $500. The pharmaceutical companies were by then agreeing to differentiate the prices between the rich world and the poor world. At the same time, generic, nonpatented drugs that cost much less were appearing on the market: $1,000 in 1998 and $350 in 2000. As soon as the triple therapy came into existence, they started being produced in Brazil, India, and Spain. Other countries soon followed.

Generic drugs represent a complex question that should not be oversimplified. It was reasonable to fear that the large pharmaceutical industry, discouraged by insufficient payment for their patents, would stop investing in AIDS. Scientific research had to be supported in order to create new antiretroviral drugs—it was not enough to copy the existing ones. On the other hand, the UN moved cautiously within a framework of political and economic powers, which also included the wealthy multinational pharmaceutical companies that each produced a part of the antiretroviral therapies. (Every molecule used in the HAART regimen has a lucrative and jealously guarded patent that is valid for twenty years.) The UN preferred to negotiate with the pharmaceutical industry instead of unleashing the competition from generic drugs, whose quality, moreover, had to be checked on a case-by-case basis, unlike branded drugs.[4] To devalue or omit patents would be to sabotage the existing economic system. The senior management of the UN did not feel they could offend the large American, German, and Swiss interests. It should be remembered that the United States is the UN's largest financial contributor.

In 1997 South Africa started producing generic antiretroviral drugs in order to avoid the patents of the Western pharmaceutical industry. The United States government immediately proceeded with commercial retaliation, and South Africa had to give up. In the same way, in 1998 Thailand tried to produced generic antiretroviral drugs, and the United States carried out a similar trade war, and Thailand also had to give up.[5] South Africa and Thailand could have turned to international law courts because since 1994 the intellectual regulatory treaties within the WTO,[6] as well as regulations protecting patents from being economically exploited, also included exception clauses in the case of emergency health situations.[7] Nothing prevented the United States from attacking the two countries and forcing them to stop. This was purely a question of strength. Brazil, however, which was much more powerful than South Africa and Thailand and had millions of people with AIDS who could not be left to die, had started producing generic drugs in 1997 and proudly resisted the American threat by engaging in a long battle with the United States. India had done the same. In 2002 what the media interpreted as a clash between humanitarian rights and international business started cooling off. Bill Clinton and Al Gore, convinced that the world AIDS pandemic threatened the very safety of the United States, had stopped waging war against the generic drug industry. An agreement was reached: the patented drugs would have profitable prices in the rich countries and affordable prices in the poor countries, in order to be able to face the competition from the generic drugs. The patents continued to be profitable, less so than before but also less blatantly.

In any case, the UN's approach had always been to negotiate a compromise with the multinational pharmaceutical companies in order to obtain reductions in prices or other facilitations without causing rifts and by respecting the patents, which were considered an essential stimulus for scientific research. No patents, no profits—therefore, no funds for research, no discoveries of better drugs, no vaccine. This was true, but in the meantime people in Africa were dying. The UN wanted to bring down the cost of the antiretroviral drugs but without upsetting anyone. Kofi Annan, Peter Piot, and Gro Harlem Brundtland all made a huge effort. For years they met with the top managers of the pharmaceutical industry. After all, it was a general issue that not only concerned countries with limited resources but also developed countries, considering the exorbitant prices of the antiretroviral drugs. If there had been a political intention to reduce the patents, the UN would have been able to concentrate more on the generic drugs, whose prices came down in relation to the scale-up in orders. However, the UN was not seriously interested in this aspect and what reigned instead was skepticism regarding the capacity of the Africans, and of the people of the third world in general, to set up mass antiretroviral treatments. So, those in Africa who really did want to treat poor people, after carrying out the appropriate controls, used generic drugs without waiting for the Western pharmaceutical industry and were careful not to be noticed.

The second argument in favor of prevention alone: inadequate health care systems. Mass treatments for AIDS would take the African health care systems to a point of total collapse. How could AIDS be treated in run-down hospitals with underqualified staff? Outside major towns in Africa, there were very few health care centers. Primary health care was neglected, and endemic diseases such as malaria, tuberculosis, dysentery, and typhoid that killed millions of people a year also had to be dealt with. The old diseases had by no means disappeared. Even though the sub-Saharan countries refused to treat AIDS itself, the high prevalence of opportunistic infections related to AIDS meant that crowds of people with AIDS were trying to get treatment at the health centers, which were totally unable to cope with so many people. Moreover, in those days people often said there were more Malawian doctors in Manchester than in Malawi or more Guinean doctors in Paris than in Guinea. It was difficult to imagine treating AIDS in conditions like that.

Nonetheless, although the situation was briefly acknowledged by the international development agencies, practically nothing was done to improve the health care facilities, particularly the poorest ones outside the towns, or to train new staff and encourage them to stay in the country. It was as though being resigned to this situation was the only option—as though it was impossible to do anything about it. The tiny amount spent by the African governments on the health sector (e.g., around $2 per person in Mozambique, Malawi, and Guinea) was obviously discouraging, and yet it was accepted without looking into the contributing factors, which were very embarrassing for the UN and for the international community. These factors included public spending cuts, privatization of medical centers, and injunctions against providing treatment free of charge, which represented the outcome of the reorganization imposed on African economies in the 1980s and 1990s by the Bretton Woods institutions. The endogenous shortcomings of the African public health care system were caused by corruption, disorganization, and bureaucracy. This situation was also conditioned by exogenous factors, such as the international donor policies that encouraged the privatization of medical centers and turning health care into a free market, less influence of governments in health care services, and the fact that the already low number of African medical staff moved abroad to work in Western nongovernmental organizations (NGOs) that were prepared to pay double or triple their salary (when these professionals had no choice but to emigrate abroad because there was no suitable work for them in the public hospitals). It did not sound strange that the patients of national health care systems in rich Europe were provided with the antiretroviral drugs free of charge, whereas the patients even in the poorest parts of Africa had to pay for the therapy themselves. Neither did anyone wonder whether, in providing aid for development, it would have been more appropriate to channel funds to the poor African health care budgets and check that they were then invested in infrastructures. Not to mention the responsibility of the former colonial powers for having created centralized, vertical health care systems that depended on large hospitals in the capital cities and ignored the outskirts and the vast rural areas where many sub-Saharan Africans live. It was obvious that treating AIDS required the horizontal infrastructures that were lacking in the system passed down from colonialism, which was only partially compensated for by missionaries and international cooperatives. As for HIV opportunistic infections causing the collapse of the health care centers, it was precisely therapeutic inertia that caused this situation. Treating AIDS would have prevented the onset of these diseases in the first place.

It was true that in order to treat AIDS, there had to be a health care system. However, this is exactly the point: if there was no health care system, it had to be set up. At an international level the public health community complained, but it did not actually do anything at all: it had a weird desire to affirm its helplessness. When the idea of therapy was finally accepted, in 2002, it was not associated with the need for a health care system worthy of that name but with the mere distribution of medicines.[8] The prejudice remained however: Africa had no scientific culture; Africans were unable to organize anything properly; training local staff took ages; setting up laboratories was like letting a teenager drive a Ferrari. Besides, even if good health care centers were set up, they kept saying, these centers would only be able to treat a few patients, who would then unfairly become a privileged elite. It was not taken into consideration that, in order to achieve something complete, it is necessary to start from a clearly defined point It was hard to see that the HIV epidemic provided the chance to improve the African public health care system and provide it with efficient medical facilities.

The therapeutic management of AIDS also involved the treatment of many opportunistic infections. This was an opportunity to invest in public health systems that would then deal with pathologies that typically occur in Africa, such as tuberculosis and malaria, in a more systematic way. Starting from the AIDS challenge, there could be a great improvement in the medical facilities in Africa. At the same time, the advances in biochemistry and hematology required by AIDS for laboratories would have a positive effect on all the whole public health system in terms of diagnostic progress for the whole population in relation to a vast number of pathologies. The same thing would apply to investments in information technology in health care.

The third argument was that according to those in favor of prevention, Africans were incapable of adhering to the therapies for AIDS, both because of the large number of pills they had to take every day and because of all the problems regarding the contact with the health centers and health care bureaucracy. A century ago, Africans' distance from Western medical practice was considered harmlessly exotic. Karen Blixen, in her 1937 memoir *Out of Africa*, talked about the "great German doctor" who could not understand the local patients or "their deep dislike of regularity, of any repeated treatment or the systematization of the whole." The author, conversely, loved Africans' attitude: "I sometimes thought that what, at the bottom of their hearts, they feared from us was pedantry. In the hands of a pedant they die of grief."[9] Blixen also reported that Africans are able to treat themselves in a very consistent way. In the twenty-first century, this is no longer an exotic issue. Saying that Africans are by nature incapable of following a medical therapy demonstrates blatant prejudice.

When Africans had the opportunity to find out about Western medicine, they appreciated it. Hundreds of millions of people were vaccinated during colonial and postcolonial vaccination campaigns in the twentieth century. They wanted Western-type clinics and hospitals, and they acknowledged the value of antibiotics. Of course, illness is often experienced in terms of nature and destiny, instead of science. Africans, however, are pragmatic too. When AIDS patients were only offered prevention by the development cooperation agencies, they nearly all went to healers and witch doctors simply because the Western pharmaceutical companies did not give them anything to help them fight the disease. When the treatment started to become available consistently, from 2003 onward, millions of African patients focused on their adherence to the therapy, which was difficult for them more because of problems with the health care systems and drug stocks and the fact that the health care facilities were mainly centralized in towns and cities than because the patients were erratic or untrustworthy.

Nobody thought this is how it would go. Before 2003 it was speculated that African patients, given the possibility to receive the treatment, would pocket the precious antiretroviral drugs and then sell them on the black market rather than use them to get better. This did not happen, for the most part. The patients felt better after starting their therapy, so they certainly did not want to sell the drugs that were providing these results. Then there was the idea that African patients wouldn't know how to take the pills at the right time. According to Andrew Natsios, the director of the United States Agency for International Development (USAID), many Africans "have never seen a clock or a watch their entire lives. . . . They know morning, they know evening, they know the darkness at night," so they would not be able to take the medicines at the right time.[10]

It was also said that if the treatments were carried out incorrectly, this would cause drug resistances on a vast scale, which would then affect the patients being treated in the Global North, putting the whole planet at risk. If the treatments were generally carried out badly, HIV would mutate and new strains would appear, making the available drugs useless. The worst alarms came from British health care. In 2004 the *British Medical Journal* warned that proceeding in a way that was described as "random and haphazard," with "suboptimal adherence," would cause "the transmission of drug resistant virus strains"—"a disaster in the long run." The authors recommended the following: "We should stop and think about the risks of resistance, and ways of minimising them, before increasing access to antiretroviral therapy in Africa."[11] In time these fears were dispelled because the number of drugs available went from four, five, or six antiretroviral drugs to dozens of types, with completely new classes of drugs. Moreover, it was not as though Western patients were a model of adherence compared to Africans. One example was Westerners' interruptions for holidays, which were so frequent that the threshold beyond which the number of missed doses would create resistances was assessed for every antiretroviral drug.[12] This was more of an ideological than a scientific concern: the Global South was considered approximate and disorganized, and it would have compromised the Global North, which was seen as accurate and scrupulous.

The fact that the antiretroviral therapies involved taking dozens of pills a day meant that it was considered inconceivable for Africa, although the number of pills was reduced year after year. Paradoxically the therapy was simplified in poor countries before rich countries because single generic drugs for the triple antiretroviral therapy were available in the former starting in 2002, whereas in the West, because of the patents, the three parts of the therapies were separate and came from different multinational pharmaceutical companies, each with their own profit requirements. Africans demonstrated that they were just as prepared to comply with the treatment as the patients in the West—if not more so, given the greater obstacles they had to overcome. This contradicts many prejudiced approaches, which may well have been inspired by the most compassionate of intentions. To argue, for example, that even limited adherence in Africa was sufficient to justify the offer of antiretroviral drugs because it would save the life of at least some patients may have been charitable, but it was also defeatist and did not reflect the patients' real experience and their desire to save their lives.

Even when the prevention-only period was over, the objection regarding the uncertain adherence of the Africans did not disappear. For a long time, this was used to justify minimalist approaches to the standard of treatment, in addition to doubts about the economic sustainability of treating people with AIDS. In the name of aiming to achieve adherence, the therapeutic schemes were oversimplified, the patients' nutritional needs were overlooked, the necessary checkups were reduced, the extra-HIV diagnoses were neglected, and the patients' living conditions and family contexts were ignored. High numbers of patients were considered lost from the beginning of the treatment in Africa. At the beginning of WHO's 3 by 5 Initiative, which aimed to put three million patients on HAART by 2005, extremely simplified guidelines were produced for fear of the program failing.[13]

The treatment was unambitious to say the least and took for granted that it was not possible to treat AIDS patients in Africa with similar criteria of excellence as those adopted in the West. Instead of one treatment for each patient, paying attention to a whole series of parameters to be taken into consideration for long-term therapy, what was proposed was mass treatments—with no personalized approaches, no therapeutic combinations, no advanced technologies, no individual monitoring, and no geographic or social differentiation. So, even losing 50 percent of the patients because of this mass-treatment approach would be considered a success because the other 50 percent would be saved. Two Italian AIDS scholars, Daniela Minerva and Stefano Vella, write:

> In poor countries, the aim is to save as many people as possible, without worrying about individuals. . . . The conditions they live in force millions of people in the Global South to not consider life the way we do: they have a lot of children because some of them die; infant mortality is accepted with a deep sense of inevitability, nobody in India or in Africa would dream of giving an individual child the absolute value we give them. This is not because the life of an African or Pakistani child is worth less, obviously. But because everyone, mothers and children, live in a context in which death is always lurking. There is a strong sense of family, of the village in poor countries, which has to continue despite sickness and hunger. We have fortunately lost this sort of inevitability of natural selection and protection of the species, because here it is the life of the individual that has to be guaranteed, not the survival of the group. This is why mass treatment, leaving death on the streets, that brings the family, the village, the whole country out of the tunnel and from certain massacre, is certainly not a colonialist imposition.[14]

No African with AIDS would ever agree with these views. Why give them half the chance to survive compared to a Western patient?

The idea of Africans' poor adherence was not supposed to lead to an extreme simplification of the treatment, even, as some people proposed, entrusting traditional healers with distributing the antiretroviral drugs, considering the shortage of doctors and nurses. On the contrary, it should have resulted in the commitment to strengthen the health care systems, extending them to rural areas, and providing them with drugs, diagnostic instruments, and staff who were not only well trained but also adequately paid, so they would not move abroad or ask patients for extra money.

Another argument—the fourth one. The limited resources available were not to be invested in expensive therapies to treat HIV-positive people when the HIV/AIDS pandemic was not the only health emergency in Africa. There was also malaria, tuberculosis, hepatitis, various types of infections from parasites, high infant mortality, and so on. There were fundamental everyday hygiene issues, starting with water and food. However, the strengthening of the African health care systems that was hoped for in view of treating AIDS also represented a chance to fight other diseases and improve public health, especially because there is a direct correlation between AIDS and some of these pathologies. The breakdown of the immune system encourages the onset of countless diseases, starting from the most common ones in the area, such as malaria and tuberculosis. Further, it is these very diseases that encourage the morbidity of HIV since they are not only AIDS-induced opportunistic infections but also pathologies that undermine the immune system itself and create a more receptive condition for HIV. The fight against AIDS is also a fight against the other African diseases and vice versa. Basically, AIDS is a multiplier of pathologies, but it is also encouraged by Africa's endemic diseases. The treatment of AIDS does not compete in any way with the treatment of other diseases: they are both necessary aspects of a comprehensive health care system, inspired by the need or by the concept of—to use an expression that was not yet popular at the beginning of the twenty-first century—global health.

As with every mainstream idea, the argument for prioritizing prevention brought together many zealous supporters who were not satisfied with demonstrating that prevention was irreplaceable. However, nobody—not even the most enthusiastic advocates of the therapeutic approach—questioned prevention, if carried out seriously. These supporters of prevention also tried to somehow invalidate the competition that treatment programs represented. Nothing but this kind of atmosphere can explain the alarm, totally out of proportion with the clinical evidence, regarding the toxicity of the antiretroviral drugs, particularly in Africa. It was as though they appeared to be less harmful at other latitudes.[15] It was true that antiretroviral drugs were new and their long-term effects were not known. That they had dramatic side effects, as claimed, had not been demonstrated. Monstrous deformations of the body, distorted faces, dramatic cardiovascular consequences, and cases of diabetes were reported, but none of this was true. Every drug has its side effects, but that should not discourage their use when necessary. Antibiotics can have negative side effects—the name itself implies it—and in the short or long term they can cause resistance, especially if abused, but in many cases they save lives. Their toxicity will not make the world of medicine go back to the age before antibiotics.

In the case of AIDS, Western patients considered antiretroviral drugs to be miraculous, and the fact that they might be harmful was not one of their first thoughts. Antiretroviral drugs saved lives, and that was enough, even if they had severe side effects, which in any case were very rare. The discussions on toxicity and resistance were inconclusive and destined to vanish even in developing countries at the same rate that the antiretroviral drugs continued to guarantee the patients good health, with only marginal side effects. There were cases of lipodystrophy, a redistribution of adipose tissue in the body with undesirable aesthetic effects, and rare cases of Stevens-Johnson syndrome, a sort of autoimmune disease caused by Nevirapine, one of the drugs that can be used in the triple therapy, in subjects with particular genetic predispositions. (This syndrome occurred in one in one thousand patients.) It was right to worry about the possible toxicity of the antiretroviral drugs, each of which, like any other drug, had side effects and had to be selected on the basis of its tolerability for the patient. It was normal clinical practice to prescribe antiretroviral drugs that were compatible with each patient's condition, bearing in mind whether the patient had hypertension, kidney failure, liver diseases, or other problems. In fact, the alarm regarding the toxicity of the antiretroviral drugs in Africa was mainly empirical and very general and was suggested by those in favor of prevention alone to be one of the reasons for not taking the HAART regimen to Africa. This was echoed by those who denied the role of HIV in immunity depression, such as South African president Thabo Mbeki.

Actually, what happened when the treatment was not carried out properly was far worse than the result of any degree of toxicity. People simply died, and the cause of death was the opportunistic infections induced by immunodeficiency, which were, moreover, sometimes concomitant. These people suffered terribly and for a long time. Mothers also died more easily during childbirth. Around 50 percent of children born HIV-positive died within their second year of life, and 60 percent of them before they were six years old.[16] In contrast, in the West since 1996, the treatments had really been resurrecting patients, and compared to that any side effects were of secondary importance.

Last but not least, an ethical principle was invoked in order to prevent even beginning the antiretroviral regimen in Africa. It was claimed that the presumed scarcity of pharmacological resources and the undeniably inadequate hospitals and medical centers would unfairly lead to treatment only for a select elite. Selecting the patients to treat appeared to be immoral in itself. A minority of patients would receive the therapy, whereas the majority would not. It was to be either everyone or no one; any other option would be absolutely unjust: "The use of public funds to subsidize the treatment of patients in the poorest countries who are most able to comply—who are better educated and have access to better health care—would be highly inequitable, and would shift health resources from the poor to those who are not poor."[17]

This pseudomoral position was very popular and cast a shadow over any attempt to do anything to treat AIDS in poor countries. When UNAIDS tested the drug-access initiative, Piot felt it was necessary to confirm its moral integrity, as though it were illicit to give some patients a chance to survive when others were dying: "tough decisions" in determining the limits of participation would only be justified by the need to carry out the experiment.[18] From the "tough," it can be understood that it would have been better not to do anything at all and not create a caste of saved patients, leaving everyone to die democratically. Is death not the maximum expression of equality? In fact, if anything was "highly inequitable" and "tough," it was giving patients in the Global North the antiretroviral drugs and therefore their health and not letting the infected people in the Global South access this same benefit.

This attitude was ideological. In Africa it was not possible to treat some people and not everyone; neither was it possible to introduce the triple antiretroviral therapy in one country and not in all the countries at the same time. On the other hand, the history of medicine shows that progress has always come from partial initiatives that then became general practice. The initiatives carried out against malnutrition have always been partial, depending on the funds available, the geographic context, and the populations affected. Tuberculosis and malaria, which are still endemic in Africa, were fought country by country and area by area in other continents. In the West, the prevalence of tuberculosis was practically eliminated even before antibiotics were available, thanks to the improvement in people's diet, which certainly did not take place at the same rate everywhere but depended on general economic factors. Moreover, malaria, which a century ago was still widespread in industrialized countries was virtually eliminated gradually thanks to the recovery of land, water regulations, distribution of quinine, and use of DDT, all of which benefited people but not all at the same time or to the same extent.

Saying "everyone or no one" meant denying the Global South what was being done in the Global North. It also meant not wanting to see what was already happening in the Global South. Rich Africans were already receiving the therapy according to the best Western standards in the clinics in Johannesburg, Kampala, and wherever else this was possible. They were not blamed for this, and "everyone or no one" did not apply to them.

From a rational point of view, it was difficult to understand this ethical objection, which blocked the beginning of treatment in Africa. Increasing the number of patients in therapy, to the point where all of them would be treated, had to be a gradual process. Universal access to therapy could not be instant but had to be the consequence of the multiplication of many single initiatives. Whoever wanted to take the antiretroviral therapies to Africa necessarily had to start from a specific geographical place, with an inevitably limited number of HIV-positive people. Did this mean all the other infected people were discriminated against? The way it was carried out was actually by starting from one place, with the aim of rapid scaling up. The moral objection was unsustainable because history showed that progress always consisted of gradual developments, but it was ideologically fascinating and was useful for the people who opposed treating AIDS in Africa.

## PREVENTION ALONE: THE OUTCOME

What was involved in incorporating AIDS in all the aspects of human development and of economic planning, as requested by UN-AIDS?[19] "Multisectorial" meant all-encompassing, but how could this "everything" be described? The area of multisectorial prevention as established in the public discussion on AIDS was partially medical (e.g., regarding transfusions, microbicides, and sexually transmitted diseases), but according to its promoters it also had to be extended indefinitely both socially and culturally. This was an open field for any proposal, like the one by two illustrious AIDS scholars, who in 2002 praised the potential benefits of electrification: "Electrification raises people's standard of living and gives them access to a range of recreational activities in addition to sex."[20] As it gradually slipped away from the scientific medical anchor, multisectorial prevention lent itself to countless debates among experts from all areas of the humanities and even more among many people who did not work in the name of science: opinion leaders, politicians, lobbyists, businessmen, swindlers, and people just full of hot air. In the United States, the prevention of AIDS became the subject of a culture war during the presidency of George W. Bush between supporters of the condom and supporters of sexual abstinence. Insofar as prevention did not involve a scientific path but an indistinct "everything," anyone could imagine practicing it their own way.

But let us begin at the beginning. Prevention of AIDS in African went through several different phases. The first one, maybe the most serious one and certainly the least ideological one, went from the first identified cases of AIDS in Africa (Uganda 1982) to the start of UNAIDS in 1995. This phase was rather anarchic, not well supervised or regulated by common sense. The aim was mainly to modify the behavior of individuals. It was during these years, in the country most badly affected by AIDS, Uganda, that the slogan ABC— "Abstain, Be faithful, Condomise"—was coined. This imitated the way the rich world appeared to be combatting AIDS, but there was more to it than just the use of condoms. In the West there was the idea that sex in Africa was totally unrestrained. This is a myth that misrepresents the relationship between sex and poverty and shows no knowledge of women's lack of property and rights. In the 1980s an American journalist even suggested that Africans were infected by HIV because they had sex with monkeys.[21] Racist stories like this would have been even more damming if it had already been known at the time that HIV had likely come from chimpanzees in the forests of Central Africa at the beginning of the twentieth century, as explained earlier. It was extremely likely that the pathogen was passed from these animals to man before it formed the critical mass that turned into an epidemic, but in the 1980s the genesis of HIV was a mystery. It was obvious that HIV was mainly transmitted in Africa through heterosexual, not homosexual relationships, like at the beginning in the rich part of the world. The first phase of prevention in Africa concentrated on sexual behavior—the risks of sexual infidelity, having a lot of partners, casual sex, not using condoms in unsafe contexts—and advised caution through educational campaigns.

There was another medical aspect. This concerned the treatment of opportunistic infections, which, during the first phase of the fight against HIV/AIDS, were still considered separate pathologies, even though they resulted from immunodeficiency. At the time there were no triple antiretroviral therapies. There was azidothymidine (AZT), which was introduced in the West in 1986 and for a long time was believed to be useful in delaying full-blown AIDS. It was later demonstrated to be basically ineffective on its own (whereas it is very effective in antiretroviral cocktails). In any case, AZT never reached Africa because it was too expensive. Regardless of the myth of unrestrained African sexual customs, the idea of curbing HIV by influencing sexual behavior was reasonable, especially since there was no therapy.

The second phase of prevention coincided with the beginning of UNAIDS, which believed that what had been done up to then was not enough and considered it a "narrow response" to the epidemic. UNAIDS had other far-reaching ambitions, as can be seen in the language used in its documents, in which prevention was always by definition multisectorial, intensified, expanded, accelerated, comprehensive, coordinated, strengthened, increased, integrated, enhanced, enlarged, reinforced, sustained. Prevention unquestionably implied involvement, commitment, progress, implementation, empowerment, advocacy, challenge, mobilization, priority, leadership, and so on. Moreover, it had to evoke new social models, new coalitions, new synergies, new alliances. According to UNAIDS, the "complex environment" in which Africans lived had been underestimated as well as the cultural obstacles to any change in their sexual behavior. Individual behavior is a result of social and cultural influences, and this was the aspect that UNAIDS wanted to work on in order to warn people about AIDS. It was the question of AIDS having to be dealt with in social terms, as mentioned above, like a challenge for human development, and removed from its medical context. Fighting AIDS this way, the governments and civil society were supposed to involve far more than their medical institutions alone. This meant that society as a whole also had to take part, including all kinds of communities and associations. UNAIDS insisted on the multisectorial aspect in order to commit all the areas of society to fighting AIDS. In the same way, every ministry in every government was to develop its own specific fight against the epidemic, not only the medical approach, and likewise every successive branch of public administration.

In line with the so-called KAPB (knowledge, attitudes, practices, behaviors) studies, prevention basically consisted of information and propaganda, sex education, and distributing condoms. Nonetheless there were medical factors that could not be ignored. UNAIDS knew what opportunistic infections were, even though in Africa they were not often acknowledged as a consequence of HIV. UNAIDS included these infections in its consideration of HIV/AIDS, and since it excluded treating this immunodeficiency a priori, it would consider treating the opportunistic infections for the diseases they were, assuming that the African public health care systems had the resources to do so. From a practical point of view, it did not make any difference: an HIV-positive patient with tuberculosis continued to be treated for tuberculosis, even if the African medical staff had started thinking that there was a connection with HIV. UNAIDS then recommended the prophylaxis and treatment of sexually transmitted diseases. It also sponsored some mother-to-child prevention projects, without going beyond the usual minimalistic standards for poor countries, which were basically ineffective because they did not involve using any funds for a HAART regimen.

While in the rich part of the world AIDS was treated with the triple antiretroviral therapy, the representatives of UNAIDS in African countries claimed to achieve great results against AIDS by administering cotrimoxazole (Bactrim) as a prophylaxis. However, cotrimoxazole is a long-term sulfonamide that was actually ineffective against HIV, since it is a virus and not a bacterium, which can be treated with sulfonamides. It was believed that cotrimoxazole prevented AIDS infection by protecting the immune system from opportunistic infections. It was like giving a leukemia patient a remedy for a secondary disorder, which may well have been annoying but was certainly not the main cause for concern. Cotrimoxazole had no effect on the progress of AIDS itself. As an antibacterial it is very effective, but its efficacy is very limited if the immune system is compromised: cotrimoxazole fought one opportunistic infection, but another one would appear and then another. The CD4s, the lymphocyte cells that make up the immune systems that are used and destroyed by HIV so the virus can reproduce, continued to decrease to lower and lower levels, and new opportunistic infections appeared, caused by microbes that did not provoke infection in healthy subjects but took advantage of the weakened immune systems of people with AIDS. This condition led to pathologies such as fungal infections, dreadful mycoses, then diarrhea, meningitis, pneumonia, tumors, and so on, until the patient died. The lower the CD4 levels, the more difficult it was to treat the patient, and cotrimoxazole did not work. As soon as the antiretroviral drugs arrived in Africa, the role of cotrimoxazole was once again to support the etiological therapy, and it was no longer used as essential protection. Around 2000, however, it was administered to treat HIV. Western NGOs sang its praises and organized petitions for

HIV-positive Africans to obtain universal access.[22] Ultimately, HIV/AIDS cannot be successfully treated with cotrimoxazole.

Instead of treatment, the UN agencies mainly talked about care, support, mitigation—basically a compassionate palliative approach—referring to the solidarity of the resources of civil society, which were praised and exalted. These resources were considered infinite, like reservoirs already there in order to be exploited. The United Nations tended to give civil society a role that replaced the African public health system, which was considered useless. It was taken for granted that the health system had gone off the rails because of corruption, lack of funds, a bureaucratic mentality, a dramatic reduction of staff because of AIDS, and overcrowding due to the opportunistic infections caused by HIV in the first place. The only other option was to count on the various aspects of civil society: the family, village community, all sorts of informal groups, possible NGOs, seropositive activists, and so forth. This issue could obviously only be addressed in very general terms, and at the same time it could only be carried out from a sociopolitical point of view.

It was believed that the health care system could not defeat AIDS, so the fight against the pandemic was entrusted to society and popular culture at a grassroots level. Civil society was not asked to save people who had already been infected, since it did not administer the drugs, but it was considered decisive in reducing the incidence of AIDS by preventing new cases. It was therefore civil society that had to deal with making people aware, confronting the stigma, countering denial of HIV/AIDS, and demystifying the disease. The main aim of the agencies coordinated by UNAIDS was to increase awareness. This was the right aim, but it was cultivated as an alternative to treatment instead of an integration within the context of the global fight against HIV.

All kinds of theories and practices were adopted: the participation of influential local people, media information campaigns, communication technique courses, sex education in and out of schools, programs for prostitutes and for their clients, propaganda in the workplace, psychological support, and even a brilliant idea that never came about, which was the local production of condoms to provide both work and prophylaxis. In the end, even traditional healers and their remedies, practices, plants, and potions were acknowledged and included in the fight against AIDS. This represented total surrender: the African health care system was considered so ineffective that people were actually encouraged to go elsewhere. The UN publication *Community Realities and Responses to HIV/AIDS in Sub-Saharan Africa* had sections headed "Deteriorating Public Service," followed by "Local Responses—No Other Alternative."[23] The local response amounted to very little, apart from the help that AIDS patients received from their families, if they were lucky enough not to be thrown out. There were the healers, of course, but not much else, so in the end the highly praised grassroots action turned out to be just hot air. More from *Community Realities and Responses*:

> Local responses are, ultimately, the most immediate and direct intervention strategies, and despite devastating impact, HIV/AIDS can have a positive influence on social cohesion as communities organize initiatives to address this urgent crisis. Vulnerability, such as HIV/AIDS, can foster a collective response among community members, which, in turn, fosters personal empowerment and social change.... "Collective action might be stimulated in the face of a community-wide threat before that threat begins to undermine the ability and incentive to act collectively." ... In sub-Saharan Africa, "Communities are mobilizing themselves, showing great resilience and solidarity, despite their vulnerability to external shocks such as premature death of their most productive members." ... Effective community-centered action can initiate an empowerment cycle, a counterweight to the poverty cycle, in which a community's success engenders more positive feelings, solidarity, and momentum for another successful cycle.[24]

These were simply abstract statements. The reality was very different. AIDS did not create social capital—it destroyed it. It did not encourage a sense of community—it led to exclusion, isolation, and death that was social before it was physical. The stigma reigned. The patients did not receive solidarity from the community at all. On the contrary, it was easy to see they were sick because AIDS was known as "the slim disease," and they were very thin. The fact that grandparents had to take care of their orphaned grandchildren may well have been a heroic way to resist AIDS, but it was first of all a sad necessity, not something to be pleased about. It was part of a family's responsibilities to take care of any members of the family who were ill, but that did not always happen because the stigma often prevailed over pity, even at home. It was crazy to talk about social cohesion, collective action, great resilience, and empowerment cycles when families were falling apart because the most productive young people were dying and families were left with no breadwinners, when funerals took place one after another, when everyone was in mourning, when there was no scientific health care, or it had nothing to offer. What was the point when people turned to traditional healers, there seemed to be no future, and people hanged themselves from trees as soon as they found out they were seropositive, when people who were HIV-positive left the towns they were living in to die in the villages where they were born? The dominating characteristics of the epidemic were desperation, escape, and suicide—not flexibility, participation, and solidarity. UNAIDS officers, perhaps because they were thinking of the old Western myth of the "noble savage," imagined African communities that guaranteed care, support, and mitigation. However, those were just dreams. It was within this context that, as mentioned above, the figure of the traditional healer was reconsidered.

The UN was shocked by how popular the traditional healers were in Africa and planned to recruit them as collaborators in the fight against AIDS. They were to be offered basic health education, training, and roles in prevention activities.[25] Since they were part of the grassroots of Africa, which was considered positive, they were bound to play a beneficial role. It did not work out like that. Traditional healers do not follow scientific logic. Africans with AIDS went to them for various reasons: because of their age-old traditions, because going to public health centers meant revealing that they were HIV-positive and risking being ostracized, because Western scientific health care turned out to be inaccessible. Traditional healers had their own ideologies, their practice was not scientific, and they were expensive, although less so than a HAART regimen carried out privately. A traditional consultation, treatment, or potion might cost a month's income. Furthermore, many Africans were not aware of the existence of germs, bacteria, viruses, and microorganisms. When children drank dirty water from a puddle and were told it was dirty, they might say that it was not dirty—it was brown.

There was also often the idea that diseases have supernatural causes, that they depend on malignant spirits, or that they are the consequence of sin.[26] Animist culture, with which even Christians and Muslims also partially identify, presupposes that behind any disease there is guilt, witchcraft, a curse, magic, or voodoo. There is a widespread alternative culture from Togo to Kenya, from Namibia to Tanzania. When you go to the traditional healer, he asks you, "What have you done? Who have you hurt? Your mother-in-law, your wife, your children?" Otherwise, if he wants to be kinder: "Who is angry with you? Who might have put a curse on you?" The cure goes in one of two directions: atonement if the ill person is guilty; retaliation if someone else is considered guilty. In the first case, the person takes herbs, potions, and often toxic mixtures to drive away the evil spirits related to the event. In the second case, the people believed to be the cause of the evil may even be killed, and they are usually chosen because they are different from everyone else. They may be weak or behave unusually or look different. They could be relatives who left the family, single women, other ill people, albinos, old people, or outcasts of any kinds.

Healers were also greatly responsible for the spread of AIDS in Africa. Their practices often involve cutting the skin, and they always use the same blade or razor to spread various essences on the cut. It is the healers, who, using the same instruments on everyone, perform male circumcision or female genital mutilation, which is still widely practiced in many sub-Saharan countries. None of the instruments used for these procedures are ever sterilized. AIDS in Africa, unlike in the West in its first decade, was related to heterosexuality more than homosexuality, and it was related to these traditional practices. That the international agencies tried to provide the healers with information about AIDS was certainly commendable. However, the healers remained in their magical/sacred sphere, in which they were legitimized in the eyes of the ordinary people. They also continued with their risky therapeutic approach. Why would they not? They really believed in traditional practices, and many of them were infected by their own blades. Besides, even if they had not wanted to treat people who it was thought had AIDS, the situation forced these people to turn to them. Otherwise, they would have been cast from their communities and died alone. It was clear that Western medicine did not provide any remedies for the slim disease and that the African health care systems were helpless against AIDS. In 2001 Sachs observed,

> In many parts of Sub-Saharan Africa the AIDS pandemic is having a double effect. It is not only killing people by the millions but is also leading to a massive rise in social conflict because the disease is interpreted within a social conflict framework. The sick and dying are seen as victims of witchcraft, poisonings, unhappiness of the ancestors, and other malefactions. You find communities where for every person dying there is also a person being accused of witchcraft for having killed that person. It is often supposed that the dying individual must have done something to offend the spirits of the ancestors, to undermine the harmony of the family, and so forth. Thus, the pandemic is ripping society apart at the same time that it is causing individual human tragedy.[27]

Many actions and strategies inspired by UNAIDS were like the ones adopted during the first phase of prevention, before 1995, and the aim was basically the same: to make people aware of the risks of irresponsible sex. There was an increase in the importance of the ideology behind prevention, and society as a whole was involved to a greater extent. Large sums were spent on raising public awareness of the danger of AIDS and ways to avoid infection. It was all about providing information, communication, education, and talking to people. One headline in the French monthly *Le Monde diplomatique* was "Contre le sida, l'arme du débat"—"Against AIDs, the Weapon of Debate."[28] The aim of UNAIDs was to "create a favourable context in which people were motivated and capable of safe behaviour."[29] The indisputable remedy was the condom. The UN agencies looked as though they had turned into advertising agencies: they advertised condoms, they filled African towns with billboards and posters on the subject, they bought radio and television time to talk about condoms so they would become familiar to people. There were discussions on taboos and on what was forbidden and on the characteristics of sex in Africa as the main spreader of AIDS: transactional sex, precocious sex, promiscuous sex partners, sex work, and so on. This was so that all Africans, from puberty to old age, would receive sex education as it was taught in the West, in particular by becoming familiar with the condom. At the same time, the UN tried to overcome the stigma, which was seen to be hindering the rational, collective prevention of infection.

Around 2000 "Break the silence" was a very popular slogan, together with "Beware of AIDS. AIDS kills." There were also some for francophone Africa: "Le sida est ici. C'est réalité"; "Je ne serai pas victime du sida"; "Combattez le sida, pas les gens avec le sida." Presenting the disease as a killer, however, helped establish the stigma, which is exactly what they wanted to undermine. The towns were covered with billboards with images of miners saying, "I was a miner. Now I'm dead," or images of truck drivers saying, "I was a truck driver. Now I'm dead," or images of mothers with their children: "I was a mother. Now I'm dead." These messages spread terror. The reaction could not be anything but discriminatory against those who were ill, and it made them run away from anything to do with AIDS, starting from the tests that the advertisements were trying so hard to encourage. Other slogans for men only were sarcastic, without making them feel anxious, such as "Zero grazing," which was an invitation to avoid indiscriminate, free-ranging sexual relations, and "Stick to one partner," which could not be more explicit about the use of their "stick." Together with the classic "Abstain," "Be faithful," and "Condomise," there were soft ones like "Love carefully," "Love faithfully," "Un ami sidéen reste un ami" (A friend with AIDS remains a friend), and "Aimez-les assez pour en parler" (Love them enough to talk about it). In socialist countries, the slogans associated people's health with the political revolutionary process; in other countries, they were more psychological.

Prevention also meant ensuring the presence of activists—people with HIV who would talk about their disease in public. Except in South Africa, a prosperous and well-organized country, there was little desire to talk about or hear anything said about AIDS at all. The role of the activist was created ad hoc. The international officers sponsored associations, movements, and groups of patients and their relatives in an attempt to encourage everyone to carry out a cultural fight against AIDS and talk about the disease and to promote the test. HIV-positive people trained in communication techniques were paid to say they were HIV-positive in public places, in hospitals, and in places where people were working, in order to fight the stigma. The UN agencies funded projects to pay HIV-positive people not to hide but show that they were anything but worried and depressed. So, more people, it was supposed, would be brave enough to take the test and, if they discovered that they were HIV-positive, would start having safe sex in order to protect other people from infection. This sounded as though sex was simply a rational and not also an emotional issue. These activists, who were themselves HIV-positive, tried to reduce the stigma, and with their willpower they succeeded to a certain extent, but it was not enough to encourage people to take the test with no prospect of therapy if they turned out to be HIV-positive.

At the end of the 1990s UNAIDS was inclined to consider community engagement to reduce stigma in Africa and encourage solidarity toward HIV-positive people as decisive. Community engagement was also seen as decisive in encouraging people to take the test without being afraid of being isolated and of dying an outcast before the disease itself killed them. It was the local community that was held responsible for the sexual culture, so it was the local community that was asked not to put HIV-positive people in quarantine or expel them and to accept these modern plague victims. But the effects of these attempts were totally insignificant. In many parts of Africa, not only were HIV-positive people excluded and made outcasts, but people were also actually hunted down for presumably being HIV-positive, for being considered witches, and for being from other areas and of various minority groups.[30] As explained above, diseases in Africa are often interpreted as being the patient's fault or as a disaster brought upon them by someone who wants to hurt them. So, the UN talking so much about civil society did not really lead to anything. This is also why the condom was frequently presented as the favorite option for a solution.

The world of advertising and entertainment liked talking about the condom, in particular with men of the church, and they compared the rational, secular approach with religious dogmatism: "If only the Pope authorized. . . ." This sounded as though, as far as their sexuality was concerned, people obeyed the Pope, even in Africa. It was also as though they were just waiting for permission from above to use the magic shield, the condom. If the Catholic Church was in any way to blame for the pandemic, it was not in terms of doctrinal doubts regarding the use of the condom, which did not make much difference to the way the faithful behaved, but because it did not fight hard enough against the widespread Afro-pessimism that made people believe it was impossible to treat AIDS in Africa. The missionaries, who ran many of the health care centers, felt helpless, and prophetic messages about therapies were few and far between. There was almost a cultural block caused by the need to conform, which prevented the compassion for people with AIDS from becoming active treatment and not just general emotional support. What happened in Northern Europe was surreal, when the discussion about the spread of AIDS led to Pope John Paul II being accused of genocide because he opposed artificial birth control methods, in accordance with the doctrine established by Pope Paul VI in 1968.[31] A similar accusation could have been made against those who made that accusation in the first place since they did not appear to be equally outraged by the fact that Africa was being denied antiretroviral drugs. This therapy saved lives and in addition prevented infection, much more than the erratic use of the condom, which was generally considered by Africans as an unnatural obstacle to sex and to having children.

The religious institutions were a scapegoat for the rich countries' lack of action with respect to AIDS in poor countries. It was the efficacy of the triple antiretroviral therapy itself in countries with limited resources around 2010 that was never challenged again and ended the arguments about the use of condoms, which gradually fell into the background with the same secondary function as before. In the years around 2000, however, there was an ideological reaction against religions in general and the Catholic Church in particular, which was seen as traditionally opposed to science. This was because the public opinion was unaware of the effectiveness of the treatment, because condoms were believed to have worked in Europe and in North America,[32] and because condoms meant safe sex at a minimal cost.

People in the West did not understand why Africans did not want to use such an excellent object. It looked simple: 100 percent use of condoms, and the pandemic is solved.[33] Clare Short, the United Kingdom's secretary of state for international development, stated, "Condoms should be as easily available as Coca-Cola if the world is to tackle the global Aids pandemic.... No human being should be more than 300 yards from a condom."[34]

Male condoms and female condoms too. It was believed that gender inferiority prevented many African women from insisting that their partners used a condom. With no rights in general and even less in the area of sex, they were totally dominated by their partners. This led to a continuous international debate on condoms (incorporating vaginal microbicides) that African women could use without their partners knowing. However, scientific research never patented any effective products for Africa. Condoms, helpful in preventing infections, were frequently rejected by the female population. They depended on the men, they were oppressed and often infibulated, and they needed children in order to exist socially and to feed themselves, so there was no way they would even think about using vaginal microbicides. Beyond the restricted urban elite, there were the people of the villages for whom it would make more sense to suggest going to the moon than to a gynecologist.

As far as male condoms were concerned, Western analysts were trying to work out how to spread their use in Africa. A study published in July 2001 called "Condom Gap in Africa," about the supply of condoms in sub-Saharan countries, found that 724 million condoms were available in 1999, which corresponded to 4.6 for each male between fifteen and fifty-nine years old. The study results suggested a larger need: at least seventeen condoms a year for each man. It was added that it would have been enough to spend just $47.5 million. As an argument against those who talked about antiretroviral drugs for Africa, it was underlined that the pandemic would have been fought much more effectively with this small amount: "Providing condoms is cheap and cost effective. All aspects of HIV control are important, but a first priority must be prevention."[35]

Africans did not seem interested. In their culture and anthropology, children, happiness, and health all go together. This is why they want to have so many children. In the rural areas, where polygamy is normal, not only among Muslims but also among Christians and animists,[36] the condoms did not reach men or women. There, having a lot of children is a kind of public guarantee for women. Fecund women are preferred over women who have few children, and they receive more food because they satisfy the virile pride that requires men to have a large number of children. In general, the more children that African women have, the greater their social security. Being mothers gives them their identity and protection. Barren women risk being repudiated, abandoned, driven out of their villages, and left with no way to support themselves. In this context, it is not exactly the women who are dominated by the men who do not want to use condoms, which is what the people in the great UN health organizations think. It is the women themselves who do not want condoms because condoms would go against their social and practical interests. The culture of condoms is also alien in African towns. Sex and planning did not generally go hand in hand.

According to data of 1992, if an African worker had wanted to use condoms regularly, he would have had to spend 40 percent of his annual income on them, compared to 1 percent spent by a European worker.[37] Later Africa was inundated with stocks of this highly praised commodity that were free or nearly free of charge. Whether it was so-called condom social marketing, or simply free distribution, it was a failure. As the UN agencies found in 2001, the use of condoms in sub-Saharan countries was less than 5 percent.[38] The female condoms were practically ignored, and the male condoms were not appreciated. They are not part of the African mentality. People did not spend money to buy them, and when they were free, they were used maybe a couple of times in a new relationship and then no longer. A young man from Ivory Coast once said, "No, a man who doesn't have lots [of women] wouldn't be normal. . . . Fidelity? What for? You use condoms once or twice and after that you know each other. Besides, they're very thick here, they're not like the ones you get in France. Anyway, it's a question of habit and in any case, if the person isn't thin, they definitely don't have AIDS. So it's better to go with big fat ones, it's safer."[39]

The *Economist* wrote ironically, "Sex is fun. Many feel that condoms make it less so. Zimbabweans ask, 'Would you eat a sweet with its wrapper on?'"[40] Africans are not prepared to go without skin-to-skin sex, and many people in the West are not either. Moreover, in Africa, material conditions, the climate, and not storing them properly makes it difficult to keep condoms intact. Not to mention that there were so many around they were used for other purposes—for example, as balloons in villages festivals.

With one of its typical broad-ranging statistics, in 2002 UNAIDS forecast that 68 million HIV-positive people would die by 2020.[41] Such apocalyptic figures made even the most serious institutions fighting AIDS, such as the Global HIV Prevention Working Group, say that "some 29 million of those new cases could be prevented through better education about HIV, the virus that causes AIDS, the distribution of condoms and other programmes, such as testing."[42] Of course, in 2002 only a few people connected treatment with prevention, and most people still thought that billions of condoms would make the difference in Africa.

Similar misconceptions regarding the emancipation of sub-Saharan women were considered valid, since in the Western way of speaking they were supposed to become empowered. That was easier said than done. African women depend on men for organizational reasons. This is how an anti-AIDS activist answered an English journalist on the reasons for the failure of condoms in northern Mozambique: "Because men are not expected to be responsible, women were expected to buy condoms and encourage their men to use them. This might work in the West, but in Africa women have much less power. Women depend on men for food, and that puts them in a position where it is hard to say no to sex. Women give life. But men give food."[43] Huberte Bashwa Ngangwa, the coordinator of an AIDS health center in the DRC, said something similar: "Men are afraid of the disease. They have to show that they are strong, and they accuse the women of giving them AIDS, when instead they are the ones who are infecting people. There is nothing scientific about this—it is always the women's fault. Women are dominated; they have not studied. Men beat them. Marriages are often forced, and the women do not react. In fact, they even justify their men. That's the mentality."[44] People who study gender issues in Africa know this:

In contemporary sub-Saharan Africa (SSA), women are facing human rights abuses unparalleled elsewhere in the world. Despite the region's diversity, its female inhabitants largely share experiences of sexual discrimination and abuse, intimate violence, political marginalization, and economic deprivation. Consider the following: a woman in South Africa has a greater chance of being raped than she does of learning how to read (BBC 2003); seventy percent of women in Niger report being beaten or raped by their husband, father or brother (UNOCHA 2007); maternal mortality rates in SSA are the highest in the world. SSA is home to 20% of the world's births but has 40% of the world's maternal deaths (UNFPA 2008); in SSA, about half of the population lives below the poverty line; over 80% of the poor are women (UNFPA 2008).[45]

Hawa Sangaré, a Muslim Malawian doctor, explained the following:

In Africa the man is traditionally the king. The woman does not do anything alone. Men always have *leur mot à dire*. Women have to have permission to get treatment. They do not take the HIV test if their men do not want them to. Many children are born HIV-positive because the men do not allow prevention of mother-to-child transmission with the antiretroviral drugs. If you treat uterine cancer, the woman has to abstain from sex for four weeks, and how can one make men accept this? HIV-positive women only take the drugs if the men want them to. If they go to the maternity center on their own initiative, their man will kick them out and divorce them. Women do not have the strength to argue because the men support them, and if they are abandoned they are left with no way to support themselves. This is why the message has to come from the chiefs. It is the village chief who decides here. In order to convince the men to let the women get treatment, one has to turn to the traditional authorities, the village chiefs, the church pastors, the imams, men who talk with other men. They get together and sit under a tree and have discussions. Once the chief agrees, one will first be able to flatter the men and tell them that they are saving the women. And then the negative part comes, and he shows them the negative consequences of a refusal: the fact that the women will die and that they will have to look after the children. The men do not care about HIV for themselves, but they are gradually bombarded with more and more information: they see concrete cases, they listen to the radio, to the speeches of the pastors at church or of the imams at the mosque, who all encourage people to get treatment, and they say it seriously in the house of God. So, these men receive information at different levels, and in the end they are convinced.[46]

The result of prevention alone was tragic for Africa. AIDS continued to spread and was only held back by the natural saturation of the areas in which most of the people at risk had already been infected. The preventive approach was not combined with a therapeutic approach, and the more "multisectorial" it was, the less integrated it was with the medical aspect. Since it was separated from health and treatment, however well-intentioned it was, it was bound to have very little effect. The educational campaigns themselves would have been more effective if, as well as talking about safe sex, which was very relevant, they had also dealt with basic hygiene, nutrition, microorganisms, and circumcision. This last aspect was only included in the prevention programs later on, and actually until the early 2000s circumcision had been considered dangerous,[47] whereas its efficacy could be proven statistically. Without circumcision, there is an increased possibility of lesions of the foreskin and therefore the transmission of HIV as well as other infections. Despite its considerable academic competence, UNAIDS seemed to ignore the fact that many great disastrous epidemics of the past were eradicated by combining prevention with therapy because the therapy itself acted as prevention.

Bent Steenberg Olsen, who studies social stigma, wrote,

> Until around 2002 . . . international agencies, donors, and national health systems planned exclusively for preventive measures in their struggle against the disease. Concerning this narrow focus on prevention as a choice of operative minimalism by African governments, I posit that this approach caused serious harm, especially in sub-Saharan Africa, by way of fuelling a profoundly negative moral experience of AIDS in this region and by contributing to AIDS' social stigmatisation. Financed largely by Western foreign aid, preventive

campaigns attributing HIV transmission to sexual intercourse alone stipulated sexual abstinence and condom use as the sole preventive means by which to halt its "deadly" proliferation. Designed out of their African contexts, these advertising campaigns largely ignored other central avenues of infection such as mother-to-child transmission, unsafe medical practices (transfusion with infected blood and the use of unsterilized hypodermic needles), and, perhaps most importantly, practices of African traditional healers.[48]

The years dedicated to prevention alone, which aimed to reduce the number of new cases and gave up the people who were already infected as lost, were terrible. Of course, the idea of prevention was in itself valid. It was not unreasonable to fight the stigma, state the existence of HIV/AIDS, encourage people to take the test, raise the awareness of the people with AIDS, distribute condoms, and promote sexual fidelity. The strategies adopted were taken from the Western world: information campaigns (in countries where many of the people were illiterate); the use of the condom (considered by most people as going against nature); social resilience (in societies destroyed by the epidemic). This was all carried out without understanding that giving hope to HIV-positive people was the most effective form of prevention. The idea of trying to frighten people into taking the test had the opposite effect and strengthened denial, the stigma, and lack of trust in the public health system. What was the point in taking the test if there was no hope of a cure? Why say you were HIV-positive? Why fight the stigma? It was better not to know and to deny it in order to continue living in the community and not die before your time as a social outcast. The stigma could only be overcome by showing that you were healthy thanks to antiretroviral drugs. Instead, despite the availability of the test, there was no intention to treat people. It is a well-known general rule in medicine that screening is unethical unless treatment is available.

## UGANDA AND SENEGAL

Two success stories were brought up for years, one actually much more than the other one, to prove that prevention could work.[49] These stories were about Uganda and Senegal—in particular Uganda, the English-speaking country on Lake Victoria that was affected by such an early and massive spread of AIDS as to make it into a laboratory for the whole of Africa. For twenty years Uganda was the subject of scientific and media interest, involving both praise and criticism that had political consequences. The case of Senegal, although it was also mentioned as a case of health care success, was not always as outstanding and significant as that of Uganda, but they were both important for the history of AIDS in Africa.

Unlike Uganda, where AIDS decreased after having devastated the country, in Senegal the epidemic was stopped at the beginning, with prevalence rates that were never over 2 percent of the population of not more than ten million people. Various circumstances helped Senegal fight AIDS, including the fact that the HIV strain throughout the country was less virulent (HIV-2 and not HIV-1, which was more common in the rest of Africa). Almost all of the men were circumcised and therefore less exposed to sexually transmitted diseases (Senegal being 95 percent Muslim). There is strong control over the behavior of young women by its consolidated Islamic society. The public health system was not rich, but it was well organized, with qualified and up-to-date staff. Senegal was much more politically and socially stable than most of the other countries in Africa. Civil society was organized, with millions of people involved in associations, Islamic brotherhoods, political parties (dominated by the Socialist Party), trade unions, and enviable freedom of speech. The sex industry was highly regulated, and there were constant bureaucratic and health controls. It is worth pointing out that HIV-2 was discovered in 1985 by Senegalese researchers, which brought prestige to the country and made the government in Dakar proud to be fighting AIDS rather than try and hide the epidemic like many other African governments did. In a certain sense, at an international level HIV-2 promoted an exemplary scientific image of Senegal instead of undermining its reputation.[50]

With characteristics like these, Senegal was able to quickly prevent HIV from spreading, although in a different way from in English-speaking Africa. Multisectoral prevention was carried out in the Senegalese way, with strong government leadership and by involving religious organizations, stimulating a collective spirit, controlling practices performed in hospitals that used blood derivatives, and the above-mentioned controls on prostitution. Prevention in Senegal did not include sex education in all the schools, alarming slogans, propaganda with images on billboards, or advertisements for condoms.

The description of this situation would not be complete without mentioning again, to give credit to the Senegalese politicians, the fact that in 1998 the government launched an antiretroviral therapy pilot program. This project was small, but it was a trailblazer because it was the first public health initiative of its kind south of the Sahara, where the triple therapy was just a figment of people's imagination. The program did not affect the prevalence rates (a little over 1 percent in 1998) since they were already low due to the prevention described above. Nonetheless, the decision to treat the people who had AIDS in an African country was at the time challenging for most people's way of thinking in Africa and throughout the world. The foresight of this decision was only acknowledged later, with the switch from prevention alone to the administration of therapeutic treatment.

The case of Senegal, because of the limited extension of the epidemic and the characteristics of the country, which could not really be compared with anywhere else, was considered less representative than that of Uganda by the international community. Uganda was soon seen as a way to fight AIDS with prevention alone, which could be replicated. Uganda was studied carefully, discussed, and praised almost as though it were a precious experimental workshop. There was a long international debate on "what really happened in Uganda."[51]

The epidemic broke out violently in this country in East Africa at the beginning of the 1980s and was partially due to a long and devastating civil war.[52] Later, from the late 1980s to the 1990s, both the prevalence and the incidence decreased—that is, the overall number of HIV-positive people and the number of new cases. In other words, many people died, while the epidemic itself diminished. The statistics on this arrived late and were taken from incomplete surveys, so they were only approximate. For a long time in Uganda, like in other countries in Africa, the data on AIDS mainly came from sentinel sites in maternity wards or from studies on sample areas, not from systematic tests for HIV, which were either unavailable or had not even been performed, which was usually the case. Uganda was full of orphans, empty villages, and terminally ill patients, worn-out ghostly figures who could hardly move. AIDS was clearly visible in the country, but it was impossible to quantify it with mathematical data. The statistics on Uganda were therefore variable, with a prevalence of HIV/AIDS hypothesized at 15 to 30 percent during the 1980s, which then decreased to under 10 percent toward 1995 and later stabilized at 4 to 8 percent, depending on the years, with spikes and dips that were difficult to decipher. In Uganda in 2016, according to UNAIDS, which modified the methods for collecting and processing data several times, the prevalence in the adult population was 6.5 percent (1.4 million cases, fifty-two thousand in the last year). This figure was not far from those in other African countries. One could not talk about Uganda being on its way to eradicating AIDS.

Incidentally, data regarding prevalence has to be interpreted if one wants to correlate it to the strength of an epidemic. An increase in prevalence can be good news if it implies that people who are ill survive; if the number of new cases is lower than that of the previous year, the good news is even better. An epidemic decreases if the incidence rate decreases, whereas the prevalence rate is less indicative. In Uganda, despite the vast number of estimates performed, there seemed to be a decrease of the incidence, together with the dramatic fall, a dismal event, in the prevalence. It was difficult to understand some people's enthusiasm about the fall in the prevalence rate in Uganda. The figures vary from one source to another: one claims there was a fall from 18.5 percent in 1995 to 8.3 percent in 2000,[53] one from 30 percent in 1990 to 6.1 percent in 2001,[54] one from 15 percent at the beginning of the 1990s to 4 percent in 2003,[55] another from 30 percent to 10 percent in five years,[56] and so on. This kind of "success" implies that in any case hundreds of people died.

It should be pointed out that this was inaccurate data, based on limited categories or small samples of the population. It was similar to that in other African countries that produced equally unreliable statistics. Sometimes the data was underestimated, such as for the registration of the birth of children that in many countries did not include over a third of the children, and sometimes it was overestimated, like when the number of vaccines exceeded the population in order to try to make a good impression, as a country, on the international agencies that were providing funds. At the same time, since the Western experts did not have established evidence and were not prepared to resign themselves to not having enough data, they produced the figures as hypotheses and through somewhat unscientific projections. There seems to have been a considerable decrease in the incidence of AIDS between the late 1980s and the early 1990s, if only in the numerous sources that confirm it and because of the lower number of deaths over time in people with full-blown AIDS years after they had been infected. So, was this a success story? Yes and no. The epidemic was stopped, but more than one million Ugandans died before the triple antiretroviral therapy arrived in their country.

Be that as it may, Ugandans were infected less and less from 1986 onward, and this was due to a political turnabout. In January of that year, Yoweri Museveni took power in Kampala after seven years of guerrilla warfare carried out first against Idi Amin and then against Milton Obote and Tito Okello. This was the beginning of an *ad personam* regime that has lasted right up to the present day. Museveni, a tough guerrilla leader, has shown great political skill. From the very beginning, the new Ugandan leader fought AIDS very energetically. He said it was everyone's patriotic duty.[57] Museveni did not behave like most African leaders, who denied the reality of AIDS in their countries for decades. On the contrary, he talked about it a lot and wanted people to talk about it. What drove him? His political fortune came from arms, and the basis of his party was the military organization with which he had conquered Kampala; many of his men were HIV-positive, and the army was under threat.

Museveni had just started operating as a civilian, but he decided to continue fighting in a different way and against this new enemy, HIV. He fought with the only weapon available at the time, prevention, in which, with the authority to do so, he involved the government and society. This was all he could do. At the time there was no therapy: the government propaganda against the epidemic warned that "AIDS has no cure." Museveni mobilized the government bureaucracies, civil authorities, religious leaders, village councils, NGOs, hospitals, health care centers, and social centers. He regulated the categories at risk, from the sex workers to the truck drivers, the shopkeepers, fishermen, soldiers, and students. Tens of thousands of people were ordered or recruited to be activists to carry out prevention throughout the entire country—towns, villages, schools, meeting places, and public places. Museveni mainly achieved his aims from 1988 to 1994, after which less progress was made in the fight against AIDS and alternated with phases of regression. In 2012, for example, Uganda was ashamed to be one of the two African countries (the other being Chad) with increasing AIDS incidence rates.[58] The stigma had been lessened but never really defeated, and it could not be as long as AIDS was an irrevocable death sentence. The stigma only became less harsh when the antiretroviral drugs became available.

Ugandan prevention had three important characteristics. The first was the fact that Museveni was like a leader on the battlefield. The media and press were under his control, with no dissenting opinions allowed. The second characteristic concerned the type of prevention, which concentrated on a change in sexual behavior. The results were excellent because Ugandans were put under pressure to reduce the number of their partners and avoid unsafe sex. "Zero grazing" hit the mark. Sex before marriage in men from fifteen to twenty-four years old decreased from 60 percent in 1989 to 23 percent in 1995, an unthinkable figure in the African context. During the same period, casual sex decreased among young people from 35 to 15 percent in men and from 16 to 6 percent in women. The percentage of people with several casual partners decreased dramatically. The age of young people's first time rose. Museveni did not promote condoms, but he accepted them as a second-line remedy. The famous Ugandan ABC campaign underlined abstinence and being faithful in particular, and condoms were there for an emergency: it was "zero grazing" first of all "and using condoms if you're going to move around."[59] Abstinence, marital fidelity, and fewer partners were the first options adopted; condoms were there just to fall back on. (In 1995, at the end of the most intense and effective fight against AIDS, only 6 percent of sexually active Ugandans were familiar with condoms.) This was Museveni's approach for decades, and it was approved of so much that in the 2000s Bush's PEPFAR invested nearly $2 million in Uganda in the name of marital fidelity and at the same time alienated those who were in favor of condoms.[60] In this sense, the case of Uganda was one of the topics of the American culture wars.

The third characteristic concerns the interest in Uganda at an international level. Hundreds of international development agencies, both governmental and nongovernmental, were working in the country, and most of them were British or American. (There were over seven hundred altogether in 2001.)[61] Uganda was a former British colony and was one of the Anglo-American world's favorite foreign aid recipients in sub-Saharan Africa. Museveni himself received support from North America the moment he came to power, after he cooled down his previous third-world tone of voice and erased the image of himself as a friend of Muammar Qaddafi, which had led the United States to support Okello against him. For the United States, he was no longer a revolutionary but an ally. The presence of so many Western organizations fighting the epidemic meant plenty of investments in the Ugandan health care system, money flowing in various directions, well-paid work for thousands of people in information and educational campaigns, the public promotion of talented activists and their associations, and a widespread feeling that HIV/AIDS was a crucial issue.

As of today, though, there is still no happy ending to the situation in Uganda. A reconstruction of the prevalence, incidence, and mortality rates in graphs during the 2000s does not show any lines or curves that clearly go up or down but only irregular trends. The current data on Uganda is close to the averages of many African countries that are dealing with AIDS. At the turn of the 1990s, the sexual behavior change, understood as the only chance to escape infection, was probably also due to the terrifying vision of the effect of AIDS in action: gardens full of tombs, bodies transported as though they were just bundles, coffins stacked up high, desolate areas, abandoned fields, hospitals overwhelmed with all their incurable patients, multitudes of orphans. After this awful period, the Ugandans started taking fewer precautions. From 1995, when the emergency situation was over, concentrating on condoms did not give the desired results, just as after 2002 the renewed insistence on abstinence and being faithful sounded weary, despite the attractive financial support from PEPFAR.

Museveni found out about the antiretroviral drugs as soon as they appeared. In Kampala there was a luxury health clinic that had been administering the triple therapy since 1996. Nonetheless, because it was so expensive, the government considered that it was unthinkable to offer antiretroviral drugs to even only a small part of the one and a half million Ugandans who were HIV-positive at the end of the 1990s. Precisely because Uganda was considered at the forefront of the fight against AIDS, in 1998 it was selected by UNAIDS for the first therapeutic experiments with antiretroviral cocktails.[62] The results were not very good, with high numbers of deaths, resistances to the drugs, and people abandoning the treatment. Fifteen months after the beginning, only 54 percent of the patients treated were still alive and in treatment. The pilot project was also not free of charge: the patients had to pay for their medicines, diagnosis, medical examinations, and whatever else was necessary. One such drug, Combivir, alone cost $60 a month. Although the patients who enrolled were wealthy and had an income well over the average Ugandan's $26 per month, they were unable cope with the costs, which were also subject to the devaluation of the Ugandan shilling. The pilot project did not understand the patients' personal and family difficulties because its approach was just technical and economic and was dictated by protocols written in a Western context. The Ugandan Ministry of Health, in a final report on the experiment in March 2000, made no objection to the way the project had been carried out, and its conclusion that it was unrealistic to consider antiretroviral drugs was well received. This opinion confirmed the excellence of the decision to carry out prevention alone, for which up until then the country had been so highly praised:

> Efforts to expand access to antiretroviral therapies must weigh the benefits and costs to the health sector. Even if patients meet the costs of their medical care, costs of training, development and implementation of treatment guidelines, and expanded access to laboratory diagnostics require substantial investment. Although newly-reduced drug costs have been announced, scaling up of antiretroviral treatment programs will be limited by the rudimentary laboratory infrastructure in the periphery and the median $300 annual per

capita income. In this context, the importance of HIV prevention must remain the cornerstone of programs to prevent AIDS-related morbidity and mortality in Uganda.[63]

This pilot project had supposedly been conceived in order to explore the possibility of providing HIV-positive Africans access to the same drugs and same therapeutic chances as HIV-positive people in the West. It ended, however, with incongruous expressions of satisfaction from Ugandan health authorities and local UNAIDS representatives that the administration of these therapies in countries with limited resources was economically unsustainable: "Promotion of AIDS care, and not just AIDS drugs, has been an important component to the success and evolution of this pilot program. . . . In these ways, improved AIDS care can be expanded to reach more of those in need." The report expressed the dichotomy, which at the time was usual, between care (treatment for opportunistic infections and palliative treatment) and treatment (the life-saving antiretroviral drugs—the HAART regimen). What made the difference was the fact that the treatment had not been free of charge. The report said that it was impossible to think of scaling up the therapy if its overall costs were higher than the average income in Uganda. However, there was no sign of offering the treatment free of charge as an alternative. The report even went so far as to suggest that administering antiretroviral drugs to patients who wanted to recover at any cost could compromise the well-being of their families: "Extending survival for a matter of months might drain family resources needed for living expenses and education of surviving family members."

There was also the factor of the patients selected to treat. Their condition in most cases was so bad that it was extremely unlikely that the triple therapy would be effective. Eighty percent had fewer than 200 CD4 cells, while the mean of the whole cohort was only 67 CD4 cells; 34 percent had full-blown AIDS. The pilot project seemed designed to fail, as though its whole purpose had been to justify the refusal to treat AIDS in poor countries.

The logical consequence was that the antiretroviral drugs would only be available for wealthy Ugandans. According to a leaflet published at the same time, in March 2000, by the report's authors—that is, the Ugandan Ministry of Health and UNAIDS–Uganda—the antiretroviral drugs were good and bad news at the same time. The good news was that the virus would stop multiplying itself in the patient's body and the patient would get better; the bad news was that the virus would stay in the patient's body and that the treatment would be very expensive—over $750 a month, plus further costs for the various tests that had to be carried out. Those who had enough money could go to the clinic in Kampala, which had the drugs.[64] As mentioned earlier, the average monthly income in Uganda was $25. A farmer hardly earned anything, and Uganda was 87 percent rural.

The WHO, with its 3 by 5 Initiative, soon changed the prospects of the treatment for AIDS in countries with limited resources like Uganda. The patients had the opportunity to survive. In Uganda, which provided prevention alone, this was only available for the rich.

To finish with Uganda: Museveni did not save the AIDS-afflicted Ugandans, but he controlled the epidemic with an aggressive, widespread, and thorough campaign. When UNAIDS made the multisectorial aspect the fundamental criterion for prevention, it based its approach on the Ugandan model. However, this model was difficult to replicate because of the peculiarities of the country: its authoritarian leader, his insistence on sexual fidelity and not on condoms, and the strong support from the Anglo-American world. Besides, the timing of the UNAIDS initiative did not coincide with the experience in Uganda. UNAIDS was set up in 1995, exactly when the heroic and incisive phase of the Ugandan fight against AIDS was coming to an end. After 1996 there was the triple antiretroviral therapy, which worked as both the treatment and protection from infection. Uganda could have become part of a second phase in the fight against the epidemic and kept its role in Africa as a pioneer if it had combined the therapy with prevention, but it did not make the most of that opportunity. It continued to replicate the prevention model, giving more or less space to condoms depending on the president's frame of mind. It ended up demonstrating, despite its best intentions, that prevention alone is not enough. Prevention does not eradicate the virus, and it shows only contempt for those who are already infected. Fighting HIV/AIDS with prevention alone gave HIV-positive people no hope, and in fact they died.

## PREVENTION AND TREATMENT ARE INSEPARABLE

The 3 by 5 Initiative was the beginning of a mass antiretroviral therapy regimen in Africa. Prevention was no longer the only regimen considered. In July 2002 authors of a letter in the *Lancet* claimed, "Treatment and prevention are inextricably linked, offering treatment strengthens prevention measures, and prevention is less effective without treatment."[65] These words were soon put into practice everywhere in Africa.

Therapy and prevention provided support for each other in a virtuous circle. The therapy transformed AIDS from a deadly disease into a chronic pathology and increased the sense of responsibility of HIV-positive patients, who would otherwise be desperate and tempted to behave recklessly. Only the possibility of receiving treatment encouraged people to do the test because without treatment, if the result of the test was positive, it was seen as a death sentence. The therapy reduced the viral load—the amount of virus in the body fluids—making it very unlikely that the virus would be transmitted to other people, which drastically reduced its morbidity.

These facts were clear for those who were fully aware of the history of AIDS in the West, and yet, until 2002, for Africa they were totally disregarded. Insisting on prevention was an alibi for the lack of a commitment to the therapy, which required greater economic and human investments.

In fact, making the therapy available was exhausting because it implied being responsible, it required the health care system to be made efficient, it needed a huge financial outlay, and the results had to be monitored scientifically—in short, it was all blood, sweat, and tears. Prevention was far less demanding. It consisted of speeches, messages, information and educational programs, and reports, which did not involve much anxiety; delegations for activists and local authorities were purchasing condoms; and comfortable appeals to personal and collective common sense. From an ideological point of view, prevention was gratifying when it referred to human development, civil rights, and the promotion of women's rights. It was also unfortunately (and this was easy to establish) much more vulnerable to money being siphoned off and to corruption. Prevention was just a matter of talking to people and spreading words; who checked the actions and the results? Prevention filled the pockets of the ever-present dishonest officials, who in poor countries, without close supervision, managed the funds that came from multilateral or bilateral cooperation.[66]

One of UNAIDS's policies was to create an AIDS national committee in every country, with the intention of leading the fight against the epidemic instead of the ministries of health, which had given up. With their abundant international funds, in Africa these committees became spending centers and often centers of corruption. Money disappeared into thin air or was used for other purposes. In the center of Lilongwe, the capital of Malawi, which was very poor, a futuristic glass building was constructed for the local committee, as though it were for the United Nations itself, and became the symbol of AIDS-related corruption throughout the country. The therapies, when they were introduced, were subject to regular checks, clearly visible and controlled investments in drugs and infrastructures, and the results were compared from place to place, with evaluations of staff and other aspects. The therapies were not generalized, like the concepts of care, support, and mitigation, with which the promoters of prevention piously filled their speeches.

Until 2002 it sounded politically correct and prudent to say that administering the therapy in Africa was unthinkable for medical, technical, and financial reasons. It was also politically correct to avoid criticizing the concept of prevention. Of course, the concept of prevention was always positive in itself, but if prevention was the only instrument available in the fight against AIDS, then nothing at all could be done for those who were already ill. However, from the end of 2003, the percentage of HIV-positive people in treatment increased with the 3 by 5 Initiative. Although it did not completely achieve its aims because it took longer than expected to adopt the antiretroviral therapies everywhere, the 3 by 5 Initiative was achieving good results in terms of both therapy and prevention. The patients stopped being infectious. Those who suspected they might be infected had a good reason to do the test and, if need be, change their behavior. A book published by Stephen Lewis in 2005 explained why the 3 by 5 Initiative was to be considered successful:

Instead of three million people in treatment by the end of 2005, there were only 1.3 million. It seemed to some a setback, even a failure. I regard it as a qualified triumph. It's important to remember that before the impetus for treatment was launched by the World Health Organization, the virus was in the ascendant. But with treatment comes hope, and with hope comes testing, and with testing comes prevention, so that what we now have, in country after country, is the single-minded pursuit of keeping people alive. When historians look back, there is no doubt in my mind that the "three by five" campaign will be seen as a turning point. Everyone is now talking of "universal access" to treatment, prevention, and care by 2010. That would never have happened without the "three by five" initiative. There is of course a lot of carping about treatment dominating the response to AIDS at the expense of prevention. For what it's worth, I've had the view throughout that playing one against the other is often (although by no means always) the product of neurotic rivalry. In some quarters, there was so much resentment at the way in which the WHO had grasped the nettle, that it became important to sully the accomplishment, in however sly and subtle a fashion. It's all such nonsense. Treatment and prevention are absolutely inseparable; one fortifies the other. We'll never break the back of the pandemic unless both are given primacy.[67]

The 3 by 5 Initiative marked a watershed. It represented the end of inactivity and the awareness of the race against time to save lives. Whether it was one, two, or three million patients treated by the end of 2005, most of them had been plucked from certain death. There were some people who saw the treatment as a chance to finally control the pandemic and maybe even eradicate it. Then there were people who were anchored to the dogma of prevention alone and considered the 3 by 5 Initiative a risk that was bound to fail and that at the same time would damage the prevention activities by using up their resources. In theory, everyone seemed to agree on starting the treatment, subject to a commitment not to stop prevention. This was wanted by Kofi Annan, the senior management of the WHO (Gro Harlem Brundtland and then Lee Jong-wook), the world of humanitarian aid and the NGOs, the international public opinion after the

Durban conference, and above all the people in Africa. Those in favor of prevention alone fell in line in the end, but they sometimes tried to condition the implementation of the new political approach that supported treatment by insinuating doubt and complaining about the obstacles.[68]

After it had been proved that Africans were able to adhere to the treatment, the objection of severe side effects caused by the therapeutic treatments had been silenced, it had been verified that resistances to the first line drugs could be dealt with in Africa with second-line antiretroviral drugs, and it had been ascertained that Africans' bodies reacted to the drugs exactly the same way as those of North Americans and Europeans, new reservations were presented to try to slow down the 3 by 5 Initiative. It was said that access to the therapies would medicalize the prevention activities to the detriment of their community and cultural aspects and would encourage an increase in the incidence of the epidemic—that is, new infections. In other words, access to the treatment would decrease prevention at a social level. Moreover, it was pointed out that access to the treatment reduced safe sex: since people did not die anymore, they would go back to behaving recklessly—to sexual promiscuity, sex without condoms, and the enticement of the sex industry. If the disease was no longer deadly, people would be less careful to avoid it. "AIDS kills," the favorite slogan of the prevention of the 1990s, would no longer be effective.

Then there was the financial question. The Global Fund, which bore the main burden of the 3 by 5 Initiative, promised to be, at least in the medium term, the great health care treasury for the developing world. Together with the streams of funding from bilateral cooperation, the Global Fund spent $40.2 billion on the fight against HIV/AIDS from 2002 to 2010.[69] Around $10 billion a year was planned, but in the end it was less, although it was enough to attract all the actors of the international health community. In 1999 the bilateral and multilateral donations for all the health care programs for sub-Saharan Africa came to an overall figure of $865 million. With the Global Fund the donations suddenly multiplied. The situation changed from the miserable equivalent of $1.30 per African to what Annan called a rich war chest.

The proponents of prevention alone had never complained much about the lack of resources and had exaggerated the cost-effectiveness of their prophylactic theories, but when it came to the distribution of the war chest, they all rushed in and tried to get as much as they could. The previously mentioned article by Schwartländer of UNAIDS and other experts published in *Science* in June 2001 at the beginning of the Global Fund asked for a greater share for prevention and a smaller share for treatment. One year later, the same German epidemiologist, together with some of the same experts as before as well as some new ones mainly funded by UNAIDS, reiterated the request in the *Lancet*, claiming that if the success achieved in preventing HIV in some countries could be extended on a global scale, around twenty-nine million new cases out of an estimated forty-five million could be avoided by 2010. The article was based on poorly explained simulations and mathematical models, developed by the authors. Why twenty-nine million cases and not twice as many or half as many? Why forty-five million new cases estimated over the following eight years? These figures were to a great extent hypothetical.

With such imaginative mathematics applied to the benefit of prevention, Schwartländer and his colleagues intended to warn their readers that "the effect of care programmes—e.g. drug treatment—on new infections was not included in this exercise, because there is little empirical data available on the magnitude of the preventive effect of treatment (reduced viral load and hence infectiousness) and care."[70] Moreover, in 2002 the reduction of the viral load as a result of the triple antiretroviral therapy had already been widely demonstrated by six years of clinical practice on around one and a half million patients in countries with a medium to high income. The article confirmed the request made the year before: $4.8 billion for prevention. It also warned that the total cost of a serious and "expanded prevention response" would come to not less than $27 billion by 2010. If this did not take place, the above-mentioned forty-five million new cases would hit the world. The results calculated afterward, based on the 2010 figures (the last year considered in the article), showed that the promoters of prevention did not obtain those funds, but there were not forty-five million new cases of HIV.[71]

But what treatment did the 3 by 5 Initiative guarantee? The antiretroviral treatments can be administered according to very different modalities, with different standards and very different costs. The regimens can be optimum or mediocre. Here a second important battle took place regarding the destiny of African patients. The 3 by 5 Initiative started in December 2003 as a major event, though its guidelines were quite minimalist. For example, the therapy was prescribed when the patient's CD4s dropped below 200 (not below 350 like in the West), which is when the immune system has very few lymphocyte cells. Consequently, the mortality was higher, and when the patient's immune system did manage to recover, it did not recover completely. This saved on the number of treatments, but the number of deaths increased. And then, monitoring the viral load was considered optional. (It was not even considered essential before the therapy.) The diagnostics were limited to just the CD4 lymphocyte count. This meant that it was impossible to notice the onset of resistance in time and then switch to a second line of antiretroviral cocktails. Money was saved on diagnosis and on improving the infrastructures, with the risk of wasting it on expensive second-line drugs, and the patients died. The WHO was heavily criticized for promoting the 3 by 5 Initiative, and there were heated discussions even within the organization, so it was not prepared to produce avant-garde guidelines demanding the medical excellence provided in the West. In the end this was done too but gradually, and it took years.

The 3 by 5 Initiative had a time limit, a numerical goal to reach, a planned rhythm to keep to, and this took place through many different channels. The WHO and the Global Fund acted through national governments, local public health systems, all sorts of NGOs, ad hoc projects presented by various organizations for funds, and so on. Even with the best intentions, it was not easy to control this heterogeneous combination of organizations and associations. The treatment was often reduced to simply distributing the drugs. In Africa the patients were given some information at the beginning, and then they had to manage on their own. However much they intended to adhere to the treatment properly, they were not looked after adequately, not encouraged enough, not monitored enough, and not supported enough from a nutritional point of view. Moreover, the antiretroviral drugs were not always given free of charge. The governments pursued various strategies: sometimes they wanted the treatment to be paid for, sometimes they offered subsidies to help cover the costs, and sometimes they decided to provide it free of charge. When the treatment had to be paid for, men had easier access than women, and in families where more than one person was HIV-positive, it was sometimes only economically possible for one person to be treated.

Even the best NGOs tended to interpret the 3 by 5 Initiative in terms of quantity rather than quality. This was the emblematic case of the Médecins Sans Frontières (MSF), the glorious European secular humanitarian organization set up in 1968 that over the years acquired tens of thousands of health professionals and logistic and administrative staff. At the time of the 3 by 5 Initiative, MSF represented the good and the bad aspects of a typically Western approach to Africa: the courage, the clinical science, and the well-organized logistics but also the deference to the current popular standards of health care and intolerance of long-lasting projects. MSF had been set up and developed during emergencies and wars—dangerous operations in which the aim was to save as many lives as possible as quickly as possible. In fighting AIDS in Africa, MSF learned that the epidemic could not be addressed as an emergency: it was necessary to stay in a country, learn about its culture, and train local health staff. In a certain sense, MSF changed its identity by fighting AIDS in Africa. It discovered that it had to provide a long-term commitment after saving patients' lives. Normally it would have left when the situation was back to normal, but with AIDS there was no return to normality. The patients were chronic and had to be treated for their whole lives, even when they recovered and could lead an ordinary life. The fight against AIDS required setting up a health system and supporting it over time.

The solution that MSF would have liked to adopt consisted of the idea of passing on the medical know-how of both staff and patients to the African health care systems: "It is not our role to treat everyone. We showed ART [antiretroviral] is feasible: we can train others, but we cannot substitute for the government.... Local solutions are needed—there is no other choice."[72] What could be done, though, if there were no local solutions, or if they were unreliable? MSF did not avoid the question, and it transformed its very nature in order to support therapeutic continuity. The value of MSF lay in the fact that every now and then almost everywhere in Africa it announced that it would close one or another AIDS health center, but it never did, in order not to compromise the patients' health. In contradiction of its original emergency-based, adrenaline-fueled vocation, MSF gradually and sensibly started to calculate the extent of AIDS in Africa. For the first years, it followed the approach indicated by the UN agencies, with a large-scale distribution of drugs and simplified diagnostics. By verifying the results of this approach, it realized that it was worth setting up optimum-level treatment. This way it rewarded the adherence of patients, many of whom would have died if they had abandoned their treatment.

Meanwhile, experts from developed countries advocated pragmatic shortcuts, such as the above-mentioned proposal of intermittent antiretroviral therapies in order to save on drugs and make it easier for the patients to adhere to their therapy. One area in which improvised remedies seemed to be particularly appealing was the mother-to-child transmission of HIV. For a long time during the 1990s, it was confirmed that AZT provided therapeutic benefits, whereas in fact it was ineffective unless administered within the triple therapy in Africa as much as anywhere else. In 1999 Nevirapine became popular, and in the early 2000s it was the standard therapy in vertical prevention in countries with limited resources. This was a miracle antiretroviral drug when administered to pregnant women during labor. Nevirapine was particularly appreciated because of its cost-effectiveness—$4 compared to AZT, which cost $280. In practice, though, both AZT and Nevirapine were disappointing. At the time of delivery, they seemed to reduce infection, but the effect did not last. During the first months of life, the infections increased due to the limited effect of the drugs on the virus and to breast-feeding, through which the virus was transmitted. Not to mention the fact that giving the mothers single doses of antiretroviral drugs affected the successive therapies needed to save their lives, assuming a HAART regimen was within their reach. Many infants, if they managed to survive, ended up in orphanages, with everything that implied in Africa. So, in Europe and the United States the regimens included three drugs for pregnant women but in Africa only one or two. In the West the triple therapy for pregnant women meant that almost all the newborn infants were immune to HIV, whereas in Africa the approach using Nevirapine had practically no effect on the percentages of vertical transmission of the virus (if these percentages are considered not at the time of administration but during the period between pregnancy and the end of breast-feeding).

The economic sustainability of the 3 by 5 Initiative was also considered to be very unconvincing because it was suspected of gradually introducing the concept of universal treatment or universal access. Who would pay for the treatment for HIV-positive patients who had been saved and had become chronic patients, year after year or, rather, decade after decade? The objection regarding the long-term costs referred to the understandable reluctance of any donor to take on long-term commitments, which, moreover, were always the same. How was it possible to present philanthropic commitments to the board of directors of banks or companies when they were repeated year after financial year? The donors preferred projects that achieved their aim and ended with everyone congratulating each other, so they could then think about different initiatives that would satisfy new requests. Donors were horrified when they were told their money had to be channeled in the same monotonous direction for decades. Besides, if once the funding was underway, they were made aware that interrupting this commitment would cause many people to die, they felt they had been blackmailed.

The antiretroviral drugs, and the way they were administered, were claimed to be unthinkable for Africans, first by putting forward the objection of the economic burden. Up to 2000 the problem was explained in just a few comments: "Paying for even basic treatment depletes private savings and places huge demands on public health-care systems. According to the World Bank, in any given country, one year of basic medical treatment for one person costs about two to three times the national GDP per person. . . . In the short term, the focus will be on preventing the disease's spread by changing behaviour."[73] Then, fortunately the Global Fund and PEPFAR arrived and provided tens of billions of dollars that had not been there before. People started receiving treatment. However, the Global Fund and PEPFAR were new initiatives, and it was impossible to say how long they would last. What would happen to the millions of patients being treated when the public and private donors supporting the Global Fund got tired or George W. Bush was no longer president and consequently the two safes would be empty? Who would provide them with their therapies?

As soon as the discussion turned to universal access to treatment, the question of sustainability was talked about, in an alarming tone of voice. A lifelong outlay for tens of millions of patients living in the Southern Hemisphere was expected. Why start spending so much for drugs that did not kill the virus and needed to be taken for life? Since the HAART regimen did not cure the disease, even though it did eliminate the symptoms and make the patients fit again, it was said that turning AIDS into a chronic disease would cause African societies to suffer an unsustainable burden. If the international community did not take responsibility for it, the continuity of the treatment would mean bottomless pits for economies that were already in dire straits and that would be forced to support tens of millions of chronic patients who would die naturally of old age. The rich West, which was always worried about its finances, would have to cover the costs of the treatment forever. In November 2006 the World Bank organized a large international conference in Washington with the aim of acknowledging the new situation with respect to the treatment of AIDS in developing countries. Its name said it all: Sustaining Treatment Costs: Who Will Pay?

The fact that the antiretroviral treatments implied a long-term commitment weighed heavily on the development agencies and donors. They were worried about having to continuously finance the treatment for tens of millions of patients for thirty, forty, if not fifty, years—for as long as people were expected to live in each country. The international cooperation normally worked with fixed-term projects: help was brought in, technicians were trained, infrastructures were set up, and the work was started. At the end of the day everyone just went home. What was particularly appreciated was the intense but short vaccine campaigns. Treating AIDS was something else. Having a new AIDS patient was like adopting a child.

In 2010 the *New York Times* wrote, "The last decade has been what some doctors call a 'golden window' for treatment. Drugs that once cost $12,000 a year fell to less than $100, and the world was willing to pay." But now, it added, "the golden window is closing. . . . The collapse was set off by the global recession's effect on donors, and by a growing sense that more lives would be saved by fighting other, cheaper diseases. Even as the number of people infected by AIDS grows by a million a year, money for treatment has stopped growing." The *Times* explained the withdrawal of the donors who provided funds for AIDS, with a calculation regarding Uganda, a country that benefited from support from North America, where 88 percent of the anti-AIDS drugs were paid for by US taxpayers: "The lifetime bill for treating one Ugandan AIDS patient, counting drugs, tests and medical salaries, is $11,500. Donors have decided that is too much, that more lives can be saved by concentrating on child-killers like stillbirth, pneumonia, diarrhea, malaria, measles and tetanus. Cures for those killers, like antibiotics, mosquito nets, rehydration salts, water filters, shots and deworming pills, cost $1 to $10."[74]

The article in the American newspaper touched a sore spot. Donors' support for treating AIDS in poor countries was unpredictable. They were intimidated by the fact that they were taking on lifelong commitments for chronically ill patients. Added to this was the equally volatile public spending for health by the developing countries, especially in Africa. Programs for treating AIDS could only work in conditions with stable resources. The patients only began the treatment if they were assured that it would continue over time. The slightest breakdown on stocks because of a lack of funds could frustrate so much effort made and increase the need for more funds for second-line or subsequent therapies. Year after year the donors were more keen on finding a way out, whatever that might be: a vaccine, a drug that would eradicate HIV, new types of condoms that men and women would like, local governments taking responsibility for the treatment, or the unspoken abandonment of and escape from their commitment. Maybe they regretted not just sticking to prevention without treatment. Prevention alone was relatively cheap.

June 2006 was the twenty-fifth anniversary of the first scientific report on HIV/AIDS by the CDC.[75] For the occasion a new UNGASS was dedicated to AIDS, commemorating the one of five years before. It was time to take stock and be satisfied with the development of the five-year period, which opened up universal access to treatment and marked a decrease in the incidence rate of the epidemic. It was also the time for some calculations, as pointed out by the British press:

> The message now is that AIDS can be contained if you are prepared to spend the money to contain it. . . . Some of the news is unambiguously good. . . . More people are being treated with anti-retroviral drugs. The figure at the end of 2005 was 1.3m. That was less than half the target of 3m that UNAIDS had set itself, but is nevertheless not negligible. Some optimists believe that the stated aim of making these drugs available to all who need them by the end of the decade is still within reach. That number, by the way, is nowhere near 39m, the number infected today. . . . But there is a harsher calculus, and the meeting in New York needs to confront it. AIDS is still incurable. The treatment works only as long as you take the drugs. The more people who take them, the bigger the cost. And that cost lasts as long as the patient lives. Even if humanity wised up tomorrow, stopped sleeping around and stopped taking drugs, those already infected would still remain infected for life. Treat them, and you create a body of dependents for whom you have assumed indefinite responsibility. . . . [It is] a mission without an end. If this week's meeting in New York can tackle the question of how that mission can be financed—and without a cure that means indefinitely—and start groping towards answers, then the 50th anniversary of AIDS may yet be more cheerful than the 25th.[76]

These were crucial points. The 2006 UNGASS decided to move onward universal access to the antiretroviral therapy. It was increasingly obvious that treatment also meant prevention and that HIV/AIDS was being brought under control. It was necessary to think about stable and lasting forms of sustainability. "A mission without an end" had been started. How would the cost be borne? Actually, it was a provocation with respect to the international community's sense of responsibility. Less money given, fewer lives saved. It had to be understood that the fight against AIDS in poor countries could not be compared to building public works, such as roads, bridges, hospitals, and dams, which took a few years, after which the construction sites were closed with congratulations all round. On the contrary, it meant establishing long-lasting partnerships for financing treatment and developing human resources together, for more solid infrastructures, and for cultural and social processes, such as positive bilateral influences of the Global North with the Global South, of the rich world with the poor world.

## NOTES

1. Freedberg et al., "Cost-effectiveness of Combination Anti-retroviral Therapy," 824–31.
2. Data taken from the World Bank, https://data.worldbank.org/indicator/NY.GDP.PCAP.CD?locations=ZG.
3. UNAIDS, *Accelerating Access to HIV Care.*
4. *UNAIDS*, 75–76.
5. Sweeney, "U.S. Push for Worldwide Patent Protection, 445–71.
6. These were the trade-related aspects of intellectual property rights negotiated within the World Trade Organization.
7. On this issue, see Gostin, *AIDS Pandemic*, 301–9; Gehler, *Un continent se meurt*, 141–48; Martine Bulard, "Les firmes pharmaceutiques organisent l'apartheid sanitaire," *Le Monde diplomatique*, January 2000; and "Brains v Bugs," *Economist*, November 8, 2001.
8. Years later people realized that by fighting AIDS seriously on a vast scale, the African health care systems were renewed and revitalized or created from scratch, but in 2003 they were still far away from seeing it this way.
9. Blixen, *Out of Africa*, 30.
10. John Donnelly, "Prevention Urged in AIDS fight," *Boston Globe*, June 7, 2001.
11. Stevens, Kaye, and Corrah, "Antiretroviral Therapy in Africa," 280–82.
12. Smith, "Adherence to Antiretroviral HIV Drugs," 617–24.
13. Fortunately for African patients, the unusual proposals put forward by Mark Dybul, a brilliant American diplomat, whose career took him from the National Institutes of Health to being the head of PEPFAR and then of the Global Fund, did not see the light. In 2001 Dybul, in contrast with the still popular prevention-only line and with a certain Afro-optimism, wondered on the basis of some studies whether it would be possible to reduce the dosages of the patients on HAART without risking getting the symptoms of AIDS again. His idea was that the halved or in any case reduced antiretroviral doses would work like a vaccine,

leaving limited viral loads in circulation. The immune system would then get the better of the viral loads and become stronger as a result. Dybul hypothesized administering the antiretroviral drugs on alternate weeks—an intermittent therapy. According to him, the advantages would be found in the considerable reduction of the toxicity of the antiretroviral drugs ("highly exaggerated toxicity," as it was fashionable to describe it in the medical literature) and then, since the HAART regime would be made possible in Africa, the cost and the number of pills would be halved. Mark Dybul et al., "Short-Cycle Structured Intermittent Treatment," 15161–66. See also "AIDS Drugs: Alternative Therapy," *Economist*, December 6, 2001.

14. Minerva and Vella, *No AIDS*, 67–68.

15. There is a constant echo of this alarm in the literature and in the media on AIDS in this period. It is worth noting that South African president Thabo Mbeki, famous in Africa for denying HIV/AIDS, contested the use of antiretroviral drugs on the basis of their alleged potential toxicity. See van der Vliet, "South Africa Divided," 48–96.

16. See, among others, Spira et al., "Natural History of Human Immunodeficiency Virus," and Newell, Brahmbhatt, and Ghys, "Child Mortality," which report mortality rates in children born HIV-positive at 45 percent and 54 percent at two years and 62 percent at five years old.

17. Ainsworth and Teokul, "Breaking the Silence," 58–59.

18. Schwartländer, Grubb, and Perriëns, "10-Year Struggle," 542.

19. Knight, *UNAIDS*, 42.

20. Barnett and Whiteside, *AIDS in the Twenty-First Century*, 334.

21. This episode occurred during the First International Conference on AIDS in Atlanta in 1985. Knight, *UNAIDS*, 13–14.

22. Gehler, *Un continent se meurt*, 43–50, 79–87. This book is an example of what people thought of Bactrim and AIDS in 2000.

23. United Nations Office of the Special Adviser on Africa, *Community Realities and Responses to HIV/AIDS*, 29 and 34 of the English text.

24. United Nations Office of the Special Adviser on Africa, 34.

25. UNAIDS, *Collaboration with Traditional Healers*.

26. From Caraël, "Face à la mondialisation," 48: "In many African ethnic cultures, a deadly disease is never 'natural' even if it is caused by a virus. A chronic disease or early death are punishments for having done something wrong."

27. Sachs, "Links of Public Health and Economic Development."

28. Dominique Frommel, "Contre le sida, l'arme du débat," *Le Monde diplomatique*, December 2000.

29. Knight, *UNAIDS*, 41.

30. Some examples are found in Colson, "En quête de guérison," 141–64; Dilger, *Leben mit Aids*; and Thomas, "'Our Families Are Killing Us,'" 279–91.

31. With the encyclical *Humanae Vitae* of July 25, 1968.

32. The statistics on new cases of HIV in Western Europe and North America

from 1990 to today show quite a stable incidence. The condom, supported by adequate sex education, slowed down the spread of HIV, but it does not seem to have been decisive in reversing the epidemic in the Western world. See the historical data on this issue in UNAIDS, *UNAIDS Data 2018*.

33. This is said with reference to Thailand's 100% Condom Program, often touted as a success story. See, e.g., Sonntag, *AIDS and Aid*, 25.

34. "Condoms 'Should Be as Easily Available as Coca-Cola,'" BBC News, November 24, 1998, http://news.bbc.co.uk/2/hi/health/221114.stm.

35. Shelton and Johnston, "Condom Gap in Africa."

36. In the words of a man from Mozambique who felt like joking: "You just don't feel that you're a man until you've had your fourth wife." Steenberg Olsen, "Structures of Stigma," 73.

37. Williams, *AIDS*, 12.

38. United Nations, "Countries Most Affected by HIV/AIDS Are Least Able to Pay for Prevention and Treatment," press release, June 11, 2001, https://press.un.org/en/2001/aids18.doc.htm.

39. Gehler, *Un continent se meurt*, 68.

40. "A Global Disaster," *Economist*, December 31, 1998.

41. "The Menace of AIDS," *Economist*, July 8, 2002.

42. "Menace of AIDS."

43. Austen Ivereigh, "The Elixir of Hope: Why Africa Need Not Die of AIDS," unpublished manuscript, 2004, filed in the DREAM Archives in Rome (hereafter DAR).

44. Interview with Susanna Ceffa, Kinshasa, June 23, 2018, text in DAR.

45. Kathryn Birdwell Wester, "Violated: Women's Human Rights in Sub-Saharan Africa," Topical Review Digest: Human Rights in Sub-Saharan Africa, University of Denver, 2009. https://digitalcommons.du.edu/cgi/viewcontent.cgi?article=1447&context=hrhw.

46. Interview with the author on May 21, 2018.

47. See in UNFPA and UNAIDS, *Report of the Planning Meeting on Strategic Options*, 13, 42, in which male circumcision is criticized because only the risks of performing it in a traditional context are taken into account.

48. Steenberg Olsen, "Structures of Stigma," 104–5.

49. Piot insists in his memoirs on his need to find some success stories in order to make the UNAIDS message credible: "I started scouting for success stories.... Uganda and Thailand reported—basically, anecdotal evidence—that programs to shift people's sexual behaviour were working.... So now I jumped on it.... Uganda became a core part of our political and communications strategy." Piot, *No Time to Lose*, 235–38.

50. Delaunay, "Le Programme national de lutte"; Becker, *La recherche sénégalaise*; ONUSIDA/Sénégal, *Lutte contre le sida*; Putzel, "Histoire d'une action d'état, 245–70.

51. This started with Hogle, *What Happened in Uganda?*

52. The first cases of HIV/AIDS were diagnosed in Uganda in 1982, before the rest of the continent.

53. Uganda Aids Commission, *Twenty Years of HIV.*

54. "Was the Miracle Faked? No, but Possibly Exaggerated," *Economist*, August 15, 2002.

55. Green et al., "Uganda's HIV Prevention Success, 335–46.

56. Government of Uganda, Uganda Aids Commission, UNAIDS, *Draft National Strategic Framework*, as well as the critical comment in Parkhurst, "Ugandan Success Story?"

57. For a history of Museveni's fight against AIDS, see Putzel, "Politics of Action," 19–30, and Putzel, "Histoire d'une action d'état."

58. Josh Kron, "In Uganda, an AIDS Success Story Comes Undone," *New York Times*, August 2, 2012.

59. Green et al., "Uganda's HIV Prevention Success."

60. Kron, "In Uganda, an AIDS Success Story Comes Undone."

61. Kirby, "Presentation on USAID's ABC Study."

62. The drug-access initiative mentioned in chapter 1.

63. Uganda Ministry of Health, UNAIDS, and CDC, *HIV/AIDS Drug Access Initiative.*

64. Gehler, *Un continent se meurt*, 210.

65. Goemaere, Ford, and Benatar, "HIV/AIDS Prevention and Treatment," 86.

66. See Johnson, "Abuse of HIV/AIDS-Relief Funds," 523–24: "Widespread corruption involves HIV prevention. Prevention activities necessarily occur in remote villages, where they are difficult to monitor. A growing trend in Mozambique has been to request grants for rural education programmes (such as taking a theatre group to a rural primary school). However, because of a lack of monitoring—almost a technical impossibility in a country as vast and as lacking in infrastructure as Mozambique—it is common practice to pocket the money and falsify reports of having done prevention work. Not only is aid money misspent, but the data collected on the number of people reached by prevention programmes are inaccurate. The process of monitoring and evaluation is confounded by false data and an inaccurate picture of the progress in HIV/AIDS prevention results. NGOs have outreach targets and require statistics to report to donors, so there is little motivation to investigate fraud. Money remains available because the total funds available outpace the amount being spent."

67. Lewis, *Race against Time*, 199–200.

68. Supra in chapter 1.

69. The figures rose progressively from $1.2 billion in 2002 to $7.7 billion in 2008 and 2009. They fell to $6.9 billion in 2010 and then rose again up to $8.6 billion in 2014. Kates, Wexler, and Lief, *Financing the Response to HIV.*

70. Stover et al. (who include Bernhard Schwartländer), "Can We Reverse the HIV/AIDS Pandemic?," 74.

71. It is not easy to produce credible figures regarding new cases of HIV worldwide from 2002 to 2010. The main source is that of the totals reported by UNAIDS in its yearly reports, alternated with its regular AIDS epidemic updates. Sometimes the data does not correspond in the same year. Up to 2006 the figures on new cases were four to five million a year, understood as averages within very wide fluctuations, of between four and seven million hypothetical new cases. The approximation was easy to explain, especially since the figures were halved from 2007. That year 6,800 people a day were said to have been infected—that is, 2,482,000 people on an annual basis—after it was explained that the data had to be revised because of "methodological improvements" and new information provided by some countries. Incidentally, for the same reason, estimates on the prevalence of the pandemic were reduced from 39.5 million in 2006 to 33.2 million in 2007. From 2007 onward, the new cases varied between 2.5 and 2.7 million. Assuming that the figures provided by UNAIDS before 2007 were far too high, the new cases from 2002 to 2010 should be around 20 million. The variability and confusion regarding the statistics on HIV/AIDS were not necessarily due to the incompetence of the statistics staff of UNAIDS and other institutions working on them but on the fact that the highest rates were found in countries with a low income, with a badly organized public health care system, and therefore also no sentinel sites. Data collection generally depended on maternity centers, but this ended up being limited to just checking for HIV in young pregnant women, not to mention that in many poor countries women never even used the public health care system. Regarding the question of statistics, which has always plagued the history of AIDS, there have been plenty of exaggerated estimations and terrifying projections, which strangely enough went hand in hand with inertia and resignation from an operative point of view. See the notes on the update of the methodology scattered throughout the various annual UNAIDS publications. There are also some useful observations in "Twenty-Five years of AIDS," *Economist,* June 1, 2006, and Denis, "Pour une histoire sociale du sida," 29–30. An example of how vague the statistical projections on HIV/AIDS were, which was particularly evident in the period before the treatment in countries with a low income, can be seen in statements given to CNN by Sandra Thurman, who was copresident of the Office of National AIDS Policy in the Bill Clinton administration: "AIDS poses the greatest threat to mankind since the Bubonic Plague in the Middle Ages. And with no vaccine and no cure in sight, certainly in the next couple of decades we will have literally hundreds of millions of people dying of AIDS around the world." "Clinton Administration Declares AIDS a New Threat to National Security and Global Stability," CNN, April 30, 2000, http://edition.cnn.com/TRANSCRIPTS/0004/30/sun.02.html.

72. Patrick Wieland, MSF general coordinator, quoted at UN Office for the Coordination of Humanitarian Affairs, "Africa: Focus on Mozambique; ART in Africa," press release, PlusNews, December 16, 2004, https://reliefweb.int/report/mozambique/africa-focus-mozambique-art-africa.

73. "Aid for AIDS," *Economist*, April 27, 2000.

74. Donald G. McNeil Jr., "At Front Lines, AIDS War Is Falling Apart," *New York Times*, May 9, 2010.

75. See the beginning of chapter 1.

76. "Twenty-five Years of AIDS," *Economist*, June 1, 2006. The question of the exit strategy from indefinite treatment for AIDS patients, considered unsustainable, appeared frequently in the Western press during the first decade of the prospects of therapy for countries with limited resources. A typical example is the above-mentioned article from the *New York Times*, McNeil, "At Front Lines."

# 3

# DREAM

How did most of the African governments react to the lack of therapies for their AIDS patients? They were not shocked, nor did they rebel. The prevention-only policy did not raise any doubts. It was the position of the international organizations, of the development cooperation agencies, and of the most accredited scientific experts. How could African leaders challenge this mainstream opinion? Besides, they believed that they had good reason to avoid taking action against AIDS. Even if they did acknowledge the AIDS emergency and the need to deal with it, they did not have the means to do anything about it. International aid to Africa had reached its lowest levels at the end of the 1990s. It had been cut back by Western countries, reduced to zero from the Soviet world that had collapsed, and was only just tolerated by the International Monetary Fund and the World Bank, which demanded adjustments, meaning a reduction of state budgets. It certainly was not advocated by neoliberalism at the height of the Bill Clinton era.

It should also be said that many African countries had only recently become democracies after years of dictatorships, Marxist regimes, apartheid, and civil war. The neophyte democratic political classes were afraid that if their people saw how widespread AIDS was, it would cause uncontrollable uprisings among them, to whom democracy had just given an unprecedented say in matters. Even though the civil societies were weak and badly organized, the governments were afraid that once people realized that they needed treatment, they would react.

At the end of the 1990s, the perception of the epidemic varied from country to country. In many capitals in Africa, people had doubted for a long time that HIV even existed. Many deaths caused by AIDS were blamed on the much better-known opportunistic infections.

They were recorded as not caused by AIDS but by tuberculosis, cancer, malaria, or other ubiquitous diseases. The immunodepressive effects of the virus were very similar to those caused by severe malnutrition, explaining why many Africans blamed their country's poverty and considered that it was the fault of the colonialist and racist West, when in fact the problem was AIDS. There was a scientific reason for their thinking: looking at the whole world, the main cause of acquired immunodeficiency (that is, not genetic immunodeficiency) was severe malnutrition, not HIV.[1] In fact, however many HIV-positive people there were, the number of undernourished people was vastly greater, according to the FAO—at least 850 million in 2000—and most of them were in Africa.

This passive approach to the epidemic also came from the fact that African societies, with a few exceptions, did not think in scientific terms. The traditional healers downplayed HIV/AIDS and provided rather unempirical explanations (guilt, curses, magic, bad spirits). The same happened in the various neo-Protestant or neo-Pentecostal communities, which were often guided by a "prophet" who indulged the popular beliefs by explaining people's troubles in terms of guilt or superstition: AIDS was caused by the ill people themselves, who were then called to make amends for or atone for their sins and mistakes. From a medical point of view, African societies did not ask to fight HIV/AIDS with scientific means any more than their ruling classes intended to do.

Nonetheless, the disease existed, and one after the other African governments had to surrender to the evidence. They had no intention of dealing with it with treatment programs. However, neither did they want to give themselves up to civil society and set off debates about how to save millions of people, with public opinion inevitably prompted to wonder who was responsible for the delay in the fight against the epidemic. They were even less in favor of mobilizing activists, who were instinctively seen as opponents because of African governments' frequent conviction (and even more so if they were in an uncertain, learning phase of their democracy) that most decisions should be made from the top down and only a few should be grass-roots decisions.

Acknowledging AIDS as a national emergency frightened the

governments because of the enormity of what was involved. The reasons for their lack of action were different from those of the international Afro-pessimistic community, which was persuaded that Africans were not able to adhere to antiretroviral treatments. African countries were afraid of serious social and political upheavals if the treatment were given the go-ahead because their public health systems would only be able to provide a minority of ill people with the therapies. How could the patients be selected without causing a revolution by the people who were excluded and their families? It was better to ignore the therapeutic possibilities and continue to frighten everyone with the deadly spectrum of AIDS if they did not practice safe sex, which was what the UN agencies wanted. African governments gave the impression that they hoped the epidemic would somehow sort itself out on its own over time, with the inevitable death of sick people and healthy people taking increasing care to avoid being infected. Even importing the drugs for the triple therapy was prohibited in many countries, except that private treatment channels were set up for the countries' few wealthy people.

This rigid antitherapy approach had been the most politically correct international position since 2002 and was the position adopted by international development cooperation agencies and Western governments. African countries had an interest in maintaining good relations with the multilateral and bilateral global aid community, which sent them development aid for various initiatives and, in the specific case of AIDS, mainly funded prevention projects. In turn, international agencies and donors had an interest in keeping good relations with the single African governments since they could expect a political return in exchange for the funds they provided. Ultimately UN agencies depended on all the member countries, even the poorest ones. And donors expected political returns in different locations and contexts from those covered by development cooperation. A poor country that was supported financially was in some way obliged to take sides with the donor country in the various international disputes.

That said, the responsibility for the lack of action with respect to the therapy was not comparable: agencies and institutional donors were fully aware of the efficacy of the triple antiretroviral therapy, unlike many African leaders. Those who know are to be held more responsible than those who do not know very much.

An emblematic example is that of the richest and most powerful country in the continent, South Africa, where thousands of people were dying from AIDS every year. Thabo Mbeki came to power there in 1999 after Nelson Mandela, who was already unsure about whether to engage in the fight against AIDS.[2] Mbeki ended up denying that HIV/AIDS existed at all, blaming the deaths on the poverty in Africa and obtaining sweeping pan-African consensus. According to him, an uncompromising fighter of apartheid, what people in the West called HIV/AIDS could be prevented with a good diet containing plenty of garlic. In the same years, his political rival Jacob Zuma argued that a shower after unprotected intercourse with an HIV-positive woman eliminated all risks. (Later, as president, he no longer insisted that this was so.[3])

In any case, the whole of Africa seemed to find it hard to believe the scientific explanations of HIV, with politicians recommending particular foods and miraculous plants, "prophets" preaching special propitiatory rites, healers guaranteeing everlasting immunity to men who had sex with adolescent virgins, gurus recommending spending a long time in the sunlight, and charlatans "inventing" molecules that were said to destroy the virus through the "production of oxygen."[4] These superstitions and scams were tolerated by governments because they were useful for distracting people from the antiretroviral drugs. The governments were afraid that introducing the antiretroviral therapies would have uncontrollable consequences: people would demand treatment en masse, health care centers would be invaded, and there would be civil disorder and political crises. Giving the treatment to some people but not everyone, because they would have to start with a few groups of patients and then extend the treatment, looked dangerous. Dealing with the question of AIDS was like touching something red-hot.

These concerns could not be dismissed in a hurry: the feasible per capita health care costs in almost all the sub-Saharan countries was a few dollars a year, and once AIDS patients started treatment, it would have to continue for their whole life. After people realized how widespread HIV/AIDS really was, if the government then admitted there was a lack of drugs, which were known to be expensive, it would be very unpopular, and there were bound to be riots. If generic drugs were imported, this might lead to political and trade reprisals from countries producing the brand drugs.

Nonetheless, African governments were not forced to fall in line with the dominant international trend. One way or another, with a sense of responsibility, they could have raised the question of the lives of tens of millions of HIV-positive Africans: they could show the developed countries how their people were suffering, ask for help, and negotiate for more than just prevention. This might be politically inconvenient but not impossible. However, the governments preferred to repeat the large development agencies' slogans and programs in order not to appear out of line in the eyes of the donors of funds for development. In 2000 almost all the requests from African governments to fight AIDS insisted on prevention, multisectoriality, human rights, and gender inequalities. This was out of respect for the language adopted at the time by the UN and WHO, which depended on the variations in the debate on global health, whose continuous innovations in terms of vocabulary and whose projections into the future only appeared to be useful to those with a short memory of what had not been implemented or achieved.[5]

## THE BEGINNING OF DREAM IN MOZAMBIQUE

Mozambique's attitude regarding AIDS was no different from that of most African countries, despite the fact that its rulers were among the best qualified and most unified in the continent. The president, Joaquim Chissano, had vast international experience. He had lived in Europe for a long time as a representative of the Liberation Front of Mozambique (FRELIMO), the Mozambican liberation movement. With independence in 1975, he became foreign minister; in 1986, after the death of the father of the nation, Samora Machel, he succeeded him as president. He acquired worldwide prestige with the peace agreement signed in 1992 ending the Mozambican Civil War and the simultaneous transition from a single-party Marxist regime to a democracy. Chissano had studied medicine at Lisbon, had extensive knowledge of HIV, and did not believe in unscientific fantasies. In public he solemnly affirmed his "commitment to the fight against AIDS"[6] and even appeared on television with a condom showing in his breast pocket. Nonetheless, he did not ask for the antiretroviral therapies. He was aware of the international line, and he also was afraid of taking the lid off a seething social cauldron. He was a pragmatic statesman who saw any mass treatments for AIDS as a danger because of the social unrest that he imagined they would provoke.

In this context something new came about at the end of the 1990s. Mozambique had reached peace in 1992, after the civil war that started in the aftermath of its independence. Peace was achieved thanks in particular to the work of an Italian secular Catholic movement, the Community of Sant'Egidio, which had carried out the mediation between the warring parties. Sant'Egidio, founded in Rome in 1968, had large groups of volunteers in several countries, most in Europe and Africa. The movement is characterized by a spirit of prayer and service to the poor, according to the inspiration of the Second Vatican Council. Its commitment to peace in Mozambique, where it was performing humanitarian activities, derived from the conviction that war was, almost by its very nature, the "mother of all poverty." In 1997 the Community of Sant'Egidio learned that some of its members had died from AIDS in Mozambique, where it had thousands of members. For an association based on providing support, it seemed unacceptable that whether people would live or die depended on geography. European doctors from Sant'Egidio went to Mozambique and started systematically screening people, and they had no other choice at the time than to send the blood samples abroad in refrigerated suitcases (which the customs officers were afraid to even look at). The prevalence rate in the country was over 10 percent, so it was not surprising that many of the blood tests were positive. Apart from the limited number of cases among its members, which were themselves alarming, Sant'Egidio felt involved because after contributing to restoring peace in the country, there was now the threat of an even worse scourge, if that were possible, than the sixteen-year civil war.[7] One million people died during the war between the FRELIMO government and the RENAMO guerrillas. The exponential spread of HIV, which started with the return to peace and the possibility for people to travel again, brought with it the fear that there would be an even higher number of victims. In 1997 more than one million people were infected.

The idea of treating AIDS free of charge, according to the best standards applied in the West, came about in this African context and specifically in Mozambique. Sant'Egidio organized a series of missions to check the feasibility of what was to become DREAM, then the auspicious acronym for Drug Resource Enhancement against AIDS and Malnutrition. Mozambique is a large country (around eight hundred thousand square kilometers) and is very poor. In those years it was always one of the last ten of the 180 or so countries assessed statistically in human development indices.[8] However, the country was not in chaos. FRELIMO had been leading the country with a political-administrative ruling class that was established by winning the elections after independence in 1975. This ruling class, previously loyal to Marxist ideals and to the strictness of the Soviet bloc, of which Mozambique was part, did not trust private initiatives. During the 1990s, however, it saw that the free market offered its first opportunities to become rich. Some leaders were more easygoing than before and were already turning into a *compradora* middle class,[9] without denying the statism learned from Marxism but adapting it pragmatically for business purposes. Sant'Egidio had to come to an agreement with the Mozambican public administration on every step it took. Everything was cumbersome and very slow. An institutional driving force was needed, and this was found in the projects developed within the context of Italian cooperation. The DREAM project was defined and improved for three years without members ever explicitly mentioning it in public: visits were made to the Mozambican health facilities, the situation was studied, and meetings were held with local officials and international NGOs. The aim was to look for a way to treat AIDS.

This was the beginning. It was practically forbidden to talk about therapies, but it was possible to deal with AIDS. The staff worked at the nighttime clinics to help prostitutes at least by treating their gynecological infections and providing condoms. (The women could go there during the night without being seen, to avoid being stigmatized.) Improvements were made in the blood transfusion centers, a continuous source of infection, where the Mozambican health staff worked but not at professional standards—with no gloves or other personal protection and no awareness of the risks for themselves and for the patients. A home care service was set up for AIDS patients. This was officially approved for tuberculosis patients, but actually most of these patients had AIDS, with tuberculosis a consequent infection. ("Opportunistic" would be the word for such infections if AIDS had been acknowledged, but this was not yet the case.) Nutrition centers were opened, which found that they were receiving many obviously sick people, even though they had not been tested. These centers saw the tragedy of the children sent by pediatricians from hospitals where malnutrition and HIV overlapped and were confused. Child mortality was so high that they started being tested for HIV and treated with antiretroviral drugs flown in from Italy in personal luggage.

Then there were the laboratories. The agreements with Mozambican health authorities included improvements in activities carried out in the diagnostic laboratories. There were basic microbiology laboratories in Mozambique that were useful for opportunistic infections, but there were no molecular biology laboratories, which were needed for the antiretroviral therapies. In 1999 the laboratories performed two types of tests. One was for tuberculosis, with a microscopic test that was a very simple basic test to assess the presence of the microbacterium responsible for tuberculosis in the patient's sputum. The other test consisted of counting the red blood cells in a drop of blood under the microscope, and there could be hundreds of them. Many people did these tests every day, and by the end of the day they were exhausted and counted more or less the same number of red blood cells for everyone. There were no automated cell counters.

The Mozambican Ministry of Health (MISAU) was very interested in improving the laboratories, which did not even have gowns for their staffs, in order to do more than basic sputum and blood tests and to reach the stage of having their own molecular biology laboratories. One might ask what the point was of having these laboratories if AIDS therapies were not allowed in the country. The fact was that the HIV-positive Mozambicans who could afford it, including members of the government, were treated in South Africa or in a private clinic in Mozambique's capital, Maputo, which, however, did not have any laboratories that could count the CD4s let alone molecular biology laboratories that could measure the viral load.[10] An express courier called Blue Panther traveled regularly between Maputo and Johannesburg with samples and drugs at a price established for a monopoly service. Having molecular biology laboratories in Mozambique would be a practical way to save money.

Sant'Egidio started talking about possible antiretroviral treatments, both with the international officials who dictated Mozambique's health policy and with the country's health authorities, but their reactions were negative. The idea of bringing treatments for AIDS to Mozambique at the same level of excellence as those offered in the West sounded impractical and even harmful.

The people most against the idea were the representatives of the international development cooperation agencies. Treating AIDS would have revealed their inertia and resignation. The intention to officially introduce the triple combination of antiretroviral drugs, the highly active antiretroviral therapy (HAART) in the Mozambican health care system was ridiculed. It would have been like a slap in the face for most people, who would be excluded from the treatments, and at the same time a luxury for the few privileged people who would be able to benefit from it. It was considered ethically unacceptable. A sarcastic representative of the World Bank compared giving HAART to Mozambicans to Marie Antoinette suggesting that French peasants lacking bread should eat cake.

Mozambican health officials were skeptical too but less hostile. They were worried about tackling AIDS head on. They wanted to receive funds from abroad for their public health system but not necessarily for fighting the HIV epidemic. The highest public health administrative director, Avertino Barreto, repeated that AIDS was not a tragedy or a priority for Mozambique, which was very badly afflicted by tuberculosis and malaria. He also insisted on focusing on other emergencies, in particular on the periodic cholera epidemics. How can you propose an expensive program to treat AIDS, Barreto said, when you cannot even cope with the seasonal crises that cause thousands of deaths from diarrhea? In order to start collaborating, the Sant'Egidio doctors agreed to deal with cholera during floods. Barreto explained that the treatment for AIDS was forbidden because that was what the large international development agencies wanted.

They, the Mozambicans, had to pragmatically adapt because half the state's budget depended on foreign aid (which covered up to 70 percent of the health care costs).[11] In order to grant at least something, Barreto asked for palliative treatment for terminally sick AIDS patients and training for the staff accompanying people at the end of their life.

Sant'Egidio's first meetings were discouraging. The minister of health, Francisco Songane, said he did not agree with the international development agencies that saw treatment as taking away something from prevention, but at the same time he refused to open up to the therapy. He did not say he was against treatment but emphasized that it was so complex that this would make it impossible to provide mass treatment. The fact that not everyone would be reached at the same time would create a minority of privileged people, which in his socialist view was unacceptable. Since it was impossible to treat all HIV-positive people immediately, it would be better to avoid the injustice of a draw for life in which most people would lose. Songane feared the expectations that the population might have regarding individual treatment programs for AIDS because the health system was far from being able to guarantee treatment at a national level. He overestimated the cost of the antiretroviral drugs, whose price, especially considering that generic drugs were now available, was actually falling month by month and would be even lower if large volumes were purchased and consumed. When contradicted on this point, Songane still believed that the fact that it was impossible to guarantee the therapy to everyone from the beginning was decisive and that it was better not to do anything and avoid giving people illusions.

The positions of Prime Minister Pascoal Mocumbi and President Chissano were almost identical. According to them, the therapy had to be made available for everyone with HIV/AIDS, but nobody had the resources for this mass offer. Giving the treatment to only a few people would not have been fair. Mocumbi and Chissano emphasized how poor Mozambique was, also in relation to the fact that the treatment for AIDS lasted a lifetime and required very long-term investments. On the other hand, in those years there were not even treatments for AIDS in South Africa, which was extremely advanced in terms of health care. (The first human-to-human heart transplant in the world was performed in Cape Town in 1967.) Those years South Africa's per capita income was over $3,000, whereas that of Mozambique was less than $300. If South Africa did not contemplate universal treatment, why should its miserable neighbor? The Mozambican health care personnel kept saying, with almost friendly resignation, "They don't do the therapy in South Africa, and you want us to do it when we are the poor neighbors?"[12]

In their antitherapy obstinacy, the representatives of the international development agencies and the donor countries were even more adamant than the Mozambican government. As was customary, it was the UNAIDS delegate who led the way in the UN Theme Group on HIV/AIDS, which was formed in every country by the resident UN agencies in order to inspire the policies of the African governments on AIDS. In Mozambique this delegate considered the DREAM project to be utopian and dangerous because he was convinced that bringing HAART to Africa would mean provoking massive phenomena of resistances since the Africans would not be able to adhere to the treatment. In other words, DREAM would not be helping Africa but would be putting it in danger. There are various testimonies that describe this negative atmosphere:

> We were against the double standard that gave the therapy in the West and condoms in Africa. But in all the international meetings in Maputo, between 1998 and 2000, we were told that we were crazy because there were over a million sick people in Mozambique and one treatment cost $10,000 a year. They wanted to ignore the fact that there were already low-cost generic drugs. Furthermore, they argued that the resources invested for AIDS would take away resources from other diseases and would not encourage the development of the health systems. But money for AIDS was being added, not taken away, and it was precisely with the resources for AIDS that the health systems would then improve enormously. And then there was the ideology that you cannot give something to someone and not to everyone.[13]

The accusation of creating health care for the few went together with another point, regarding the fact that the treatment was free of charge. According to the prevailing opinion at the time, the African patients were supposed to pay for all or part of their antiretroviral therapies. Otherwise, it would be morally bad for them. It was said that some people would even speculate on the fact that they had AIDS and sell the drugs they had received free of charge. In any case, the criticisms regarding elitism and free treatment did not make sense. Health care provided free of charge, the way that DREAM conceived it, aimed to treat the poor in particular and not the wealthy elite. It was the opposite of health care for the few. In addition, the fact that it was free of charge guaranteed adherence to the treatment to such an extent that it would create a critical mass of patients who were no longer infectious, which would be an enormous benefit for everyone and not just for the elite. But let us continue with the testimonies:

> The World Bank delegate argued that treatment was out of the question because Mozambique did not have the facilities, the doctors, the laboratories, etc., and in any case the guidelines for AIDS only indicated prevention. And then if we did treat someone, we would have created inequality. We said that if a ship is sinking and there is only one lifeboat, it has to be used to save at least some people. The WHO representative was adamant: we should not have even been talking about treatment because it was ethically deplorable. It would only create illusions. The UNICEF representative treated us as though we were naive.[14]

The political and cultural pressure that aimed to nip the DREAM program in the bud was very strong. It was said that the treatment would take away resources from prevention, which prevailed in the sacrosanct National Strategic Plan to Fight AIDS for 2000–2002, approved in September 1999 by the MISAU under the supervision of international development agencies. In reality, the objective data reported all the ineffectiveness of prevention. Every year in Mozambique, the HIV prevalence rates and the deaths from AIDS increased. Yet prevention alone, the symbol of the mental stubbornness of the development cooperation agencies, for whom prevention and therapy were obviously different and distinct, was unmovable.

Many of the doctors promoting DREAM were epidemiologists,

hygienists, and infectious disease specialists. Therefore, because of their studies and their culture, they tended to be prevention supporters. However, there was the real situation in Africa that blatantly belied prevention alone and showed how it was failing.

Although its attempts had been unsuccessful, Sant'Egidio decided to continue insisting on its line of action. If the Mozambican public health system was falling apart and lacked personnel and resources, nothing could be done to counter AIDS. This aspect had to be dealt with, and DREAM had to be planned in such a way as to allow for a considerable improvement in the health care infrastructure and offer models that would be functional for the conditions of the country, starting with efficient diagnostic procedures. In the same way, if there were only four hundred doctors in Mozambique, 80 percent of whom lived in Maputo, where there were patients who could pay for their treatment and where there were administrative resources, intensive training would have to be provided for extra health personnel. In short, since there was no system, DREAM was going to have to create one.

Both the MISAU and the international development agencies represented in Maputo would have liked a DREAM program that distributed palliative treatments and drugs for opportunistic infections and operated in public facilities. This would have been a minimalist, makeshift solution with respect to its original intentions that aimed to offer Africans the same standard of antiretroviral treatment as in the West. The international aid community justified its impotence in Africa with the lack of health facilities, diagnostic instruments, and specialized staff. Sant'Egidio did not deny this reality, but it interpreted the fight against AIDS as an opportunity for African health care as a whole. The following point was made by Italian doctor Leonardo Palombi, among the first volunteers of DREAM:

> Prevention cannot be the only answer. If we let it be so, it will be a word that condemns everyone who is infected. There is an alternative. The knowledge acquired about the virus has led to effective pharmacotherapies whose cost for developing countries does not seem to be insurmountable today. The scientific data shows that the multi-antiretroviral therapies that have been used in Western countries since 1996 have clearly increased the possibility of survival.

... On the other hand, in Africa people die on average seven to eight months afterward [after full-blown AIDS]. To people who object that malaria, tuberculosis, and malnutrition should be treated before AIDS, we cannot but say that the only right answer is to take on the health care systems completely so they are able to provide health, at least in relation to the main causes of death and disease. The fight against AIDS can become a testing ground for responsible globalization.[15]

Too ambitious? Sant'Egidio started in 1968 and had a sensitivity tinged with the utopianism expressed in May of that year by French demonstrators: "Soyez realistes, demandez l'impossible" (Be realistic, demand the impossible). It also honored the teaching of the gospel, according to which "nothing is impossible for God." Resigning was not in its nature.[16]

Sant'Egidio was socially rooted in Africa. It knew the weaknesses of the continent but also its vast human resources, which were generally underestimated by people in the West who were not familiar with the everyday life of African men and women. Over the years it had developed a particular aptitude for working with little means, especially for peace, by cultivating synergies and collaborations with people that went beyond any form of prejudice. In particular, it knew that Africa had many people who were in love with their land and wanted to improve its destiny.

The resolve to take action was strong. It was now a question of starting. The DREAM project did not receive any support from international development agencies, so it had to obtain consent directly from the Mozambican government. The government had to overcome its own resistance but also to a certain extent stand back from the international setting. A step forward in time helps reconstruct the history of this consent, which in the end was achieved with difficulty. In 2008 in Maputo, Chissano, who by then was the authentic leader of the country, remembered the work carried out in order to achieve with Sant'Egidio the 1992 peace deal, in particular Andrea Riccardi and Matteo Zuppi, who had a vision but also the capacity to interpret the various phases of the negotiations. And so, the peace agreement was signed in two years:

This was how we found out that Sant'Egidio was an organization that was able to bring about peace. Later, we began to understand that Sant'Egidio was much more than that because it also helped us preserve and defend peace and help the Mozambican population live better. And I remember a big discussion, almost a negotiation, about Sant'Egidio starting a program here to fight AIDS. It was a question of introducing the antiretroviral drugs to Mozambique. Our public health service was panicking because it looked as though there was no way it could start. I was on Sant'Egidio's side, and I tried to convince our government that it was necessary to start. The right conditions could not be created in a day—they had to be created a bit at a time. After a long time, we agreed to start, very timidly. Today Sant'Egidio has this program called DREAM. And we would like to thank Sant'Egidio for fighting AIDS because there is no peace when there is a disease like this. With AIDS, peace is not complete.[17]

The "big discussion, almost a negotiation" that Chissano mentioned corresponded to the work that took a long time in order to convince the Mozambican authorities to allow AIDS to be treated. Faced with the refusal of the government systems to open up to the treatment, Sant'Egidio had turned directly to Chissano as president of the country.

In May 2000 an opportunity arose that led him to think again. It was a state visit to Rome. A private meeting about AIDS was organized at Sant'Egidio, with Riccardi, Zuppi, and the Italian prime minister, Giuliano Amato, in attendance.[18] The situation occurred when Amato strongly reminded Chissano about Italy's great contributions to the good of his country, adding that if Maputo opened up to the antiretroviral treatments, Italy would be even more in favor of cooperating in the development of Mozambique. In other words, Italy's "yes" to Mozambique was connected to Mozambique's "yes" to the treatment for AIDS. Chissano was impressed by the meeting, by how motivated Sant'Egidio was, and by how determined Amato was. Collaboration with Mozambique had been demanding and costly for Italy since independence, not to mention its role in the peace negotiations.[19] Chissano was a flexible and pragmatic politician, but he had not yet accepted the antiretroviral drugs because he was well aware of the international unwillingness to promote the treatment for AIDS patients in Africa. The antitherapy approach of South Africa, his powerful neighbor, had further discouraged him from taking action. Could poor Mozambique do what not even South Africa itself dared do? But now an important figure in international cooperation was now asking him to change his mind. Italy's official support for the introduction of the antiretroviral drugs to Mozambique gave Chissano a glimpse of a different health policy for his country.

When he got back to Mozambique, the president set up a review of the nation's approach to AIDS. The conditions for a political turnaround in favor of the treatment were put in place, despite the strong resistance of the MISAU and representatives of the international development cooperation agencies in Maputo. Chissano intended to gradually overcome this resistance. It took a year for the MISAU to communicate its official approval of DREAM's preparatory work.[20]

This was how the building of the molecular biology laboratories in the country's three main hospitals began, laboratories that were necessary for diagnosing the virus and for monitoring the therapies, which would start as soon as possible. At the same time, funds were raised, training courses for local staff were carried out, the purchasing channels for the drugs were perfected, and a home assistance network was set up for AIDS patients. On December 18, 2001, a government decree canceled the ban on importing antiretroviral drugs to Mozambique. The drugs that inhibited the replication of HIV were finally authorized, and in February 2002 DREAM's first "authorized" patients came to the Machava-Maputo health center—that is, after the center had treated patients informally case by case in previous years. The people who came were mainly in poor condition, desperate, isolated, and stigmatized. They arrived dragging themselves along or carried by relatives. Some were even brought in wheelbarrows.

Those who were not too sick did not come yet, wanting to avoid manifesting their disease, which was perceived as a social death sentence. There was no mass assault on the therapies, which the politicians had so feared. What prevailed in people was stigma, shame, and fear of showing that they were HIV-positive. Gradually more people started coming because the patients who started the treatment recovered so surprisingly. Late-stage patients were transformed: they were walking again, and some even went back to work. The results went beyond all expectations and were clearly visible to everyone. Representatives of the development cooperation agencies, journalists, South Africans passing through, and all kinds of curious people took photographs of the antiretroviral drugs on the shelves in Machava-Maputo, an unusual sight in Africa. The government, however, was still afraid:

> Prime Minister Mocumbi told us several times that it was our responsibility alone and that the government had nothing to do with the project. Mocumbi was afraid of the political impact of this move. AIDS was a controversial topic and a nightmare for the population. People who tested positive often committed suicide. The case of South Africa, which did not propose any treatment for AIDS, was a model for Mozambique. They wanted treatment centers to be invisible. This is exactly what happened with Machava. When it opened there was the fear of an assault, but nothing like that happened. There was a constant, regular flow of people, even from far away, from the whole of Mozambique. After a short time, Machava became famous throughout the country with none of the feared social unrest.[21]

Soon, in 2003, the Mozambican health authorities changed their minds, probably following the new international approach to AIDS, which was now in favor of treatment, even for countries with limited resources. The MISAU suddenly made it known that "Mozambique has a strong primary health care system" suitable "to both serve chronic disease and to manage active tracking of healthy HIV-positive individuals."[22] In reality, apart from what was surprisingly happening in Machava, without social peace being jeopardized as feared, practically nothing had changed in the public health system. Internationally, however, everything had changed: the Global Fund, PEPFAR, and the Gates, Clinton, and other patrons' foundations led to the hope for a flow of money for the antiretroviral therapies, since clinging to prevention alone was no longer politically correct or advantageous when negotiating with donors. In the meantime, the MISAU reception areas were full of representatives of various international cooperations and NGOs, who were all suddenly eager to take care of the treatment for HIV/AIDS. The fast change in opinion of the potential of the public health system, which up to recently had been complained about because it was considered so fragile,[23] led to ironic comments: "This U-turn represents little more than a political stage act in favour of the introduction of ART in Mozambique. This can be taken as an example of what happens when a recipient country is just as eager to attract funding as the donors are to step on each other's toes to be let in."[24]

In any case, a change had taken place. Chissano had been pragmatic and cautious, and now Mozambique was one of the few African countries dealing with HIV/AIDS not just with words but with action.

## ANA MARIA MUHAI

The Mozambican media called her a *gladiatora*, and that is what Ana Maria Muhai was. In 2011 she won one of the Women of Courage Awards of the US Department of State, directed by Hillary Clinton, an honor reserved for women who have distinguished themselves for their leadership in human rights. "I didn't learn about AIDS in associations or in books. I learned about it the hard way. I am AIDS!" was how she spoke on the television, on the radio, in the schools, in the hospitals, and in other public places.[25] Luísa Diogo, Mozambique's prime minister from 2004 to 2010, grew fond of her and took her with her when she traveled abroad. Muhai, with her broad face and deep eyes, a charismatic but ordinary person, semi-illiterate but an excellent communicator, got to know the world.

In 1998, at forty-one years old, Muhai, whose only ambition had been to give her children a beautiful life, discovered how fragile she was. Two months after giving birth to her eighth child of different fathers, she felt unusually weak. She did not get any better. A year later she was coughing day and night and covered in sores. Her hair fell out. She lost a lot of weight. It was the slim disease.

Muhai was treated as well as possible in Mozambique at the time. She did not have a formal diagnosis of AIDS because those years people there preferred to avoid talking about the disease. Opportunistic infections, on the other hand, connected to the progression of HIV, which destroyed the immune system, were acknowledged as pathologies in their own right. For the local doctors, tuberculosis was tuberculosis, a malaria attack was a malaria attack, parasitosis was parasitosis, and so on. The possibility that AIDS was behind that frightening loss of weight was something people imagined but then dismissed. Politicians denied it, and the public health system adapted passively, all the more so because there were no therapies. The hospitals were full of patients with diseases that could be traced to AIDS, but there was no diagnosis for it. What was seen was what was treated, if possible. It was not pointless, it eased suffering, but it did not solve the problem. AIDS did not appear to be a deadly disease because it did not kill directly, but by destroying the immune system it made the body susceptible to the most ruthless pathologies. The fact that it was hidden meant it lent itself to misunderstandings and to misrepresentations and encouraged it to be dismissed by the African governments that were afraid of opening the doors to hell. Muhai also had one infection after another without anyone studying their cause, which was easy enough to imagine: for years she was told in the hospital that she had malaria. In the meantime, her worn-out immune system predicted an imminent pathology that would be fatal.

Muhai was as poor as most people in Mozambique and spent her days lying on a mat in her plastic-roofed hut on the outskirts of Maputo, where she lived with her mother and three youngest daughters. Her last partner left her as soon as he understood that she was HIV-positive. She was used to that. For her, men had been a form of survival: her beauty and vitality in exchange for sustenance. Above all, many African women used men to obtain what they consider essential for their social identity—children. Her mother had eleven children, the same way: Muhai was brought up without a father. The sociologists call it transactional sex, and they connect it, rightly so in countries with limited resources, with poverty. In sub-Saharan Africa, it is a frequent form of exchange and is not at all shameful for women, who have few rights and resources.[26]

Muhai no longer had the strength to eat. AIDS takes away one's appetite, almost as though in order to accelerate the wasting. As long as she was strong enough, she sold things at a stall in front of her home. Cassava, tomatoes, traditional drinks. But nobody would buy from her anymore because she was sick. People pointed at her on the street, and even though she felt she was just the shadow of herself, she turned toward them defiantly "so they could see my face, I had nothing to lose, I was only worried for my children."[27] Muhai was part of a sect, the Zion Church, which sent her away at the first mention of her being HIV-positive. In her neighborhood, people expected her to die at any moment and avoided her like the plague. Sometimes people came to her hut and danced and sang songs about AIDS, as a form of exorcism. Muhai suffered from the typical stigma of people with AIDS in Africa, which extended to her family. A neighboring family had a television, which very few people had. Muhai's three daughters tried to watch secretly from the neighbors' window, but they were always chased away. The same thing happened at school, where there was a vacuum around them: "Their mother's got AIDS."[28] Muhai felt she had reached the end. Sometimes she wanted to die so the stigma on her children would disappear. Other times she prayed to God to heal her.

In February 2002 a nurse directed her to the doctors of the DREAM program in a health care center for AIDS that had just opened a few days before in Machava in her own neighborhood. They offered the treatment for AIDS with HAART, which had proved to be extraordinarily effective in the Western world. HAART does not mean being healed because the virus cannot be eliminated, but it does mean surviving in a good condition. Basically, it means being well, strong again, able to work, only that the patients have to be treated for their whole lives (unless new scientific discoveries say otherwise). Sant'Egidio had a good reputation among the Mozambicans because it had mediated the peace that ended the civil war, and Muhai put her trust in it.

Her immune system had practically disappeared. The way to assess the state of the immune system is by measuring the $CD_4$ lymphocyte cells: the fewer $CD_4$s there are, the more compromised the immune defenses. A healthy person has around 1,000 $CD_4$s for every milligram of blood. The result of Muhai's $CD_4$ measurement: 11. At the time, according to the treatment protocols for AIDS in the Western world, the treatment with antiretroviral drugs started once the $CD_4$s were below 350 and in developing countries once the $CD_4$s were below

200. This was already a very critical threshold, with fewer guarantees of survival during the early stages of treatment and difficult recovery of the immune system. In the Global North, the treatment was started when the immune system had been affected but not compromised; in the Global South, in order to limit the number of patients treated, greater risks were accepted regarding the recovery of their defenses, and as a result the treatment often failed. This discrepancy came from the minimalist approach that prevailed in treating the poor compared to how the rich were treated. Muhai died tragically years later because of the delay in starting the HAART regimen.

When Muhai started the therapy, for the first four months the drugs were brought to her home. She was taken to the center by car for her medical examinations and blood tests. Then she started walking again and going out. Many people did not even believe it was her. Wasn't she already dead? She recalled,

> People who met me couldn't believe it was me, that it was the same person. Many people thought I was my sister, and when I told them I was Ana Maria, they didn't think it was true. So, I went for a walk around my area arm in arm with my sister to show everyone that it was me. At the beginning, when I was sick, they came and picked me up to take me to the Machava center, where I got my treatment. Then I started getting better, and I could go on my own. I had to go through a market to get to the center. When I went through it, everyone was amazed, and they were a bit scared. They walked around me; they thought I was a ghost. We have a custom in Africa: if you see a ghost, you touch it, and it flies away. So, a lot of people started touching me and pinching me, to see if I was real, but I didn't fly away.[29]

She recovered quickly. By the end of the first year, Muhai weighed seventy kilograms again. She looked perfectly healthy—so much so that people who did not know her story did not believe that she was HIV-positive. Her attractiveness worked against her. When she spoke in public wearing a seductive black dress, mean people said she was pretending she had AIDS just to scrounge a job.[30] For proof of her story, she started carrying photographs of herself taken when she weighed twenty-eight kilograms, the image of a dehydrated woman who was a total wreck—just skin and bones. Muhai had lived through the experience described by many AIDS patients on the HAART regimen, what in the literature is called "the Lazarus syndrome."

But hers was not only a physical resurrection. No longer afraid of anything, she gave free rein to her feelings as a true, simple, but authoritative woman. You would see her at the Machava DREAM center just after she had recovered, when she would pass time among the patients, often under a big mango tree. She had given herself a mission on her own, without anyone asking her, and she took on the work of providing a testimonial. She wanted to give something back. She felt she had been saved and wanted to communicate this to those who were trembling in the face of AIDS. She had firsthand experience of the stigma that excluded people from society and wanted to free those who were its prisoners. She knew about people's reluctance to take the HIV test and the terror of getting the result, which was seen as social death before biological death. She convinced people to face the test and accept the outcome, explaining that they could have the therapy, unlike what happened in other health centers.

The staff in the Machava DREAM center, which was just starting up, noticed the potential of what Muhai was doing. She was dealing with some of the most important problems of any approach to AIDS in Africa: the terror of the stigma, being rejected by the community of relatives and neighbors, feeling sentenced to death because of the lack of safe treatment, the silence around a disease generated by sex and blood about which it was forbidden to talk. It also concerned the crucial distance between the medical facilities and the patients, which put at risk lifelong adherence to the therapy. The antiretroviral drugs miraculously restored life and strength but were not able to eliminate the virus definitively. They were only able to limit it to some remote reservoir in the body, from where, if the treatment were interrupted or not taken properly, its attacks the immune system were even worse than before. This is how Muhai described her commitment:

> I work as an activist at the DREAM center: I talk about the treatment and give hope to the many people who go to the center. I try and remember them all. Every day I have a meeting with many other

women like me, but also with men and young people who have come for the first time. People in Mozambique are afraid of the test. Before DREAM started giving the treatment, everyone who took the test and was positive—received a death sentence. There was no medicine. Nobody even hoped that it was possible to live with AIDS, so it was better not to know you were sick. That's what I thought too. The people who come to our clinic have heard of the treatment, but they don't believe it. They're afraid of other people's prejudice and of being abandoned by their relatives. Especially the women: here, if a woman gets AIDS, it's always her fault even if it's in fact their husbands who infect them, then abandon them, and the women' relatives and neighbors insult them. I welcome these people. I explain that AIDS can be treated, and I tell them my story. At the beginning many of them don't believe that I'm sick too, so I show them the packet of medicines that are the same ones that are given. Some of them don't even believe that, so I take the photographs of me when I weighed twenty-eight kilograms out of my wallet, and only then do they start smiling. In the meeting, I also explain how they have to take their medicine, and I always tell them that they should not be ashamed of having AIDS—that it is a disease like any other disease that can be treated. Shame is people's ignorance—it's leaving sick people alone. And I ask everyone to talk about this disease and to help change the Mozambican people's mentality.[31]

When Muhai started her treatment, the AIDS epidemic affected 1.2 million Mozambicans (6.3 percent of the nineteen million inhabitants but 13 percent of adults between fifteen and forty-nine). The number of deaths was around one hundred thousand a year. There were four hundred thousand orphans of one or two parents who had died from AIDS.[32] Mozambican society struggled to acknowledge the emergency. It was said that despite occasional alarms directed at the international community, which provided most of the funds for the public health system, the political leaders were afraid that masses of sick people looking for treatment would create a risk in terms of public order. Therefore, they excluded AIDS from their operative horizons, and the result was effectively denial.

The stigma reigned in society. People who said they were sick were isolated, marginalized, and segregated. They lost all their social relationships. Sociological research on Africans' general feelings regarding AIDS showed that the great fear was not so much of physical suffering but of being excluded from their community, family, work, and friendships.[33] Letting people know that one was HIV-positive was the equivalent of social suicide. One lost all one's resources for survival as well as for fighting the disease.

But when Muhai, radiating well-being, exclaimed on television, "I am AIDS!," people's terror and prejudice dissolved, and they started talking about AIDS in less imaginary and superstitious ways. They started to think in scientific terms about the transmission of HIV and to accept the physical proximity of HIV-positive people. Muhai became a national point of reference. In the Mozambican public opinion, AIDS gradually stopped being a disease of foreigners, white people, albinos, witches, prostitutes, soldiers, and truck drivers—basically of anyone but themselves.

At the end of 2012 Muhai discovered that she had stomach cancer. By then it was incurable. This was very probably because her immune system had only partially recovered after her initial extremely low CD4 count. She died a few months later at age 55. Mozambique's highest institutions were represented at her last farewell, a sort of state funeral to acknowledge Muhai's important public role.

In the 1990s when Muhai was infected, a person with HIV had an average life expectancy of around ten years from the moment when they were infected. How long they lived depended on several factors: the initial number of viral particles, the quality of their life, their material resources, their social context, and their general health. There were cases of people who had been infected by frequent blood transfusions in whom full-blown AIDS manifested almost immediately and who died a few months later. On the other hand, there were people who lived for many years because their immune system was strong and their lifestyle was under control. In sub-Saharan Africa, where the human development indices are the lowest on the planet, full-blown AIDS tended to manifest before it did in developed countries. Above all, African scourges such as malnutrition, tuberculosis, and HIV all made each other worse and attracted each other.

Muhai was not someone who looked for whose fault anything was and for who was responsible. But it is worth wondering how and when she was infected. We can imagine, considering her terminal condition at the beginning of 2002, that Muhai was infected soon after there was peace again in Mozambique at the beginning of the 1990s. At that time she was probably with a man who was HIV-positive—maybe with one of the many Mozambicans who had been in the South African mining townships. The spread of AIDS in the southern part of Africa was connected to the mining centers with their millions of single men and the related sex work industry. Maybe her partner at the time went with prostitutes or other women who were at risk. Or maybe he was a former soldier or a former refugee. During the civil war HIV was not very common in Mozambique because it was difficult to travel, but there were big outbreaks among soldiers and in the refugee camps. For example, 80 percent of the Zimbabwean troops, who were allies of the Mozambican government and guarded the strategic corridors of the Zambesi and Limpopo Rivers, which were full of displaced people, had HIV and passed it on to the women around them. When peace was restored and the soldiers on both sides were demobilized, millions of refugees and displaced persons returned home, transportation and trade were restored, and HIV spread easily. After the end of the war in 1992, the incidence rate in Mozambique shot up.

Muhai was probably one of the first victims of this viral explosion. Even practices outside the sexual sphere could have infected her, like so many other people in Mozambique, such as surgical procedures performed without sterilizing instruments and operations carried out by traditional healers who made incisions using the same razor on everyone. Nonetheless, Muhai did not say that any of this had happened to her. Her case seemed to be the typical situation of many African women infected by unconscientious and irresponsible men. The African statistics on HIV show that the number of HIV-positive women—particularly young women—was much higher than that of the men. The men carried the infection because they traveled and had unsafe sex with the women they met. Even if she had tried, Muhai would have found it very difficult to make her partner take care and wear a condom. In order to do this, she would have had to have her own resources, a job, and not have to be a slave to the need to feed her children. Like every poor African woman, she depended materially on her man. A friend of hers, Luzete Chàuque, explains it well:

> I was born in Maputo in a very poor family. I started going to school when I was ten. I didn't understand anything the teachers said. I just thought about what I would eat when I got home. I lost my father when I was seventeen, and I'd already lost my mother. I was left alone with my five brothers and nobody to help us. I met a boy who worked in a bakery. . . . He gave me bread in exchange for sex. In 1994, without wanting to, I got pregnant. He didn't take responsibility. . . . In 2003 I got pregnant again, by another man. I went to the prenatal medical examination at Matola where DREAM does prevention of vertical transmission. They asked me if I wanted to do the HIV test. I said yes. I was positive. It was very hard. At that time all you heard was that being HIV-positive was like getting a death sentence. I was paying for all the sins of all my sexual relationships—the ones I exchanged for a piece of bread. I knew that by not using a condom I could get AIDS, but I had no choice. When you're poor, you accept anything. You accept sex without a condom; you accept sex you don't want; you accept being raped; you accept anything for a piece of bread. Being poor is a rip-off. And being a poor woman is even worse. You're like trash.[34]

In the West some people believe in a cultural stereotype of Africans as genetically inclined to be "sexually promiscuous" and indulging in "excessive copulation."[35] In reality what is specific to Africans is not their sexual behavior but the poverty that generates an unstable social context and health context. Women are materially dependent on men, and a lack of hygiene, health checkups, and prevention of gynecological infections provokes a greater incidence of diseases of the sexual sphere (syphilis, gonorrhea, herpes, etc.). When the genital tissues are less intact, this encourages the transmission of HIV.

## NO TO AFRO-PESSIMISM

In the words of the Italian doctor Cristina Marazzi, who devised the DREAM program at the end of the 1990s, DREAM originated from the intellectual honesty of not wanting to accept a widely shared but absurd reality that implicitly insisted that Africa be left with 30 million people with AIDS and no therapy: within a few years it had reached the extent of genocide. It was therefore necessary to work to show that the therapy for AIDS was also possible in Africa, when there was still the debate on unacceptable costs for the treatment, at the same level of quality and excellence that had been so very successful in the First World.[36]

In its full name itself (Drug Resource Enhancement against AIDS and Malnutrition), DREAM communicated a specific mission: to fight AIDS with the use of drugs. The program was set up at the time when the maximum emphasis was on behavior-based prevention and the idea of the condom as the main way to control HIV was in vogue. Not that DREAM was against behavioral-based prevention. However, it believed that the pharmacological treatment, by its very nature, was a decisive element, not only in treating the tens of millions of people who were already infected but also in prevention, thanks to the prophylaxis obtained by antiretroviral drugs reducing the presence of the HIV virus in bodily fluids, with the parallel decline in the probability of infecting other people. In the years after DREAM was set up, the value of pharmacological and biology-based prevention came to be acknowledged alongside that of behavior-based prevention. However, around 2000, this was not the case for low-income countries.

DREAM was devised in order to take to Africa the same medical and pharmacological excellence that had been used to treat HIV/AIDS patients in Western countries since 1996. This included setting up molecular biology laboratories for complex measurements, such as of the CD4s and of the viral load—the same diagnostics that ensured the success of the treatments in North America and Europe. If DREAM had only been conceived as a distributor of resources, drugs, and medical instruments, taking this level of excellence to Africa would not have been much use. The availability of the antiretroviral drugs as well as advanced diagnostics were essential but still not enough.[37] A new model for treating AIDS in Africa had to be found, and it had to involve Africans and understand the special conditions of African patients. These were patients who, according to the widespread idea of Afro-pessimism in the West, were believed incapable of adherence, the basis for claiming that the triple antiretroviral therapy could not be carried out in Africa.

DREAM had faith in Africans, who were considered the protagonists in the fight against AIDS. It would, however, be at least a few years before they would be able to take on this leading role. During this time the African health care system would have to be supported until it had consolidated a capacity for the autonomous management of the AIDS therapies. In setting up and developing DREAM, European volunteers took care to train as many African professionals as possible, to the point that Africans achieved complete professional independence: doctors, biologists, computer experts, nurses, and technicians, all trained on the job.

In the end, despite keeping its Euro-African characteristics, DREAM became fully African in terms of the staff working in Africa. Today all the coordinators of the DREAM centers there are African, not European—the best solution in terms of excellence and results. However, the current situation could not have been achieved without European professionals' long-term support in technical and scientific terms as well as in the communication of a culture of solidarity, female emancipation, and overcoming the stigma.

According to DREAM, in order to make it possible for the African patients to adhere to the therapy, the Western know-how had to be transferred to the African situation, not mechanically but by verifying its effectiveness in this different context. This meant first of all guaranteeing the patients a stable interaction that would make them loyal. The AIDS patients had to know that there was always a doctor or other competent member of staff they could turn to, including the so-called activists, who will be discussed later. Second, scientific research was necessary. This was a decisive part of the DREAM's clinical commitment. It was not a question of discovering clinically different antiretroviral drugs for the Africans, which did not make sense, but of devising new practical applications for an epidemic in Africa that could not be quantitatively compared to that in the West and required combining data that was certain with data that was experimental. This led to a series of scientific advances facilitated by the large number of patients who would be monitored. DREAM's scientific battles involved clinical aspects, such as the thresholds for starting therapy, drug resistance, mother-to-child transmission of HIV, and links between malnutrition and AIDS, but they also dealt with the critical aspects of the African public health systems, which looked like an unsuccessful copy of Western health care systems, with overloaded and inefficient hospitals. DREAM advocated small-scale territorial health care, easy for patients to reach, because treating a disease like AIDS required an infinite number of appointments and examinations.

The question of the treatment being free of charge was also decisive for the patients' adherence. In every DREAM center there was a clearly visible sign: "You don't have to pay." How could people who did not even have enough money to buy food be asked to pay for their treatment? How could single mothers with no source of income be asked to pay? How could sick orphans or their grandparents be asked to pay? In Africa, at the beginning of the 2000s, when mainstream health care wanted the HAART regimen to be paid for, the few fortunate people who could afford to start the antiretroviral therapy often had to interrupt it due to economic problems, which seriously compromised their condition and created resistances. DREAM wanted to avoid this. Paola Germano, DREAM's executive director, was very clear: "[Free-of-charge treatment] is a question both of fairness and of efficacy because if it is not like this, then nobody, or practically nobody, can afford the drugs. In order to reduce the infection the treatments have to be free of charge."[38]

There is not much to say on how fair it was not to charge. Many Western patients received their antiretroviral drugs through their public health systems. Should Africans, who were poorer, have had to pay for theirs? Michel Sidibé from Mali, who was the executive director of UNAIDS from 2009 to 2019, rightly observed, "The fight against AIDS is also a fight against inequality, including inequality between men and women, between children and adults, between poor countries and the other ones."[39] Regarding the efficacy of providing the treatment free of charge, it was obvious that if it were not so, the treatment would be inaccessible for most Africans. In the 2000s an ordinary HAART regimen could cost, depending on the country and the way it was carried out, between $200 and $700 a year, including the drugs, blood tests, medical examinations, and management costs. The complexity of the procedures that are part of the treatment demands a high number of appointments to check the patients' health, so there is still a cost for the patients.[40] However well distributed Mozambican medical centers are, they cannot possibly cover the entire immense country. Patients are considered lucky if they live within fifteen kilometers of a center; some must even travel up to one hundred kilometers. Their transportation costs thus can be high. People typically pay to get around in private minivan taxis, which are often old and overloaded. This is Africa: long journeys take a long time, resources, and good feet. There is an image common to every part of Africa that remains impressed on every Western visitor: people walking alongside roads or on paths at any time of day, almost like a society that has walking in its nature.

Treating AIDS, especially at the beginning, requires an extra investment from the patients in terms of food, but the disease limits their possibility to work until they recover, so they live with an even lower income. The low spending capacity of the patients also has to be considered in view of the fact that the therapy is for life. After the initial shock of discovering they are HIV-positive, patients start talking to their doctor about what needs to be done and immediately have to face the question of the duration of the therapy. They are distressed by the fact that the treatment is forever, whereas they know that malaria can be treated in a few days and tuberculosis can be treated in hopefully less than a year. Then there are the patients who have even less than average resources: women, children, orphaned teenagers, and those who already have several HIV-positive patients in their family. Offering the treatment free of charge in the poorest continent on earth is the only way if people are to take the test and, if they are HIV-positive, start the antiretroviral therapy with the aim of continuing over time and adhering to the therapy.

It was only the global aid community's gradual acceptance of authentic universal access to treatment for AIDS that led to treatment free of charge being considered politically correct. At the beginning of the 2000s, however, the international tendency was to make the patients from poor countries pay for at least part of their treatment, almost like a moral and educative obligation as well as a way to contribute to improving their poor public health systems. The agencies, donors, and governments all demanded more or less expensive contributions from the patients. It was argued that even if they only paid something from their own pocket, this would make them aware of the value of the drugs they were being given—as though coming back to life from certain death did not already give them an idea of their value. Then there was the matter of corruption. Patients were often told that even though the drugs were free of charge, they were not immediately available but could be bought privately. Desperately needing these drugs, they paid the staff, who soon came back with drugs that had been "bought." This is not to mention the *pourboires* that African patients often had to give in order to be seen quickly.

Apart from scientific excellence and apart from the fact that the treatment was free of charge, achieving adequate adherence meant that the clinical aspect had to be carried out with an understanding of the African patients in their context. DREAM defines its approach to patients as holistic. This means that the main medical approach has to be integrated with as great an understanding as possible of the person, their condition, and their social and family situations. A patient may be illiterate, stigmatized, malnourished, poor, or psychologically exhausted; they may live in an isolated place, be in bad health regardless of HIV, or have difficult relationships with their family. All this has to be taken into account. The medical (or health) aspect is fundamental, but for adherence the social aspects also have to be considered in order to build a community of care around the patient. This way the loneliness that derives from the stigma can be overcome and the patient can once again believe in the future. The guiding concept is "the patient in the center." Cristina Marazzi explains it like this:

> The first guiding idea that the other ideas all come from is the centrality of the patient. DREAM always starts from the concrete man and woman and not from the institutions. The patient is considered as a whole, with a holistic approach. In fact, the AIDS patients [in Africa] have their specific complexities, they are not a photocopy of patients who live in rich countries, they have to be known, studied, and it is important to respond to their specific needs in terms of prevention, therapy, and in social terms. They often have opportunistic

infections, including malaria and tuberculosis. They have to be assessed from a nutritional point of view and have to be offered food support, when needed, as a therapeutic treatment so that the medical treatment is not given in vain. They are often illiterate and need to be given health education; they have to be motivated to adhere to their care program and be reintegrated into their family and their social setting."[41]

Expressing herself in a different way but with similar concepts, Noorjehan Abdul Majid, a Mozambican doctor, explains: "The attention given to the patients is what makes the difference; it is the 'difference with DREAM.' If they live far away and have no way of getting here, we give them the money to pay for their journey. We walk with the patients, we fight with them, and as their hair turns white our hair does too."[42] According to this professional, treating the patient in the center means taking care of everything that might hinder their treatment.

In DREAM, the patients themselves often become protagonists in the fight against AIDS, not only because they spread hope to other sick people like themselves by showing that they are healthy again but also, after receiving ad hoc training, by collaborating with the health care staff and taking on responsibilities in terms of the organization and management of the centers. One consequence of putting the patient in the center is that they become actively involved, in various ways, in the fight against AIDS.[43] DREAM exists because of the doctors and administrators who set it up, but it also works because many patients whose health is stable have made it their life commitment.

One initial Afro-pessimistic objection to DREAM concerned the therapy adherence of Africans, and another one concerned the shortage of local medical staff and health facilities. This second objection would have been reasonable if DREAM had wanted to carry out emergency or short-term work. However, DREAM intended to create a long-term partnership and also develop the African public health systems by providing new human resources, setting up facilities throughout the country, and creating unprecedented operational solutions and a scientific culture of health among people who were attracted to traditional healers. Through this partnership, the public health systems would be strengthened and equipped to fight AIDS and consequently the other pathologies too because complex laboratories were not set up in order to be closed once the epidemic was under control and the emergency was over. And all the doctors, clinical officers, nurses, medical technicians, community health workers, activists, and biologists were not trained to be sent home when they were no longer needed to deal with HIV.

DREAM proposed working together on long-term projects with the African governments, in order to overcome HIV but also to strengthen the public health systems. The international cooperation's prevailing philosophy is to concentrate on short-term projects, works to be delivered within a limited period, and then move on to other projects in other places. DREAM, on the other hand, became part of the local public health systems, with the idea of increasing the number of qualified Africans, so they would outnumber the Europeans who were there at the beginning. The idea of DREAM in the end was to become Mozambican, Malawian, Guinean, Cameroonian, Kenyan, Congolese, and so on.

In 2000, when DREAM started, 62 percent of the population of sub-Saharan Africa lived in rural areas, in poverty, culturally isolated, with poor living conditions, very bad communication systems, not many vehicles, no public transport, and very few schools or health centers.[44] Many people with AIDS who lived in the vast African rural areas could hardly travel at all. They suffered and died alone, far away from the health centers. They do not even appear on the international statistics on AIDS, which are derived from the sentinel sites. How could they be reached?

DREAM decided to organize a system throughout the country, by first setting up its day hospitals for HIV/AIDS on the outskirts of the towns, which could be reached both from the center of town and from the countryside, and then in the rural areas themselves. Moreover, it drew up agreements with the governments so it could be present with its own staff in the village health centers scattered over vast areas, in order to carry out systematic screening after offering treatment and in particular to intercept HIV-positive pregnant women, save them and their babies, and through these women get to know their families and their local communities to be able to contact more people with

HIV. This created a kind of small-scale universal access to therapy. The complex DREAM laboratories, however, were centralized, and the rural health centers and DREAM mobile clinics sent them the samples to be tested.[45]

Unlike health care systems that were concentrated in large hospitals, DREAM organized a health care system that was spread out throughout the country, paying attention to home care for patients who were hard to reach. It didn't need huge buildings. The first center in 2002 in Machava, on the outskirts of Maputo, was very dignified—it did not leave people lying on the ground outside like the public hospitals did—and thanks to the trees and verandas, it protected the patients from the sun and from the hostile looks of the passers-by. However, it was just a tiny corner of a far bigger public hospital. It consisted of the former caretaker's house and a sheltered area in the open air—that was all.

The DREAM system was designed to prevent large areas of the country from being excluded. By "recovering" certain distinct areas and taking in patients from farther away when required, it made clear that therapy also meant prevention. When the HAART regimen was available in a community, HIV lost its momentum, became weaker, and was much less infectious. This benefit of the therapy was particularly valued by DREAM doctors in the early 2000s, when there were still people who separated treatment from prevention: "We are seeing a potential effect of the reduction of transmission in treated subjects because their viral load is obviously lower, and this greatly reduces the possibility of infecting other people. This is very important for a pathology like HIV/AIDS, which develops and is latent over many years."[46] The recovery of every area involved a mobility strategy and communications network, as Germano notes:

> It was decided not to build large hospitals, which in any case turned out to be too expensive, both because of the actual construction costs but also because of all the costs of running them. A better solution was to build many excellent reference centers for patients who would come from second-level health care centers in areas that were farther away or in rural areas, where there could be intermediate-level health care services, like checking and distributing the

drugs or doing some types of tests. In addition, there were the mobile clinics and home care, which made it possible for everyone to access the treatment. Running the centers involved taking particular care in collecting the clinical data, ensuring stable Internet connections, and in all the activities regarding support for, coordination, and management of the staff. All the services were also connected through satellite or landlines, and all the staff could receive second opinions and advice from experts working at universities and hospitals.[47]

In areas with no landlines, DREAM invested in information technology from the very beginning, using renewable energy supplies sourced locally because many DREAM centers were in areas with no electricity or with intermittent power supplies.[48] All the clinical information about the patients was put into a software program. This was a practical decision that meant not only enormous logistical savings but also the possibility to visualize complex clinical parameters immediately and share information in real time with the most highly qualified specialists during remote consultations. The vast amount of data collected also boosted scientific research.[49]

## EURO-AFRICAN SYNERGY

The characteristics of DREAM—treatment given according to Western standards, taking into account the specific African aspects of the patients, offering the therapy free of charge, in-depth scientific and professional training for local personnel, a holistic view of the patient, therapy as prevention, strengthening the African health care system by reaching people in faraway places—were all reasonable solutions, with which the international agencies and NGOs gradually came to agree. Around 2000 these solutions challenged the prevalent opinions, but in the end they were adopted because they were effective. Nonetheless, DREAM's originality was not limited to operational decisions that went against the flow.

DREAM originated from a Christian community and is rooted in spiritual and human values, which make it possible to see rare synergies between science and religious hope, between Europeans and Africans, between professionals and volunteers. This has produced extraordinary results. DREAM has forty-eight main centers in Africa, twenty-five of which have molecular biology laboratories that treat thousands of patients and provide services for patients who are looked after by mobile units and peripheral health centers around the country. Each of these forty-eight centers is divided into departments: medical, diagnostic, pharmaceutical, nursing, nutritional, storage, and home care. The centers are not run by doctors but by ad hoc coordinators. They are often patients who are again in good health, were activists, and have become coordinators after completing training and guided studies, earning them health diplomas. The coordinators are experts in many fields, and their primary function is to facilitate access for the patients to the services. So, what exactly does a coordinator do? A woman from Tanzania provides an example:

> I'm a coordinator of the Iringa center. My main job consists of understanding the patients and also every one of the staff. In our vision, all the roles are equally important, although they all involve different responsibilities. We concentrate on the patients' problems. This is why we have to work as a team. The doctor is important but also the cleaner who makes sure the center is clean and tidy and the person in charge of the food storeroom who gives the food packages to the malnourished patients and also gives them advice on how to make their meals. Putting the patients in the center means that everything is fundamental for their treatment to be successful: from the reception to the pharmacy, from the blood test room to the health education carried out in the outside waiting room.[50]

A woman from Malawi told me:

> I am the coordinator of the main Blantyre center. We have around five thousand patients. I run the center, and I try to be a bridge between the patients and the staff. Personal knowledge is essential. This is why I also go and visit the patients in their homes: I have to understand their problems. The work in the DREAM centers is organized in a circular way, while respecting the various professions. The

coordinator is the link between all the different staff members and always puts the patients in the center. None of us are self-sufficient—we are all individual members of a whole unit.[51]

Of course, the doctors play a decisive role in DREAM. Pasquale Narciso, an infectious diseases specialist at the Spallanzani Hospital in Rome, looked after the first Italian patients there with AIDS and has provided DREAM his exceptional clinical experience. Cristina Marazzi and Leonardo Palombi are epidemiologists and public health experts and have translated their experience on the field with DREAM into scientific knowledge.

However, other skills were also necessary. The natural medical leadership had to be mixed in teamwork with different professional figures, from biologists to nutritionists, from laboratory technicians to nurses, from activists to computer experts. Without this collaboration, without the respect and value given to the staff regardless of their role, it would not have been possible to run an operation like DREAM, which was conceived as a mosaic of skills and different contributions. One could say that DREAM represents medical excellence without exclusive medical leadership. The point is that DREAM's medical excellence only works in a wider humane framework built around the patients. The doctors at the DREAM centers are highly motivated because they have advanced diagnostics, they receive a decent salary, and they see results in their patients.

The African public health doctors, on the other hand, are often frustrated by the lack of even minimal personal protective equipment and instruments, the widespread ethical negligence in the public hospitals, and by the bureaucracy, where treating is less important than writing reports. They are tempted to adapt to the general tendency to accept bribes in order to make up for their low salaries, at the expense of the patients who have to pay to be looked after. In other cases, the doctors go to work in private health care facilities because not only are the salaries better, but they also have the necessary instruments and offer professional opportunities. For many African doctors, AIDS has been bitterly and painfully frustrating for a long time. This is the case even in good health care systems, as shown in this explanation by a South African doctor who in 2003 and 2004, due to

President Mbeki's policies, could not use antiretroviral drugs, even though South Africa certainly was not a developing country:

> I saw a feeling of desperation spread among the medical staff. The question everyone was asking themselves was: What on earth am I doing here? If 80 percent of the patients have AIDS and I can't do anything, what am I doing here as a doctor? One particular incident made me change my mind. One day I was doing the rounds of the patients with my team. We got to one patient's bed. We talked about his heart problems, about his treatment; we talked to him. Then I quickly looked at the next patient, and I turned to the nurse, not to the patient himself. I knew he was at an advanced stage of AIDS. We couldn't do anything for him, so we went on to the next patient. I understand Zulu, and when the patient said to his neighbor, "I wonder why the doctors don't want to see me today. I'm probably going to die," I heard him, and I was dreadfully shocked. I suddenly realized that the patient was right: this was the message we'd given him. I knew in my heart that it was true, but at the same time I'd taken all hope away from him. I immediately understood that it wasn't right. I should have stopped to greet him. It wouldn't have even taken that long. I went back to my office, sat down, and cried. I told myself that if this was all I could do as a doctor, then I wasn't in the right place. I had to leave the system or else do something to change it. And then I started working harder and looking for a way to treat people with antiretroviral drugs.[52]

Doctor Noorjehan Abdul Majid worked in the hospital of Machava/Maputo, on the grounds of which, as previously mentioned, the first DREAM center was set up. This was a referral hospital for tuberculosis for the province of Maputo. When she started working there, she was very surprised that her colleagues said sarcastically, "Welcome to the airport." She thought they said that because it was geographically near Maputo Airport. Instead they were referring to the fact that the patients only stayed in the hospital for a very short time because they all died very soon. The tuberculosis patients often died before they were even given a bed. The turnover was extremely high. In fact, it was not really because of tuberculosis: most of the patients had AIDS, and there was no treatment for AIDS. It was awful for the doctors and the rest of the staff. They felt helpless. They could only watch this coming and going of people who were dying.

The medical staff of the DREAM centers benefit from the work carried out by the local team regarding the patients' health and social problems. However, they also benefit from a wider synergy with DREAM in Europe, with its headquarters in Rome, where fundraising is carried out, the telematics aspect is taken care of, and scientific meetings are organized. The current director of DREAM, Paola Germano, who has a PhD in infectious diseases, was the first DREAM activist and coordinator, and she divides her time between Rome and Africa.[53] The European connection with DREAM, which is Italian but also German, French, Spanish, Belgian, and so forth, is a guarantee that its almost entirely African staff appreciate: DREAM's centers in Africa operate with the scientific and technical support of its European platform. Nonetheless, after years of working side by side with Europeans and after training at schools and universities in specific courses and internships, Africans now do all of DREAM's work in Africa.[54]

There are some historical and objective reasons that led to this type of partnership. For the Europeans, it was more complicated to operate in a different ethnic context. For the Africans, it was difficult to keep up to date with scientific know-how, they had less access to funds, and they tended to be more influenced by their nonscientific culture. Since the Africans working in DREAM are local, it is easier for them to carry out the work that the Europeans from DREAM started. They can try to convince the traditional authorities to eliminate the stigma; they use the local dialect to win the patients' trust; they have confidential conversations with polygamous men; they are able to reach hidden sick people in nearly impenetrable Muslim communities; they listen to the anxieties of HIV-positive adolescents about their future; as former patients, they carry out effective counseling for new patients. Nonetheless, this would not have been possible without the Afro-optimism of the founders of DREAM and without the transmission of the medical and social knowledge between Europe and Africa.

The forty-eight DREAM centers in Africa are all run by women because basically no men who would have been any better were found for this role. AIDS in sub-Saharan Africa is a gender tragedy: 60 percent of the people infected are women (worldwide 47 percent)[55]; AIDS is the leading cause of death in Africa for women of reproductive age; more than three quarters of HIV-positive Africans between fifteen and twenty-five years of age are women.[56] The victims of HIV in Africa are mainly young, poorly educated, malnourished women, who are easily discriminated against. DREAM made a bet on these socially vulnerable women, who have suffered unspeakably to the point of not even being allowed to be treated and were sometimes convinced that this was right. Even before being a question of empowerment, it was a question of dignity:

> Let's imagine what it means for an African mother to come to a center where everything is free of charge, where she is welcomed with kindness and people are really interested in her and her family. Through other people's attitude, she can finally understand the value of her own life. She finds her dignity again, which had been crushed in the humiliation of her disease and in being abandoned. Her desire for life for herself and for her children takes over, and she realizes that she has changed her destiny.[57]

Many women in Africa think they are of little value and are amazed when someone looks for them to remind them about an appointment or to give them their medicine. They feel guilty for having gotten HIV, and they do not ask for attention from the health care workers. In DREAM, however, they are the center of everyone's attention. This gives them dignity and also gives them the idea that they are part of a new type of family, where even what is fragile is of value.

From an administrative point of view, DREAM is often understood as an NGO. However, it might be better defined as a community created around the patient, as Germano observes: "In its vision and in practice the health center is the place for meeting people and breaking away from isolation. It is a welcoming place, where the patients are listened to and can talk and ask all their questions. Basically, a place where, as well as the health center and the skills related to a health care facility, the patients' relationships and social integration are also promoted."[58] A survey carried out among DREAM's stabilized patients in 2008 included a question about their experience of the disease: "What made you suffer most?" What stood out was not the answers regarding the physical aspects of the disease (pain was only indicated as a main aspect by 21 percent of the patients interviewed) but the ones about the relationships and inner aspects: the contempt of acquaintances and neighbors (24 percent), being abandoned by their family (24 percent), the loss of hope for the future (21 percent). When asked what recovery meant for them, almost half of the people interviewed (47.4 percent) said that it was having found their family again, and only a few of them (8 percent) mentioned the end of their physical symptoms.[59] Community life does not only motivate people to get treatment but it also deals with a very important problem for the patients: contempt, loneliness, and resignation.

The patients are offered counseling in the DREAM centers, not only when they take the test but also during their whole treatment. They are provided with health education and information on nutrition, and altogether a lot of time is spent talking to them. Alongside their pharmacological treatment, the questions of culture, their income, access to food and water, and very importantly the question of their relationships all also contribute to their health. The end of the stigma, of being isolated and an outcast, is not only an ethical but also a health priority. Of course, medicine based on scientific research and clinical tests is essential. Nonetheless, in DREAM "its excessive autonomy is challenged by a very old principle that is still true, that of one man who takes care of another man, because in the gestures of the treatment, in the words, in the medical examinations, and in the medical attention given, there hides an equally powerful and essential healing principle."[60] When AIDS patients are not given back their humanity and social life, they do not adhere so well to the therapy, or they abandon it completely. So, it is also thanks to DREAM's approach that the retention of their patients is high. According to a study carried out in 2009, the annual average of patients lost at follow-up was 2 percent, and fewer than 5 percent developed resistances and switched to second-line antiretroviral drugs.[61] The treatment offered free of charge, the community that the patients can become part of, and the nutritional supplementation are a result of DREAM's acknowledgment of the dignity of each person.

## A VALUABLE ADDITION: THE ACTIVISTS

DREAM works as a health care community, and the visibility of this community is provided by the activists, who are halfway between volunteers and professionals. Every DREAM health care center has a team of activists, stabilized patients who help the patients who are not yet stable and who do whatever is necessary, from tidying up their rooms to distributing food packages. But mainly they act as facilitators between the center and the patients. The activists help the patients adhere to their treatment by showing them that it is possible to live well despite having AIDS and by encouraging them to follow the instructions given for their therapy. The activists become friends with the people in the waiting areas, call patients on the telephone if they miss their appointments, go to the homes of the people who are very sick to check the effect of the therapies, make sure the patients have enough food, and carry out health education. They travel around a lot by any means of transportation in order to contact patients who live in remote areas: bicycles, jeeps, donkeys, pirogues, and so on. They often stay in the rural maternity centers to talk to the pregnant women, many of whom have HIV but are unaware of it, and they explain to them that they can save themselves and the babies they are carrying.

In DREAM 95 percent of the activists are women. Often the activists' families have been devastated by AIDS, so as survivors they find themselves having to support not only their own children but also those of their dead brothers and sisters. Their strength in leading such a demanding private and public life, despite being marked by a disease like AIDS, is astonishing.

DREAM has five thousand activists in ten African countries, and they are irreplaceable in winning the trust of the patients because they themselves are patients who testify that AIDS is not a death sentence. In fact, they show the effectiveness of the antiretroviral therapies on their own bodies. The beginning, when the test is carried out and the patient receives the result, is dramatic. When there were no antiretroviral drugs in Africa, HIV-infected people often committed suicide. Knowing the right thing to say, the activists calm the patients down.

One of the greatest problems in treating AIDS is resistances. When the drugs are not taken properly, the virus starts replicating again and mutates in such a way that it no longer responds to the therapy. The antiretroviral cocktail of drugs then has to be changed so it will be effective against the new HIV strain. In Europe there are many further lines of treatment, and new ones are tested all the time, whereas in Africa, because of the logistic problems and high costs, the patients are only given second or third lines, except for in exceptional cases. This is why adherence to the therapy is, if possible, even more important than in the West. The activists encourage the patients to take their therapy properly. This is what activist Pacem Kawonga from Malawi says:

> Consistency and punctuality are essential. How can this be explained to people who live in remote villages and don't have a radio, a telephone, or a watch? We have worked out some ways to help them. For example, on the medicine packets we draw a rising sun, the sun high in the sky, dusk, and the moon. Next to the drawing we indicate the number of pills they have to take at that stage of the day. But we always have to watch out. Sometimes the patients are sick, and we think they haven't taken their medicine, despite the sun and the moon, and that's exactly what happened. We ask them why. "It was always cloudy." Over time many people regain their strength, they go back to work, and with their first earnings they buy a watch or a cell phone. Sometimes when I meet people in rags, who live in huts, with no water, electricity, or toilets, I ask them how they are, and I'm surprised by their answer: "Fine! At the beginning I had 58 CD4s, and my viral load was over 100,000. Last month I had my tests and I had 450 CD4s, and my viral load was undetectable!" This means we've been able to pass on what we've learned.[62]

The activist is not an unknown figure in public medicine. Sometimes activists engage in DOT (directly observed therapy), the ingenious practice of having unskilled staff, either paid or volunteer, accompany patients to make sure they take their treatment properly and solve their everyday problems. Invented in Somalia by Annalena Tonelli in the 1970s,[63] DOT has spread over the past decades for treatment of tuberculosis but also for other pathologies in countries with limited resources. The DREAM activists accompany the patients, but they do more than that. Sometimes in countries where DREAM started up, they were seen by the public health system as annoying, as though they represented a form of uncontrollable "parallel health care." While it was thought that the DOT-type activists could be considered integrated into the state systems, the DREAM-type activists were seen as unusual. In fact, the stories, motivations, and aims of the DREAM activists are very special. When they talk, the idea of a kind of resurrected humanity is what comes across. This is how an activist from Kenya describes her experience: "I experienced a moment of feeling like I was in the desert. I was spiritually weak, physically weak, and not strong enough to work. I cried in my bed, and I asked God, 'When am I going to die?' This is to say that resurrection was possible in my life. And now I go out, I testify to this miracle with my life everywhere."[64] An activist from Tanzania had a similar experience: "I tested HIV-positive. I went to a witch doctor. He told me I didn't have AIDS. But then I got sick—I was in the Arusha Hospital for three months. I weighed twenty-nine kilograms. I heard my parents say I wouldn't last until the end of the week. DREAM treated me. I was born again. People on the street were asking how come I was alive."[65]

These people experienced being born again, going from desperation to a new life. They suffered for years, they spent all their money on healers, they saw their relatives and acquaintances die, they suffered from stigma, they were outcasts, they had severe opportunistic infections. In their life they experienced poverty, prostration, hunger, and discrimination—until they received pharmacological therapy and found themselves in a health care community, finally convinced that they had an important job to do for other patients.[66] This is the story of another activist:

> In 2003 I was pregnant, and I felt ill. At the health center the nurse told me I was HIV-positive. As soon as I got home, I started crying.

> I cried for over a month. . . . Then I started the treatment at the DREAM center. I never missed taking my medicine. The day I was going to give birth arrived. From that moment, I didn't cry anymore—I started hoping again. My daughter grew up healthy. When she was eighteen months old, she did the test: it was negative. That was an immense joy for me. I, an HIV-positive mother, had had a negative daughter. I started encouraging the other patients even more: if I was alive and had managed to save my daughter, the other mothers could also save themselves and save their children's lives. It was worth taking the therapy properly. My words were effective because I'd been through such a big struggle.[67]

Bent Steenberg Olsen defined the DREAM activists as members of a "stigma cult" that brought them together and mobilized them.[68] Undoubtedly the stigma they suffered from is what they have in common. But Steenberg Olsen was mistaken when, in the link created by the effect of the disease, he saw a group of people with a subculture that separated them from healthy people. Instead of a cult, stigma constitutes an element of identity and a step toward being outgoing. The DREAM activists do not make a club out of the stigma; they want to get rid of it in the families and villages and eliminate it from public opinion. These are liberated women who have acquired a civil consciousness. This is how a scholar from South Africa explains it:

> It is precisely the extremity of the "near death" experiences of full-blown AIDS, and the profound stigma and "social death" associated with the later stages of the disease, that produce the conditions for HIV/AIDS survivors' commitment to "new life" and social activism. . . . It is also the profound negativity of stigma and social death that animates the activist's construction of a new positive HIV-positive identity and understanding of what it means to be a citizen-activist and member of a social movement.[69]

These concepts are expressed in Cacilda Massango's story:

> I found out about the DREAM program, and my life was saved, and then I had to show other people how a weak life can turn into a

life of hope. Today I feel that I am a strong woman. I am afraid of discrimination, but I feel a responsibility to speak. In Mozambique's history books it says that many people fought great fights in the national liberation movement. We activists also want to show what we can do and be actors in the history of this country—actors in saving many human lives. Our story will have to be remembered in the books that children study at school, the story of strong, persevering men and women who loved life, who saved themselves, their children, their wives or husbands. I did not have an education. I didn't have any academic certificates. I started studying again, and I graduated from university. I met Mrs. Laura Bush, the first lady of the United States of America. I talked to her about AIDS, about lives saved from AIDS.[70]

A few years after DREAM's first experiments, the use of activists in the fight against AIDS was widespread among the international organizations, the large NGOs, and the African public health systems themselves. The activists were credited with representing the connection between the technical and health staff and the patients. They were also acknowledged as important because they could reach the most inaccessible people in the rural areas, the villages, the forests, and the savannah but also in the outskirts of the towns. The intuition of Ana Maria Muhai, who invented the figure of the DREAM activist in Maputo, soon became the common heritage of the public health system in Africa, although not always with her powerful existential and redemptive motivations.

### FATOUMATA SYLLA

People who meet Fatoumata Sylla remember her for her wide smile, a natural expression of her victory over adversity. In 2010, when Sylla was thirty-one years old, she became the first HIV-positive person in Guinea to fight AIDS publicly, without hiding her face. The country was turning over a new political page with the democratic election to president of Alpha Condé. The state television, the only television that existed, was launching an AIDS campaign on the initiative of the Hadja Djéné Condé Foundation, named for the new first lady of the republic. Sylla agreed to tell the story of how, as an HIV-positive patient, she regained her health. In particular she explained how she was able to have two healthy children thanks to the antiretroviral drugs. She looked good on television, she was persuasive, and she encouraged women to take the test and then have the treatment. Everyone saw her, including her own family. Many people wanted to meet her, some to thank her but some to repudiate her. Some people even wondered whether she really did have HIV/AIDS. Many of her relatives avoided her. Her older sister, with whom she had stayed for a long time in Conakry, the capital, broke off relations with her. Her father, on the other hand, was not afraid of the stigma that might affect the family and said he was proud of her. But he was an exception. In Guinean society if a woman was HIV-positive, she was abandoned both by her family and by her husband's family. And if she was not kicked out of her home, she was isolated and told not to touch anyone or anything. There was no knowledge of how people got infected. The prevention campaigns had spread more terror than awareness.

Three years previously, Sylla was in Conakry finishing her studies on *aménagement du territoire*, a combination of urban science, geography, and sociology. She came from Kindia, the third largest city, where her father was a government official. She had not been well for some time. She had a temperature, a headache, and diarrhea and was losing weight. In such cases in Guinea, everyone went to the healer, the witch doctor, for a traditional cure of potions, incisions, bloodletting, and so on. But Sylla did not go because she was better educated than most people and belonged to a higher social class. She went to a hospital, where she was diagnosed with malaria and the following time with typhus. A doctor suggested taking the HIV test:

> She waited for at least five seconds and then said, "Fatoumata, I'm so sorry, the test is positive." I couldn't help it—I burst into tears and cried and cried, but she stayed with me the whole time, she tried to calm me down, she held my hands while I cried my heart out. In the end I was tired and calm, but I thought that was the end because when people talked about HIV, they said, "When you have HIV you die." But when she saw that I'd calmed down, she said, "I know

someone. I can send you to them. They're white people. They will take care of you."[71]

She was directed to a DREAM center. But she thought it was all over: university, her boyfriend, her family, her dream of becoming a mother. All she had was the recommendation to go to DREAM. She was wary. They were Christians; she was Muslim: "Will they accept me?" She wondered what alternatives she might have. There were the two typical, large colonial-era hospitals in the center of Conakry, the Donka and the Ignace Deen, which were the referral hospitals for the whole country, but they were disorganized, the doctors were not paid, the buildings were dilapidated, corruption was common, and everything had to be paid in advance, even emergency deliveries. So, the public health system was out of the question. There was no alternative but to go to DREAM. But Sylla still hesitated. In Guinea religion is very important. People identify themselves and each other according to their religion. And Sylla had doubts about DREAM because it was Christian. She also did not believe it offered treatment free of charge, as she had heard people say. How could anything be free of charge in a country where you had to pay for everything? Not to mention Christians offering something free of charge to Muslims.

This was 2007, and in Guinea the antiretroviral drugs were only free of charge in theory. They started to become available in the country, paid for by the Global Fund, but most people had no way of getting hold of them. There were only a few doctors who could prescribe them, and most worked in the two hospitals. They knew that the antiretroviral drugs delayed certain death and were worth the price of a whole life. So, a market was created around them, starting from the prescription. People sold everything they had, even their clothes, to buy the drugs, and they cost as much as a month's salary for a month's treatment. The patients carried on for as long as they could, and when they had no more money, they stopped their treatment and went back to their village to die. It was even more difficult for women to get hold of the drugs because they depended financially on their men. And yet as far as the spread of AIDS was concerned, women were the victims of men. For years, the representatives of the United Nations agency for the fight against AIDs, UNAIDS, ended every meeting, every presentation, every appeal with the triple recommendation "*abstinence, fidélité, préservatifs* [condoms]." But families in a predominantly Muslim country are often polygamous. And wives often found they had all been infected by their husbands, who sometimes got treated in secret, without telling them anything. There were also widows who had to look after all the children—their own and those of their husband's other wives, who had also died. The women were so powerless that they were not even given the test result if no male member of the family was with them. Without their father, husband, or brother present, it was considered inappropriate to tell a woman, "You're positive."

The story of Guinea is marked by the refusal of its first leader, Ahmed Sékou Touré, to be part of the community of West African countries that maintained a close collaboration with their former colonial power, France. The "no" Touré said to Charles de Gaulle cost Guineans a lot in terms of economic isolation, backwardness, and misery.[72] Guinea had been a model colony and Conakry, overlooking the ocean, particularly loved by the French, who called it "Conakry the coquette." As a result of the break with Paris, it gradually turned into a decadent city, with colonial-era houses and buildings deteriorating under the tropical rains.[73] Shortages have the effect of producing a ruthlessly materialistic culture. By the 2000s much had gone to ruin, the government was absent, and corruption rampaged throughout society. When anyone was given a role or a position, their family put pressure on them to make the most of it. Although there were several Internet cafés in Conakry, it lacked many essential services. The only place with a stable power supply was the square in front of the airport, where one could see groups of students studying under the streetlights. Even disease and death were opportunities for making a profit. Nobody treated AIDS patients selflessly except for DREAM and Médecins Sans Frontières.

After telling her boyfriend, who was terrified, that she was HIV-positive, Sylla went with him to the DREAM center, where as expected, he also tested positive. The international guidelines, implemented by Guinea, required that a person had to have below a certain number of CD4s in order to start the antiretroviral treatment, but Sylla's levels were higher than that. In any case, she was constantly monitored at

DREAM. In the meantime, she got married, and in 2008 she got pregnant. She developed severe anemia, her blood count was 5, and her CD4s fell drastically. Every pregnancy is stressful one way or another, but for an HIV-positive woman it is much more so. Sylla started the antiretroviral treatment, but it was not immediately effective. In fact, she had opportunistic tuberculosis before she started getting better. She survived a very critical phase during which she risked dying and then gave birth to a tiny baby girl, who was negative. But Sylla was unable to breast-feed her, and she did not have anywhere stable to stay. Her relatives, who knew that she was HIV-positive, refused to let her stay with them, but her child survived and grew up on formula milk. Sylla gradually recovered.

Once she had successfully ended her dangerous pregnancy, Sylla fully trusted DREAM because of how it had treated her, and she became an activist. She was ambitious and started studying again at the university. After she had discovered she was HIV-positive, she thought she had no future. Now she felt as though she was living for the future. She was calm and optimistic, but she had a lot of questions. Although her relatives could not believe it, she named her daughter Cristina, out of gratitude for the Christians who saved her. She had a second child and named him Mohammad, as if to affirm the unity between the two Abrahamic religions within the same family. She is a convinced Muslim, but she wondered about the fact that the treatment was free of charge and whether this was a distinctive sign of Christianity. The point is that in a country like Guinea people are amazed when anything is offered free of charge. Sylla's physical and psychological rebirth as a result of the antiretroviral treatment was so astounding that people found it unbelievable that it was free. The fact that saving a life was not assessed in terms of money contradicted people's common sense. Sylla interpreted the fact that there was no charge as an invitation for her to do the same. She did this by talking in particular to the women, who in Guinea are mainly illiterate and poor. This is what she said in an interview:

> Women are the pillars of their family: when the women are sick, the whole family is sick. I advise all the women to take the test. And to come to DREAM, where everything is free of charge. I am sending

out this message: being afraid to do the test means infecting your child, if you're positive there is a treatment, and the treatment is free of charge. Some women don't immediately believe that I'm HIV-positive, and I'm proud to be able to tell them, "I'm like you, and if you get taken care of yourself, you will soon be well, like me." And who can say that I have HIV? Nobody. I don't even consider it a disease anymore, but I take my therapy every day. Every night at nine o'clock the alarm on the phone goes off because it's time to take the therapy. My daughter noticed, saying, "You and Dad take so many pills." I'll wait a bit, but then I'll explain everything to her. I certainly don't want to hide. If you're afraid, you can't save other people.[74]

Sylla was particularly motivated. She spoke easily with patients in their local language, and after a while she became the coordinator of the DREAM center in Conakry. She looks fragile, but she does not bow to anyone, and she does not promote personal interests. She likes ending her public speeches saying, "For our beloved country, Guinea." She sees her commitment to fight AIDS as patriotic work to bring together Guineans, who are divided according to their ethnic backgrounds and their religions. She refuses Wahhabi Islamic fundamentalism, which in Guinea too, because of its funding from Saudi Arabia, insists that women be dressed in black from their head to their feet. Her Islam is that of the mass brotherhoods of West Africa but also that of a person who has met and talked to Christians. She is not ashamed of the backwardness of her country and asks every Guinean to rectify the situation.

## MALNUTRITION

After completing training, every African professional in DREAM spreads the knowledge they have learned by carrying out health education.[75] During the training courses, much time is given to studying the science of nutrition. In the current acronym DREAM, the *M* stands for (against) "malnutrition." In Africa there is a strong correlation between malnutrition and infectious diseases. Malnutrition and HIV strengthen each other in damaging the immune system.

Eating enough and well, with a disease like AIDS, is crucial. A good diet, which strengthens the immune system, hinders HIV, delays full-blown AIDS, makes it possible to fight the opportunistic infections better, makes it easier to take the antiretroviral drugs, and increases their efficacy.[76] This was all well known, but in Africa the treatment programs for AIDS generally neglected nutritional support. Ensuring food was never a priority in the fight against AIDS. As Elizabeth Mataka, the United Nations special envoy to Africa noted in 2007, "people who live with AIDS often talk about food as their greatest and most important need[, but] the interventions regarding nutrition in HIV programmes are often overlooked in the international debates on HIV, and remain seriously underfunded."[77]

Because of the minimalistic therapeutic approach to AIDS in Africa, the nutritional aspect was not appreciated as it should have been. Yet the epidemiologists knew well that before antibiotics and before vaccines, the Western populations had a spectacular reduction in infectious diseases thanks to the control of famine and increased food security. And it is no coincidence that in today's global spread of infectious diseases such as AIDS and tuberculosis, the continent that is affected most is Africa, which is the one that suffers most from food insecurity.

HIV interferes with nutrition both by increasing the body's metabolic demands and by hindering the intake of nutrients. In other words, it reduces the person's appetite and hinders the absorption of food precisely when the body needs it most in order to defend itself. This leads to dramatic weight loss, which again is why it is called the slim disease. Pat Pridmore and Roy Carr-Hill explain it as follows:

> HIV impairs the human immune system leading to increased risk of infection and reduced appetite. . . . HIV also decreases absorption and use of nutrients from the food eaten and increases the body's normal energy requirements by 10–30 percent in adults and 50–100 percent in children. At the underlying and basic levels of causation, HIV and AIDS cause food and nutritional insecurity because people are frequently sick, or are caring for the sick, and unable to work which threatens their livelihoods. Food and nutritional insecurity can in turn increase risk and vulnerability to HIV infection, hasten

the onset of AIDS, prevent effective treatment and undermine efforts to provide care and support.[78]

The fight against malnutrition was decisive in reducing the mortality of DREAM patients.[79] This was carried out through nutritional supplementation based on local foods rather than on imported nutritional supplements, which could not possibly satisfy the needs of the masses of people in Africa in the context of an epidemic on such a vast scale as HIV.[80] The DREAM centers decided whether to give food to the patients or to their family too (how could the patients not share the food they received with the members of their hungry family?[81]) with specific nutritional counseling. The criteria included anthropometric measurements as well as health and social evaluations.[82] What counted was their income and where they lived, but also whether they had tuberculosis, were anemic, pregnant, underage, in prison, and so on. The final decision was up to the doctor. DREAM is very generous in providing food supplementation. The point is that antiretroviral drugs have to be taken on a full stomach; when the patients suffer from hunger, the therapy risks not being effective.

Receiving food is a powerful stimulus for good adherence. It is a powerful antidote to abandoning the treatment, especially in sub-Saharan Africa, where the question of food is a serious problem with masses of undernourished people who would be happy to eat just once a day. There was the paradox of people bursting into tears when they found out their HIV test was negative: if it had been positive, they could have been included in a food aid program provided by the NGO that tested them.[83] It was almost as though having the infection implied being privileged with respect to the rest of the hungry population. When people are suffering from AIDS in its aggressive form, they have no appetite, to the point that they die without even feeling hungry, but when they start fighting it with antiretroviral drugs, the opposite happens, and they get very hungry. This is called the immune reconstitution syndrome.

This is what an experienced DREAM doctor said:

When we give food to a malnourished child, we must consider that the mother has another malnourished child. We try to integrate [the other child] in the food programme, because we embrace a holistic approach [to AIDS care], which means to try and see the patient in his wholeness. He comes here with a real disease, but he has a series of other problems to confront: social problems, family problems. The primary problem is with food, because he is incapacitated and can't manage to work, and clearly this is a person whose family income is decreasing. So we try to minimise this [the food problem] until the person is able to go back to being an active breadwinner.[84]

So, everyday life in the DREAM centers also involves unloading sacks of beans, rice, corn or soy flour, and containers of oil. The food is then kept in a storeroom or distributed, the patients given help taking their twenty or thirty kilograms of food home in wheelbarrows or by other means. It is not surprising that many activists specialize in the science of nutrition.

## THE DREAM MODEL

Over the years, the results regarding DREAM's work have increased enormously. Around five hundred thousand patients have been treated, one hundred and thirty thousand babies have been born healthy to HIV-positive mothers (with a success rate of over 98 percent), and fifteen thousand health staff have been given training. As well as achieving these results, DREAM has also tried to give Africa a replicable model of good practices to adopt when treating AIDS. DREAM has dealt with many health matters regarding AIDS through conducting field tests, collecting data, publishing studies, and taking part in WHO panels of experts consulted to update the guidelines for countries with limited resources. What scientific progress has been made?

DREAM operations started from a standpoint that was against the antitherapy approach, which dominated internationally until 2002, despite the UN's well-intentioned Millennium Development Goals and sensational events such as the Durban conference. This standpoint was supported by the conviction, later a certainty, that the treatment itself was also prevention, in that administering the antiretroviral drugs not only assured survival and improved the quality of life of the patients but also drastically reduced their viral load. This fact, it must be remembered, was only accepted gradually at an international level. Only in 2002 did the WHO make the end of the prevention-or-treatment dichotomy official with the publication of *Antiretroviral Treatment as Prevention (TasP) of HIV and TB*.[85] That was how powerful the inertia of the ideological emphasis on prevention alone was and its effect on public opinion. For years, looking at the poor countries, condoms had been idealised and the antiretroviral drugs had been ignored, instead of them being used side by side.

The treatment for AIDS was also legitimized for countries with limited resources in 2002 and 2003, and then there was the question of its quality and availability. Faced with the therapeutic minimalism that had dominated for years, DREAM had to try to show that the advantages of a high level in the treatment and standards of excellence in health also applied to sub-Saharan Africa. DREAM worked toward universal access to the antiretroviral therapies for HIV-positive people, but there were many technical barriers in the international guidelines for countries with limited resources, which strongly restricted the number of people who had the right to the treatment (more than for the rich countries).[86]

Today the idea is to test and treat. HIV-positive people are treated regardless of the condition of their immune system or how high their viral load is. In the past, the international guidelines only prescribed the triple antiretroviral therapy when the patients were very weak, which had a negative effect on their capacity to recover and on their survival. DREAM worked on the eligibility threshold for the HAART regimen. With their experience of large numbers of patients treated and the transformation of this experience into specific scientific knowledge, they insisted on the evolution of the international guidelines toward less restrictive thresholds, in the end eliminating the eligibility thresholds altogether in order to achieve universal access to treatment.[87]

To provide good treatment, the diagnosis also has to be good. This elementary principle inspired DREAM to criticize this other minimalist approach. In order to evaluate the HIV-positive patients' immune system, the international guidelines had initially only took into consideration their CD4 lymphocyte cell count, which is inexpensive but only a partial indicator. DREAM's request was for this evaluation to be carried out together with the measurement of the viral load in the blood, a more accurate indicator of the patient's pathological condition and a timely detector of resistance to therapies. A comparison of what DREAM practiced and what was prescribed by the international guidelines also shows that for diagnostics, DREAM was ahead in adopting operative standards that were later universally accepted.

While DREAM countered the therapies and diagnosis that were inspired by just how much they cost and how easy they were to perform, it pointed out the importance of maintaining high-quality levels of care. Simplifying treatments and tests in order to save money and streamline the work and giving a little but to everyone did not look advantageous from a medical point of view, or from an economic point of view either, because the therapeutic results were not so good and were uncertain. This became extremely clear in prevention of mother-to-child transmission of HIV. DREAM considered it scandalous to prescribe only Nevirapine to pregnant women and their babies to prevent the transmission of HIV as a shortcut in poor countries because the outcome was far worse than if they had been administered a triple antiretroviral therapy. This was happening while in rich countries the pregnant women were mainly treated, with excellent results, in the HAART regimen. So, DREAM started a long scientific battle, which reverberated far beyond the specific question of the mother-to-child transmission of HIV. Moreover, it furthered the aim to question the international health policies, which, as already mentioned, despite announcing universal access to treatment, actually limited it in the guidelines with the eligibility thresholds for the therapy (a particularly low number of CD4s, a clinical condition that had deteriorated beyond a certain level, etc.).[88]

In other words, with the results DREAM achieved, overcoming the minimalistic approach to therapy for pregnant women became a cornerstone of the work involved in becoming scientifically convincing in order to obtain real universal access to treatment. The discriminating eligibility thresholds to the HAART regimen were not so strict and were easier to modify in the case of pregnant women. This was because they were a privileged category in the concept of prevention for whom medical treatment for HIV-positive people was given. The treatment with the cocktail of triple antiretroviral drugs was considered a form of prevention against new infections because it prevented babies from being born infected, so pregnant women, who according to the international guidelines would not have satisfied the requirements to be treated, could also access the treatment. This is how cohorts of women in therapy were formed in DREAM, despite the minimalistic criteria in force regarding eligibility for the treatment. The results achieved with these patients demonstrated how appropriate it was to extend the triple therapy to all HIV-positive people, regardless of their stage of the disease.

In the 2000s hundreds of thousands of HIV infected babies were born in Africa every year, condemned to die early. Only 40 percent survived up to the age of five. Preventing the transmission of the virus from the mother to her child was possible in the developed world, with success rates of up to 98 percent, thanks to the triple antiretroviral therapy that was started during the pregnancy. On the other hand, in sub-Saharan countries the single dose of Nevirapine was heavily sponsored because it was considered very cheap and simple to administer. It was given to the mother at the moment of delivery and caused a transitory reaction of the immune system but did not solve the problem of transmission of the virus if this had already happened during the pregnancy, and neither did it prevent transmission afterward during breast-feeding.[89] Moreover, administering Nevirapine like that also complicated any antiretroviral therapies that HIV-positive mothers might have been put on later, because of the onset of pharmacological resistances. It seemed logical to DREAM, as well as right, to offer their pregnant African patients the HAART regimen, as was done in the West. This would provide results similar to those in the Global North, with almost 100 percent success rates.

When the triple antiretroviral therapy is started during pregnancy, it brings the transmission of the virus down to practically zero during the pregnancy, during delivery anytime and anywhere this takes place, and in the mother's milk. This is how over 98 percent of the babies born from HIV-positive mothers in the DREAM program stay healthy. Moreover, the triple antiretroviral therapy that is started during pregnancy and continued during breast-feeding offers further advantages in African countries. Mortality rates of babies born from HIV-positive mothers are lower than the average in their countries. There is a decrease in premature births, miscarriages, and stillbirths and a reduction of maternal mortality, even to levels lower than the national average. This is despite the greater vulnerability of HIV-positive women, who are weaker, anemic, and more exposed to opportunistic infections than healthy pregnant women.[90]

Even before starting their activity, the DREAM doctors assumed that the triple antiretroviral therapy would drastically reduce the transmission of HIV in breast milk to almost zero.[91] The empirical data confirmed this hypothesis, which had not seriously been explored scientifically up until then because it was not urgent in the developed world, where breast milk could easily be replaced with formula milk. In Africa, however, this was practically impossible because of the question of hygiene and lack of safe drinking water. DREAM decided not to interrupt the triple therapy for the mothers after the birth of their babies in order to let them breast-feed safely and not have to use formula milk.[92]

The way prevention of mother-to-child transmission of HIV was carried out by DREAM was different from the minimalistic decision to give Nevirapine at delivery for another reason too: it did not only aim to deliver healthy babies but also to save the life of their mothers. In Africa the first condition for the survival of a child is the presence of the mother. When children are orphans, even if they survive HIV, they still come up against terrible risks. It was essential not to increase the dramatic phenomenon of the orphans caused by AIDS in sub-Saharan Africa, who numbered 11.5 million in 2006 according to UNICEF.[93]

DREAM's scientific progress came about as the result of a sort of health diplomacy that made it possible to bypass the international guidelines and protocols through agreements with the single African governments. Pacts and memorandums were signed, classifying DREAM's activities as experimental projects, so they could legally go beyond the WHO guidelines. The African leaders involved in this form of health diplomacy did actually have a double interest: they procured excellent health programs and hoped they would have good antiretroviral therapies for themselves, their families, and their friends. Which president or minister or official did not have an HIV-infected family member or perhaps was ill himself?

DREAM differed from, or rather anticipated, WHO protocols on many points: eligibility thresholds for treatment, diagnostics with measurement of the viral load, treatment free of charge, nutritional supplementation, prevention of mother-to-child transmission carried out with the triple therapy, the HAART regimen assured to all pregnant women without distinction, breast-feeding, and real universal access to therapy. This required detailed agreements with each government, explaining all the figures and operations. When the trial periods were over, extensions were negotiated, perhaps in order to publish the results, until the WHO revised the guidelines and DREAM's work became the norm. After all, the world of the fight against AIDS was always moving forward. Those who one year were skeptical about a solution that had never been put into practice could not be skeptical about it the following year. And the WHO was not a dogmatic institution but a forum open to various contributions.

Finally, the political and cultural movement around the DREAM model should be mentioned as an essential part of it. A civil society that did not exist before was created and came together as a result of DREAM. Women who had been denied even their basic human rights experienced unexpected empowerment. Men who grew up struggling for material well-being found the value of solidarity. Scientific education that formed the basis for civil consciousness was spread in a world with a subculture of superstition.

There is one last story that has to be told in the context of this political and cultural movement. In 2009, officially for reasons of principle regarding the reorganization of the national health system, the Mozambican minister of health, Ivo Paulo Garrido, decided to close all the day hospitals, even though they were well organized, including those run by DREAM. He had their crowds of HIV-positive patients transferred to the public health system, which was not ready to receive them. It did not have enough personnel, stocks of drugs, diagnostic laboratories, or nutritional supplements, there were no activists to connect the health staff with the patients, and the treatment was not free of charge. This was so-called decentralization. By law the AIDS patients would be treated in public facilities around the country in order to avoid, so it was said, any treatment parallel to the impartial and egalitarian government health system. The inevitable result was enormous stress for public health staffs and reduction of quality of treatment. A third of the patients soon abandoned their therapies, and there was general social unrest. Despite the semantic appeal for decentralization—conceptually equated with widespread health care that would, in theory, democratically reach people living in the most remote areas—the reform provided poor-quality treatment that was supposed to be immediately available for all the patients (which did not happen) instead of quality treatment to be gradually extended to all the patients. The result was disintegration of the system instead of integration into it, exclusion from treatment instead of inclusion, increase of the stigma instead of a decrease, and excessively complicated bureaucratic procedures instead of operational efficiency.[94]

In the second half of 2009, DREAM's women activists, supported by their men whenever possible, together with various associations and NGOs, organized protests in towns throughout Mozambique, with the participation of thousands. The power of women: in 2010 the minister of health was removed from his position and the day hospitals started working again.

Since its independence in 1975, Mozambique had been continuously governed by FRELIMO, the only party from the beginning. It believed that it fully represented the people and all their aspirations. In FRELIMO culture, whoever took to the streets was basically considered a rebel, and it was up to the police to deal with protests. However, gatherings like that, of thousands of patients and their families in the name of dignified treatment, crowds of women and fragile people, could not be repressed with violence. National public opinion was shaken by this expression of citizenship, which was unheard of in Mozambique. Although this episode was limited, it showed how many HIV/AIDS patients, if well treated and reintegrated into society, become aware of and are able to make use of their democratic rights. This was expressed by the activist Jane Mphande:

> In many African countries [DREAM] also comes to mean an expression of civil society. I am not just thinking about the courses on AIDS

that many of us activists carry out in schools, factories, prisons, and in other contexts. I think in fact that there is now a deep sensitivity with respect to all the situations of need. . . . We have noticed the children on the streets, destitute old people, the humiliation of so many women who experience sex as a way to survive, and the need to find answers for them too. All this undoubtedly represents a precious contribution to democracy: a variety of voices, grassroots initiatives that fuel the fundamental dialogue and negotiation between the state and society, which is too often forgotten when one talks about democracy. It is not and can never be just a series of electoral rules and state apparatuses. There is no democracy without a lively and organized civil society.[95]

## NOTES

1. For an explanation of this question, see Scrimshaw et al., *Interactions of Nutrition and Infection*; Keusch, "History of Nutrition"; and Katona and Katona-Apte, "Interaction between Nutrition and Infection."

2. See in Knight, *UNAIDS*, 91: "Even those leaders who recognized the dangers of the epidemic did not always act. Mandela told South African activist Zackie Achmat and others at a meeting in March 1999 that he stopped talking about condoms and AIDS 'because he was warned [about] white conservative principles and [that] African traditional leaders do not talk about sex, if you want to win the next election.' . . . I think for someone who had been in prison a long time who is really a traditional old man and a royal without being a royalist . . . having to deal with these things was not easy." See also "Mandela, militant de la lutte contre le sida," *Jeune Afrique*, December 5, 2013. When Mandela was no longer president, he acted differently against AIDS and contributed to overcome South Africa's denial and to spread the antiretroviral therapies in the country. He also lost members of his family because of AIDS, as did several other African presidents or former presidents.

3. Zuma was tried in 2006 for sexual assault on an ANC activist. The woman was HIV-positive, and Zuma knew this but had not taken precautions. He said that he had a shower afterward and that this had prevented any problem with HIV.

4. Clarisse Juompan-Yakam, "Sida et Afrique : épidémie de bêtise," *Jeune Afrique*, May 30, 2013.

5. Explained in Steenberg Olsen, "Structures of Stigma," 22: "The problem with innovative and frequently changing paradigms is that a short memory

combined with a rapid pace of constant change serves to silence or limit critical reflection and comprehension about the paradigms that are sold (or imposed)."

6. Knight, *UNAIDS*, 55.

7. See Hume, *Ending Mozambique's War*; Hume, "Mozambique Peace Process," 81–101; and Morozzo della Rocca, *Mozambique*.

8. The Human Development Index rankings drawn up every year by the UNDP.

9. Carmen Bader, "Le Mozambique dans la tourmente de l'après-guerre," *Le Monde diplomatique*, February 1993, 20–21.

10. The measurement of the viral load is a laboratory test that detects the genetic material of the virus and provides a measure of the viral replication. A high viral load indicates that the virus is replicating fast and is correlated with high mortality. The antiretroviral therapies are able to reduce the viral load to zero, which has a very positive effect on patients' survival. The test is essential for monitoring the treatment.

11. Swedish International Development Cooperation Agency, *Country Analysis Mozambique*.

12. Leonardo Palombi, interview by the author, Rome, January 18, 2018.

13. Palombi, interview, January 18, 2018.

14. Sandro Mancinelli, interview by the author, Rome, December 30, 2018.

15. Leonardo Palombi, "Sull'AIDS in Africa e in Mozambico," presentation, DREAM meeting, Rome, February 11, 2001, text in DAR.

16. In 2019, while visiting a DREAM center in Mozambique, Pope Francis compared DREAM to the Good Samaritan who stopped, unlike others, to help a half-dead man on the side of the road (the AIDS patient), without giving in to the temptation of saying "there's nothing to be done" or "fighting this scourge is impossible," and who started to "act courageously to look for solutions." Maputo, September 9, 2019, https://www.vaticannews.va/it/papa/news/2019-09/papa-francesco-mozambico-visita-ospedale-zimpeto-viaggio-aids.html.

17. Joaquim Chissano, speech of July 10, 2008, in Maputo, during a reception at Hotel Polana.

18. The meeting took place on May 2, 2000.

19. Morozzo della Rocca, *Mozambique*.

20. Letter of June 4, 2001, from Dr. Avertino Barreto, Director Nacional Adjunto (Ministério da Saúde) and Director do Programa Nacional de controle das DTS/SIDA to Dr. Giovanni Guidotti, in DAR.

21. Leonardo Palombi, interview by the author, Rome, January 18, 2018. From a note in DAR regarding a meeting in August 2001 between Gianni Guidotti and Palombi and the prime minister of Mozambique, who was also a doctor: "The prime minister has expressed various concerns [about the DREAM programme]. He is afraid that starting the program might create expectations in people for the treatment, which the ministry and the government cannot satisfy. Moreover, he is

afraid that there are not enough resources in terms of personnel, facilities, and drugs. Considering our insistence, he says we can start but without saying it was a government initiative. It is an initiative that is to be understood as a pilot project."

22. Ministério da Saúde, *Mozambique HIV/AIDS Care Initiative*, 24.

23. Matsinhe, *Tábula Rasa*, 121.

24. Steenberg Olsen, "Structures of Stigma," 29.

25. "Il premio Donna Coraggio ad Ana Maria Muhai per la sua lotta contro l'AIDS," Notizie/Italia/News, April 9, 2012, http://www.notizieitalianews.com/2012/04/il-premio-donna-coraggio-ad-ana-maria.html.

26. The term "transactional sex" refers to sexual relationships that do not necessarily involve a predetermined payment but rather a series of obligations (not usually marriage), including material benefits (food, clothes, shelter, telephones, help for studies, etc.). It is fairly common in sub-Saharan Africa and often involves older men and younger women or teenagers. It presents higher risks of infection from HIV and is an important factor in the spread of AIDS in Africa.

27. "HIV: luta contra discriminação torna Maria Muhai 'mulher de coragem' em Moçambique," Agencia Informação Moçambique, April 6, 2012, https://www.dream-health.org/2012/04/aimhivluta-contra-discriminacao-torna-maria-muhai-mulher-de-coragem-em-mocambique/.

28. Ana Maria Muhai, presentation, May 20, 2004, Rome, at the "I DREAM" meeting for African activists, text in DAR.

29. Muhai, presentation, May 20, 2004.

30. UN Office for the Coordination of Humanitarian Affairs, "Overview: Focus on Mozambique."

31. Muhai, presentation, May 20, 2004.

32. UNAIDS, *2004 Report*. The figures are a mean of a very broad range, proving the difficulty to obtain precise data on the spread of AIDS in countries with limited resources such as sub-Saharan countries. On UNAIDS and the question of statistics, see endnote 69 of chapter 2 in this book.

33. The question of stigma is found in a lot of the literature on AIDS, in particular in reference to Africa. See a scientific description of stigma and its importance with respect to how HIV/AIDS is experienced physically in Mbonu van den Borne, and De Vries, "Stigma of People with HIV/AIDS. See also Rankin, "Stigma of Being HIV-Positive."

34. "Storia di Luzete Chàuque," text in DAR.

35. The controversy on this topic, which has been revived amid cultural prejudice and racist opinions expressed during the HIV/AIDS pandemic, generated considerable literature and controversy. See Rushton and Bogaert, "Population Differences"; Caldwell, Caldwell, and Quiggin, *Disaster in an Alternative Civilization*; and Rushing, *AIDS Epidemic*. For a critical approach to the previous texts, see Stillwaggon, "Racial Metaphors," and Oppong and Kalipeni, "Perceptions and Misperceptions."

36. Marazzi, "*DREAM*," 5.

37. For an in-depth technical analysis of DREAM's clinical protocols and diagnostic resources, not fully explained here, see Marazzi et al., *Perspectives and Practice*; Germano et al., *DREAM*; DREAM, *Viva l'Africa viva!*; and DREAM, *Curare l'AIDS in Africa*.

38. Germano, "Caro Occidente, non tradire il Global Fund."

39. Michel Sidibé, interview with Claire Brisset, mentioned in Claire Brisset, "L'Afrique francophone face au sida," *Le Monde diplomatique*, June 2013.

40. Marazzi, "DREAM," 7–8.

41. Marazzi, 7.

42. "Afrique: l'Église en première ligne contre le sida," *Pèlerin*, July 30, 2009, 27.

43. Marazzi et al., "Improving Adherence to HAART."

44. Elard Alumando, "La prossimità nell'immensità dell'Africa."

45. There were also the samples received from isolated public health prenatal clinics under to collaboration agreements. DREAM's molecular biology laboratories owe much to the voluntary work of Susanna Ceffa, a biologist from Piedmont who supervised setting up the laboratories and was responsible for training the African biologists and technicians.

46. "La Comunità di Sant'Egidio e il programma globale di lotta all'AIDS: A colloquio con Leonardo Palombi," *Care*, November/December 2004, 16–17.

47. Paola Germano, "Editorial: DREAM 2.0," 2015, text in DAR.

48. Barbaglia, "Plant for Africa."

49. This data was of course made anonymous from the beginning to guarantee respect for the person. See Zimba, "In Africa con gli strumenti migliori," 29–38, 32; Bartolo and Ferrari, *Multidisciplinary Teleconsultation*; DREAM, *Curare l'AIDS in Africa*, 91–100; and Nucita et al., "Global Approach to the Management of EMR."

50. Happy Mangula, interview by Alessandra Morvillo, September 14, 2018, Iringa, text in DAR.

51. "And we were all someone's students, like I was one of Roberto Lunghi's, an Italian who spent his holidays for years in Malawi, looking after AIDS patients." Jane Gondwe, interview by the author, May 17, 2018, Blantyre.

52. Oppenheimer and Bayer, "Choisir entre la vie et la mort," 179–80.

53. Paola Germano travels frequently between Rome and Africa. From a professional point of view, she comes from a hospital for AIDS, the Spallanzani in Rome. She obtained a specialization in HIV/AIDS in California in the early 1990s, when the triple therapy did not yet exist.

54. The local training courses, but above all the pan-African courses, attended by thirty-five thousand people over twenty years, have greatly contributed to making all the operative sectors of DREAM African.

55. See R. Michael Fleshman, "Signes de progrès dans la lutte contre le sida," *Afrique Renouveau*, January 2010, https://www.un.org/africarenewal/fr/magazine/january-2010/signes-de-progr%C3%A8s-dans-la-lutte-contre-le-sida), which combines several statistical sources.

56. Maria C. Marazzi and Leonardo Palombi, "A Dream for Africa: Children without AIDS" (presentation, 3rd International DREAM Conference, Rome, May 27, 2005), text in DAR.

57. C. Marazzi and E. Alumando, "Long Live Mothers and Children! Reduce Maternal Mortality and Raise Children without AIDS" (presentation, 8th International DREAM Conference, Rome, June 22, 2012), text in DAR.

58. Germano, "Editorial: DREAM 2.0."

59. Mphande, "DREAM," 47–56.

60. Mphande, 47–56.

61. Palombi et al., "Incidence and Predictors of Death."

62. Pacem Kawonga, interview with the author, May 23, 2018, Lilongwe.

63. Oransky, "Annalena Tonelli."

64. Irene Karea, interview by Gianni Guidotti, November 12, 2018, Meru, text in DAR.

65. Felician Pambana, interview by Alessandra Morvillo, May 21, 2018, Arusha, text in DAR.

66. On this topic it is worth mentioning a PhD thesis on health education, Iasilli, "Malattia e resilienza"

67. Josefa Graciosa Jardim Madeira (presentation, 3rd International DREAM Conference, "A Dream for Africa: Children without AIDS," Rome, May 27, 2005), text in DAR.

68. Steenberg Olsen, "Structures of Stigma," 38, 247–78.

69. Robins, "From 'Rights' to 'Ritual,'" 312.

70. Cacilda Massango, presentation (fifteen typed pages with testimonies from the lives of DREAM activists from Mozambique) given during a meeting in Maputo, July 10, 2008, in DAR.

71. Fatoumata Sylla, interview by Cristina Cannelli, January 30, 2016, Conakry, text in DAR.

72. Devey Malu Malu, *La Guinée*, and Aliou Diallo, *Histoire politique et sociale.*

73. On Conakry, see Lehideux-Vernimmen, *La naissance de Conakry,* and Diallo, *Je m'appelle Conakry.*

74. Fatoumata Sylla, interview by Cristina Cannelli, January 30, 2016, Conakry, text in DAR.

75. A health education manual produced by DREAM in the main African languages provides basic information on health and hygiene, including sexually transmitted diseases. The first edition, in 1999, was in Portuguese (*Como vai a saúde?*). The manual was then also published in English, French, Spanish, and other languages, including Swahili and Chichewa. About two hundred thousand copies have been printed so far. The book has many illustrations because 42 percent of the African population is illiterate, reaching even 60 percent among the women in some countries. The aim of the manual is to counter infection, parasites, and disease, and with education it tries to counter inadequate medicine, clean water, toilets, and sewage systems. There are many pages on nutrition.

76. On the correlation between AIDS and malnutrition as a result of poverty, see Selgelid, "Ethics, Economics, and AIDS." See also WHO, *Nutrient Requirement*; WHO and FAO, *Living Well with HIV/AIDS*; and the WFP-sponsored publication Germano et al., *DREAM*.

77. "Fame, salute e HIV/AIDS: un rapporto vitale," press release, WFP and DREAM, Rome, November 28, 2007, in DAR.

78. Pridmore and Carr-Hill, *Basic Causes of Child Undernutrition*, 15–16.

79. In the early 2000s the CD4 level was generally considered to be the most reliable predictor of death from AIDS. DREAM carried out studies that included other factors: the viral load, hemoglobin level, and body mass index (BMI) . And it was precisely the BMI that turned out to be the most effective predictor of early death. See Maria C. Marazzi and Leonardo Palombi (presentation, 5th International Conference organized by DREAM, "Long Life for Africa! Fighting AIDS and Malnutrition," Rome, May 10, 2007), included in DREAM, *Long Life for Africa!, Fighting AIDS and Malnutrition*, 4–34; Germano et al., *DREAM*; and Robin Jackson, presentation in DREAM, *We Want to Live, Too!*, 110–27.

80. In the first years of its activity, DREAM had to defend itself from the accusation of promoting a dependency culture because it gave its patients food packages. Going against the tide, the World Food Programme always generously supported the DREAM centers, and it continued to do so even after its funds from the international donors were reduced because they wanted to limit UN food interventions to wars and famines.

81. Taking food home also gives them dignity and relieves the stigma with respect to the members of their family.

82. Unlike in African health systems, where nutritional support, in the rare cases in which it is provided, is normally given on the basis of one's BMI alone, which has to be below 18.5. The BMI is calculated with a formula that anyone can apply to themselves, knowing that under 18.5 is underweight and over 25 is overweight: BMI = mass (kg)/height (m)$^2$.

83. Steenberg Olsen, "Structures of Stigma," 299.

84. Quoted in Steenberg Olsen, 308–9.

85. WHO, *Antiretroviral Treatment as Prevention (TasP)*.

86. It is enough to compare the first WHO guidelines of 2002 for the treatment of AIDS patients in countries with limited resources (WHO, *Scaling Up Antiretroviral Therapy*) with the approach in developed countries at the same time. While in the West HAART was prescribed to patients whose CD4s were under 350, in the above-mentioned WHO guidelines the threshold for starting the therapy for poor countries was under 200 CD4s. Without being able to measure this immunological threshold, which was often the case in countries with poor health systems, only symptomatic patients in a serious condition could receive the antiretroviral drugs because they were the ones who certainly had only a few CD4s.

87. For one of the first contributions in this direction, see Palombi, Perno, and Marazzi, "HIV/AIDS in Africa."

88. Before the concept of test and treat became part of the international guidelines, the very popular use of the term "universal access" was misleading in that it always referred to therapies to be administered not to everyone who was HIV-positive but only those who satisfied the restrictive criteria regarding eligibility for treatment. There was nothing very "universal" about it.

89. Nevirapine achieved only a fleeting result. It reduced the average percentage of babies who would otherwise be born infected, which was 40 percent, by around half, as reported in the health care statistics. But it was a false success. It soon lost efficacy, and breast-feeding increased the number of infected children until, at the age of one year, it was again around 40 percent—the same figure that was expected when nothing at all was done.

90. Liotta et al., "Reduction of Maternal Mortality."

91. As they wrote in 2001, the triple therapy would strongly reduce the viral load in breast milk and make it safe. See Leonardo Palombi, "Sull'AIDS in Africa e in Mozambico," presentation, DREAM meeting, Rome, February 11, 2001, text in DAR.

92. Scientific arguments in this regard are found in Marina Giuliano et al., "Triple Antiretroviral Prophylaxis"; Palombi et al., "Treatment Acceleration Program."

93. UNICEF, UNAIDS, and WHO, *Children and AIDS*, 23.

94. This process is well explained in Steenberg Olsen, "Structures of Stigma."

95. Mphande, "DREAM," 51–52.

# 4

# Looking into the Future

In 2016 the two most symbolic figures of the international discussion on AIDS, Peter Piot and Jeffrey Sachs, again presented their thoughts, which had not changed for the past fifteen years. Piot, who always criticized considering therapy as the most important factor, stated the following:

> *AIDS is not over.* . . . The emergency has not finished; underestimating it would be a serious mistake. . . . Up to today we have dealt with the hardware [health care systems, drugs]. Now, however, it is time to work on the software, which means the patients [their culture, sensitivity, values, beliefs, emotions]. The drugs are not enough to fight the virus. There has to be a change in the culture. . . . For years we hoped that treating HIV+ people immediately with the test-and-treat approach, which would stop them from being infectious, would help stem the spread of the virus. Today we know that this is not enough because some patients are not prepared to follow a heavy therapy until the first symptoms of the full-blown disease appear.[1]

Sachs, on the other hand, confirmed his trust in the therapy as prevention:

> The AIDS pandemic claimed around 36 million lives between 1981 and 2016, and a similar number around the world currently live with the HIV virus. . . . Those statistics are daunting, but the startling news is that the goal of an "AIDS-Free Generation" is realistically within reach. . . . The key reason that the epidemic can be ended is a scientific finding . . . that showed that HIV-positive individuals receiving antiretroviral (ARV) treatment suppress the HIV virus in their bloodstreams so dramatically that they are very unlikely to transmit

the virus to others through sex or shared needles. This finding confirmed the concept of "treatment as prevention." If a high enough proportion of HIV-positive individuals receive ARV treatment, it is possible not only to save their lives, but also to break the transmission of the virus itself, thereby ending the epidemic.[2]

At a certain point, the story of the fight against AIDS moved in the direction indicated by Sachs, not by Piot. The prediction in 2006 by historian Philippe Denis was wrong. He wrote that "the spread of the antiretroviral therapies will make it possible to avoid suffering, but it will not change the course of the epidemic."[3]

In 2002 the point of view published in the *Lancet* was that the prevention of HIV/AIDS was "at least 28 times more cost effective than HAART."[4] In 2015 on the other hand, a UNAIDS document estimated that HAART produced an economic return of seventeen times its investment.[5] Still, in 2015 the WHO launched its 90-90-90 Initiative, which aimed for 90 percent of HIV-positive people to be aware in 2020 that they had HIV, for 90 percent of confirmed HIV patients to be on HAART, and for 90 percent of HIV-positive patients to be treated and no longer infectious, thanks to the suppression of their viral load. The abbreviation "U=U" was soon adopted (undetectable equals untransmittable).[6] The 90-90-90 Initiative meant that if the three stages were successful, the virus was no longer infectious in 72.9 percent of HIV-positive people.[7] On the basis of these mathematical calculations, it was therefore predicted that in 2030 the AIDS pandemic would no longer threaten public health because by then there would be "a 90 percent reduction in new HIV infections and deaths from AIDS-related illness (compared to 2010 baselines)."[8]

The concept behind the 90-90-90 Initiative, which represents the current phase in the worldwide fight against AIDS, is valid: the number of new cases and of deaths is undeniably inversely proportional to the extent of therapeutic coverage. The spread of the HAART regimen has had a very strong effect on the pandemic. The worldwide mortality peak of 3.0 million deaths in 2000 (2.4 million in Africa) dropped to 770,000 in 2018 (470,000 in Africa). The number of new infections in Africa dropped from 2.5 million in 1997 to 1.8 million in 2018.[9] Nonetheless, the results of the first years of the 90-90-90

Initiative were less dynamic than expected. In 2018 the executive director of UNAIDS, Michel Sidibé, wrote the following:

> The global AIDS response is at a precarious point—partial success in saving lives and stopping new HIV infections is giving way to complacency. At the halfway point to the 2020 targets, the pace of progress is not matching the global ambition. The number of AIDS-related deaths is the lowest this century, with fewer than 1 million people dying each year from AIDS-related illnesses, thanks to sustained access to antiretroviral therapy. Three out of four people living with HIV now know their status—the first step to getting treatment. And now a record 21.7 million people are on treatment. . . . The success in saving lives has not been matched with equal success in reducing new HIV infections. New HIV infections are not falling fast enough.[10]

It is more than likely that the goals that were set will be reached later on. In any case, it would be ungenerous to see the slow progress of the 90-90-90 Initiative as a failure. The 3 by 5 Initiative that started HAART on a large scale in countries with limited resources also progressed more slowly than expected, yet it was fundamental in demonstrating the therapeutic efficacy of HAART also outside the West. On a global level, after the initial failures because the treatment was denied, it was a story of semivictories or semidefeats. It is more important to ask oneself about the factors that slow down or speed up the 90-90-90 Initiative. Vast numbers of people are being treated, such as the 21.7 million people mentioned by Sidibè for 2018, but just enrolling them on the HAART regimen is not enough. What counts is how far away the patients live from the health centers, adherence to the treatment, efficacy of diagnostic monitoring, and frequency of counseling. These are decisive aspects of a local and high-quality health care system that avoids switches to more expensive second-line or even more lines of therapy, opportunistic infections and related complications, hospitalization, and tragic treatment failures. Well-designed intervention models are urgently needed as well as specific, massive investments. The 90-90-90 Initiative can be successful in sub-Saharan Africa as long as it is not carried out with the idea of simplification, minimalism, and saving time and money.

The first "90" of the three is in the process of being achieved because once the prospect of treatment is assured, people do the test. The second "90" is more difficult. Adherence is uncertain, and at the end of the first year some people will have died, and many will have abandoned the therapy. Some studies on African hospitals show therapeutic failures at 50 percent.[11] The third "90" should therefore probably be calculated by subtracting 10 from 100 and then dividing 90 by 2 to get 45. In the end, 90 percent of these 45 patients on HAART will probably no longer be infectious. This means that if the patients continue the treatment properly, there will not be more than 40.5 percent of patients with an undetectable viral load, compared to the initial ; in African settings the 90-90-90 target can be reasonably reached in the 40.5% of HIV-positive people. The fact that hardly anyone talks or writes about AIDS anymore does not help the WHO and the other international development cooperation agencies in setting up effective policies and adequate fund-raising. If AIDS is no longer felt to be an emergency, the international donors, whether they are countries or institutions, divert their funds to newer, more engaging goals.

There is, however, reason to hope. The developments with respect to AIDS in terms of technology, diagnosis, pharmacology, and so on were carried out with great enthusiasm at the beginning, and however much they slow down, they will never stop completely. In high-income countries, the fact that AIDS can be treated, the availability of several lines of therapy, and the impression that it is no longer dangerous have paradoxically led people to be less careful. The number of new cases has been basically stable at around seventy-eight to eighty thousand a year for at least the last two decades. This is an unfortunate figure, but it encourages scientific research, which is mainly a Western prerogative. More tolerable and more powerful drugs have appeared. Solutions are being studied in order to strengthen the immune system both preventively and for therapeutic purposes, to find hidden HIV in the so-called sanctuary cells when the viral load becomes undetectable, and so on. If it was not a fairy tale told continuously from the 1980s to today, one could hope that there will be a vaccine within the next ten years, which, after the necessary tests, will be available in time to meet the UN's 2030 target for declaring HIV under control. In the meantime, the virus is recorded as less virulent than before. The widespread therapy has changed HIV, and it has become weaker. Twenty years ago in Africa, people died with 100 CD4s, and now they can be saved with 10 CD4s. Even patients with only 10 CD4s can look all right.[12] The HIV-positive people who come to the health centers are different from those of the past, who could not even stand up and were emaciated. The full-blown phase comes later too. HIV-positive children and teenagers resist better. When they are treated, they recover much faster than adults and have fewer side effects. The test-and-treat approach—that is, immediate therapeutic treatment—has reduced morbidity considerably, and there has been talk of a community quantitative reduction of HIV.[13]

Another crucial aspect for the success of the 90-90-90 Initiative concerns the allocation of interventions and funds. There are issues to solve. Multilateral or bilateral? Ownership or partnership?

## OWNERSHIP/PARTNERSHIP

The previous chapters have not been kind to some of the UN agencies, in particular UNAIDS, at least as far as some phases of the fight against HIV/AIDS are concerned. It could not be otherwise because for years the fight against HIV in sub-Saharan Africa was marked by hesitation, delays, and ineffective policies that caused the deaths of millions of people. One has to agree with Stephen Lewis, who in 2005, in his role as UN special envoy for HIV/AIDS in Africa, denounced its inaction:

> All of us, myself included, who moved too slowly in the face of the viral contagion, who fiddled while Africa burned, who have spent days upon days in incestuous discussions, meetings, conferences, seminars, roundtables, with their reports, proceedings, documents, monographs, statistical compilations ad nauseam, all repeating what has been said before, all pretending to transform the obvious into revelation, all of us spending huge amounts of money on travel and accommodation, money that could have been used to save lives . . . all of us have a lot to atone for. And there's nothing quite so unseemly as the refusal to admit we were wrong, we delayed, we

conducted business as usual when we were in the midst of the most appalling emergency in the history of humankind.[14]

This accusation could refer to various areas: bureaucratic attitudes bordering on cynicism, voluntary inertia for political reasons, mediocre interventions because of corruption. Nonetheless, despite the negative aspects of multilateralism, it does have its merits. The United Nations, also in the fight against AIDS, made it possible to overcome selfish national interests and the colonial logic that still existed between rich and poor countries. In the 2000s, alongside leaders who were indifferent to anything that did not benefit them or organizations made helpless by abstract ideological progress, the UN boasted officials who took part in alleviating the suffering of countries that had limited resources and in particular African ones: Kofi Annan, Gro Harlem Brundtland, Jeffrey Sachs, Lee Jong-wook, Kevin De Cock, Margaret Chan, Michel Sidibé, the above-mentioned Stephen Lewis, and others. These were people who wanted to act, to save lives.

The United Nations is historically of great consequence because it represents the overcoming of nationalism. This aspect can also be expressed as the multilateralism that supports and sometimes replaces bilateralism in development cooperation for countries with limited resources. Not that bilateral development cooperation is negative in principle. If it is carried out well, it represents a correct assumption of responsibility by those who are rich and developed toward those who are not. Furthermore, bilateralism can express a supportive civil society inspired by feelings of brotherhood and human universality. Yet in these country-to-country relationships what often happens is an exchange of favors, decisions taken in order to satisfy specific sectors or people of the two countries. In bilateralism, development cooperation activities, including those focused on social and health care issues, are sometimes conditioned by different types of leverage.

In theory, one might say that the multilateral approach is more transparent. Bilateralism is tempted by interest at the expense of equity. Multilateralism ought to encourage equity over the interest of the parties. The UN has its lobbyists and influence groups, and the Westerners have great influence, starting with the British-American-Scandinavian conglomeration. However, there are also lively debates wherein some feel the Global South is not necessarily subordinate a priori because large numbers can sometimes overturn the power of the few. The distribution of the assignments respects a certain balance between the continents. One can complain about the quarrels between UN agencies, but these episodes are minimal compared to the serious rivalry between countries. If every initiative taken by a UN agency makes the other UN agencies worried about violations of prerogatives, this same antagonism is expressed to a far higher degree in the relationships between countries, and the development cooperation in the other country is seen in terms of political competition. Multilateralism, as indicated by the evidence, certainly involves an excessive degree of bureaucracy and disproportionate management costs. Nonetheless, it is the best guarantee against oppression by the most powerful countries. Winston Churchill allegedly said that "democracy is based on the enthusiasm of those who do not have it and on the resignation of those who have it." Even the multilateralism of the United Nations seems to be based on the desire of those who want to enjoy the benefits and the acceptance of those who cannot see any other alternative.

In any case, it should be remembered that at least in the case of the fight against HIV in countries with limited resources, the volume of aid from bilateralism has always been greater than that from multilateral agreements, above all because of the decision of the United States not to delegate its contribution to the fight against AIDS in the world to others. In 2015, despite being vigorously sponsored by countries such as France, Germany, Japan, Italy, and Canada, multilateralism donated a quarter of the total amount of aid, whereas bilateralism donated three quarters, thanks above all to PEPFAR, by which the United States financed half of the global commitment to fight AIDS.[15]

Actually, both solutions, multilateral and bilateral, present advantages and disadvantages. Much of their efficacy is connected to the most controversial question of international cooperation, that of the effects of corruption. The risks of corruption in prevention activities carried out in ways that were neither controlled nor able to be checked have already been mentioned. The many large, unwieldy national commissions set up in African countries to fight AIDS, and for this reason flooded with means and money, were a waste of resources, even more so because of the ideology developed by UNAIDS on which they were based. This ideology consisted of multisectorial, all-encompassing prevention, which allowed activities that were as varied as they were often intangible and difficult to evaluate.[16] There was then a more subtle, perverted tendency to give without sufficiently controlling the effectiveness of these actions. This is what acting in poor places with abundant financial resources led to. The staffs of the development cooperation agencies and NGOs connected with the local political classes possibly unwittingly became part of a warped system, upsetting the labor market with exorbitant salaries. They took the best personnel away from the public health system and from the organizations that took the trouble to train them and distributed money and gifts in order to obtain quick authorizations and results.

As far as corruption is concerned, it is not possible to establish whether multilateral or bilateral development cooperation was preferable. It obviously depended on each case and its circumstances. Some people blamed development cooperation as a whole, regardless of any specific country involved, and turned it into a form of accusation of the West. This cooperation was considered not only ineffective, old fashioned, and illusory but also the cause of the problems in Africa. According to the well-known Kenyan economist James Shikwati, the aid from the West was responsible for the corruption, clientelism, lack of productivity, low volumes of trade, weak entrepreneurship, and the dependence syndrome that afflicted his continent. Moreover, according to him, AIDS also contributed to Africa's problems, not as a disease but as a driver of international aid. In 2005 Shikwati considered that the reality of AIDS in Africa was overestimated based on speculation: "If one were to believe all the horrifying reports, then all Kenyans should actually be dead by now. . . . The figures were vastly exaggerated. . . . It's only about one million. Malaria is just as much of a problem, but people rarely talk about that. AIDS is big business, maybe Africa's biggest business. There's nothing else that can generate as much aid money as shocking figures on AIDS. AIDS is a political disease here, and we should be very skeptical."[17]

Shikwati was a forerunner of the far more dialectical and seductive economist of Zambian origin, Dambisa Moyo, who was firmly rooted in Oxford and Harvard. With *Dead Aid*, a book published in 2009, Moyo also became famous for claiming that aid from the West drugs, corrupts, and annihilates Africa because it deprives it of its entrepreneurial spirit and valid governance.[18] Her book was appreciated by liberalists, and for a while the *Financial Times* madefrequent reference to it. Moyo also praised the Chinese capitalistic activism in Africa because of its noncompassionate character, which taught Africans to be tough and determined to work, earn, and get rich. However, it cannot be said that Zambia, one of China's main partners in Africa, benefited from Chinese investment and even less so from the point of view of corruption, which Moyo attributed to compassionate Western capitalism. Besides, many Western companies operate in Africa purely to make a profit, and they "educate" Africans the same way that Chinese companies{ }do. In any case, the extraction and trade of oil, diamonds, gold, and rare metals, which are the most coveted activities for these companies, whether Western or Chinese, do not seem to have reduced corruption on the continent at all.

Moyo's ideas also gratified the pride of the African leaders and produced different reactions depending on the combination of political pragmatism, patriotism, and pride of each of them. Kofi Annan appreciated the call to African energy in *Dead Aid*. According to him, Moyo was proposing "a new approach. Her message is that 'Africa's time is now.' It is time for Africans to assume full control over their own economic and political destiny. Africans should grasp the many means and opportunities available to them for improving their quality of life."[19] John Kufuor, a former president of Ghana, was less diplomatic: "Moyo is not the voice of Africa. . . . She lives in an ivory tower, far away from the reality of Africa. Perhaps she should go back to Zambia to see how much that country still needs help."[20] The Eritrean president, Isaias Afwerki, was not affected by the international opinion. He was convinced that "aid cripples people" and felt that Moyo's point of view justified his hostile attitude to the international NGOs that he had expelled from Eritrea, saying, "Let us do it alone."[21] Paul Kagame, who had taken Rwanda out of the French-speaking world into the English-speaking world, was in favor of Moyo's theory and commented, "Aid is political, Markets are neutral."[22]

> The cycle of aid and poverty is durable: as long as poor nations are focused on receiving aid they will not work to improve their economies. Some of Ms. Moyo's prescriptions, such as ending all aid within five years, are aggressive. . . . Do not get me wrong. We appreciate support from the outside, but it should be support for what we intend to achieve ourselves. No one should pretend that they care about our nations more than we do; or assume that they know what is good for us better than we do ourselves.[23]

There are many more examples, but it is not worth spending time on them. What is certain is that the credence given to Moyo by the cynical capitalists of the West and by nationalistic and frustrated Africa inevitably closed the circle: the rich desiring to be at peace with their money and the poor proud to be in trouble but being themselves. It is equally certain that without international aid to fight AIDS—without the Global Fund, PEPFAR, and everything else set up through the compassion of the developed countries—Africans would not have had the antiretroviral drugs to avoid a far worse massacre and prevent mass contagion. Today vast areas of Africa would look like cemeteries.

Discrediting development cooperation and international aid is a bitter practice: one risks throwing the baby away with the bathwater. There are fundamental questions of human justice and solidarity but also of interdependence because no health system is completely independent and sustainable. There is always a limit. It has not even been easy for the United States, which has been struggling for years with crises and reforms of its health system, let alone for countries with limited resources. Despite corruption and embezzlement, the public health systems in poor countries have to be supported as decisive for human and economic development. This is why, in the end, cooperation has to be done well and honestly. A big obstacle, as if the mistakes and confusion due to intrinsic factors were not enough, came from an idea that was popular over the last decades: ownership—a sort of sovereignty. The effectiveness and transparency of development cooperation has affected the rate and intensity of this ownership, also in the case of AIDS.

Faced with the activities of the rich countries in the scenarios in the poor world, the United Nations has always echoed the cries of alarm of neocolonialism, whether real or imaginary, from the countries that were victims of colonialism, which are the majority at the UN. This dreaded neocolonialism concerned any political or economic activity, including development cooperation. Consequently, the UN as a whole, along with the donor countries and recipient countries, elaborated a defensive concept: ownership. As stated in the Paris Declaration of March 2, 2005, on the effectiveness of public aid, ownership is the first criterion of the efficacy of international aid. The ownership claimed in the meeting in Paris basically implies full sovereignty of the receiving countries over the policies, strategies, and allocation of the aid: "Donors commit to respect partner country leadership and help strengthen their capacity to exercise it."[24]

In the philosophy of international cooperation, ownership is supposed to mean control and responsibility of the local governments in the projects and programs, with the receiving countries having greater influence in defining the development strategies. However, the reality coincides with the actual meaning of the word "ownership"—*possession* of the international cooperation resources by the government of the countries for which they are intended. Ownership means that the developing countries are, to a greater or lesser extent, sovereign in the management of the funds granted to them and the activities carried out. In Africa, ownership satisfies the nationalist point of view that shrewdly blames the backwardness of the continent on the West, attributing local corruption and poorly distributed national wealth to intrusive factors from abroad. At the same time, ownership satisfies the rich donor countries that have no intention of facing accusations of neocolonialism or of carrying out direct activities in countries where their cooperation would risk failure and scandal. The hidden meaning behind "ownership" is that it is up to Africans to take care of Africa, which satisfies both the receivers' pride and their banks and the donors' sense of political correctness and the fact that they do not have to be involved practically.

In running UNAIDS, the concept of ownership was particularly relevant in the idea that "if people don't feel 'it's my problem' then they won't really move."[25] UNAIDS then further specified ownership according to the principle of the "Three Ones." The response to the epidemic carried out by the various figures present in a country has to be within a single "common HIV/AIDS Action Framework" controlled by the national authorities, it has to follow a single strategy decided by the national governments, and it has to be subject to a single national coordination and monitoring system.[26] A practical aspect of the Three Ones is that, once agreed on, many funds for fighting AIDS are managed and allocated by national governments. This system does not appear to aim to avoid corruption in the governments and administrations of the receiving countries. In Africa, where the health systems are mainly supported by international aid, the ministries of health, which receive the most aid from abroad, together with the ministries of education and of agriculture, are notorious for being at risk of corruption.

Ownership has fueled this perverse system. Actually, the international community has been questioning this ownership for the past few years. There have been too many scandals, too much embezzlement, too much money wasted, and not enough results with respect to the funds given. The trend is now toward a greater control of funded projects and direct funds for the on-site organizations. Ideally this could be called a partnership. It consists of the humanitarian agencies and the NGOs agreeing with the governments to carry out humanitarian programs under the governments' own responsibility and with their own resources. The aim is to work closely with the Africans in the country, training them if necessary, and to commit to long periods without the anxiety of an exit strategy. A partnership implies equality, mutual rights and duties, and a common destiny: Africans and Westerners in it together. Short-term, emergency cooperation does not work. A partnership means a negotiated method of intervention, respecting the local authorities and the national prerogatives but also the operative autonomy of the humanitarian aid organizations. This avoids the almost unlimited delegation that ownership granted the national governments, without, however, reducing their sovereignty—resorting, if necessary, to legal agreements between the parties. Understandably, the African governments prefer ownership because it gives them full control of the resources. In any case, the question of ownership or partnership should not be considered from an ideological point of view. When the health care sector in an African country is unable to walk alone, or does so with difficulty, an international partnership guarantees that it will be strengthened and will grow. Doing everything yourself is fine when you have the means. Otherwise it is often impossible, especially in the field of health care.

DREAM has always clashed with ownership. In every country in which it set up its activities, it has had to challenge the authorities that wanted to affirm the Three Ones and take for themselves the economic resources intended for the treatment programs. DREAM, on the other hand, has always advocated partnerships, which involve forms of cooperation that would inspire the international multilateral and bilateral aid communities, if they were prepared to adopt a less comfortable but more effective alternative to letting the governments be responsible for the funds and projects.

For example, DREAM set up some of its first triple antiretroviral therapy projects with funds from the World Bank that were allocated directly and used with no intermediaries—let's say, no deductions—by local African governments and ministries. This made the African authorities furious with the World Bank. One minister of health in southern Africa wrote that DREAM did not deserve the funds because it treated its patients like guinea pigs. He was not happy with the World Bank, despite being fully aware of how his government neglected AIDS patients. Katherine Marshall, speaking on behalf of the World Bank, made the following point: "Partnerships are absolutely vital in the fight against AIDS. Nobody can manage alone. We have to be creative and open to explore new and dynamic forms of partnerships."[27] DREAM was well aware of this and carefully negotiated its operating conditions with individual governments from a position of strength that was reinforced by its results. Some preliminary notes written before a negotiation in 2005 with the ministers of health of Ghana, Nigeria, the Democratic Republic of Congo, and Kenya demonstrate the firmness of this health diplomacy: "Not negotiable. Treatment. Tritherapy. Excellence: same standards of the West. Partnership and not Ownership. Participation and Collaboration. Quick scaling up. Joining to our protocols. Not payment."[28] The instructions given in July 2005 to a representative of DREAM who was negotiating with the DRC government in Kinshasa illustrate the recurrent key points of negotiations. Their essential aspects are as follows:

a) treatment and tests 100 percent free of charge
b) the possibility to carry out the advanced DREAM diagnostic and therapeutic protocols completely (CD4s, viral load and triple therapy). This is very important for pregnant women because by now some countries accept the triple therapy for the general population but in the field of mother-to-child prevention, almost all the countries only use Nevirapine
c) access to treatment not only in towns but also in rural and outlying areas
d) autonomy of the centres in terms of their organisation and management
e) classification of DREAM centres as pilot centres for operational research and high quality points of reference of the national healthcare programme.[29]

DREAM is present in ten African countries: Mozambique, Malawi, the DRC, Guinea, Cameroon, Tanzania, Kenya, Nigeria, Eswatini (formerly Swaziland), and the Central African Republic. It negotiated how it would be present in each country, and in most cases it was authorized to act initially with pilot projects. Although the agreements with the governments were not ironclad, they established operative frameworks within which any disagreements could be overcome—for example, regarding the fact that the patients must not pay for anything, which many governments were not happy to accept.

Until a few years ago, several African leaders considered partnerships unrealistic and as deviating toward a form of "parallel health care." At the beginning, though, DREAM did try to become part of some public health sectors. This decision soon turned out not to be such a good idea because it meant having to deal with inefficient, arbitrary, and corrupt officials. This is why partnerships were created in every country with governments that guaranteed DREAM the freedom to operate and manage its resources, with constant exchanges of information, agreed-upon therapeutic protocols, joint interventions in certain clinical cases, and coordinated health care efforts. Years later one can say that this decision has paid off. DREAM has acquired an excellent reputation, and the national health care systems have started to see it as a precious ally for consultations and second opinions, complex diagnostic tests, training activities, transmission of know-how, personnel hiring decisions, and drawing up guidelines and national strategic plans.

## SUSTAINABILITY

The future of the fight against HIV/AIDS raises an old question again. Two decades of advances and progress have created a new context, but the original challenge has not changed. What about sustainability? The economic world is reluctant to agree with science and humanity, today as it was twenty years ago. Without resources it is not possible to defeat AIDS. In the past, as mentioned, this fact meant not acting. At the end of the 1990s it seemed to be politically wrong to ask for billions of dollars to fight AIDS in countries with limited resources—almost as though it was rude. The lack of resources was useful for denying treatment in countries with limited resources and for insisting on behavioral-based prevention, which was a very low-cost activity. Soon afterward, billions of dollars did arrive, thanks to Jeffrey Sachs, Kofi Annan, George W. Bush, Bill Gates, and other statesmen and patrons. So, the money was there to be spent—the next step was all about how to spend it. The politicians and their financial parameters intended these funds to be used to achieve economies of scale, to simplify the therapeutic protocols, and limit diagnostics, and they aimed for quantity before quality. After years of mainly unsatisfactory results, it was gradually acknowledged that patients had to be given higher-quality treatments, without cutting corners in terms of how this was to be carried out, of adherence, or of diagnostics.

Today the decision to provide quality treatment is also promoted by the WHO for poor, nonindustrialized countries. It has been understood that putting money into the fight against AIDS is an investment worth the cost. Indeed, it really is an investment and not a cost. Not only are lives saved, but opportunistic infections are also avoided, as is hospitalization and the loss of workers who are necessary for society. The human capital is not depleted. Family and social stability is guaranteed. Allocating substantial resources to the fight against AIDS does not mean taking a loss because in the medium and long terms it becomes profitable. The case of South Africa demonstrates just this. Here Thabo Mbeki's denial caused the death of a large number of specialized workers and a crisis in entire areas of production. The people responsible for the economic and financial life of the country were the ones who then had to commit themselves to making sure that the country changed its approach and that vast resources were invested in fighting AIDS.

At the beginning, DREAM's programs were more expensive than those of the public health programs in the African countries where it operated. As it expanded its activities, the difference was reduced by economies of scale, but there was still a slight difference in the average cost per patient. The results, however, were vastly better in terms of retention and survival, especially in mother-to-child prevention and in pediatric AIDS. It was worth spending more to achieve a better outcome, which already in the medium term repaid the investment and made it possible to avoid far greater damage in the case of treatments carried out with the intention to save money. Medical results like this showed that HIV/AIDS could be eradicated, which was impossible with inaccurate therapies.

That said, it is obvious that economic sustainability was one of the main challenges for the DREAM program. When DREAM started up, it seemed impossible to overcome the rejection of the programs to treat AIDS in Africa because the estimated cost-effectiveness ratio did not look good enough at all. The calculations of this ratio showed how science gave up, faced with economic factors. However, the donors' governments, the development cooperation agencies, and the institutional investors considered these calculations to be plausible and binding. Therefore, no treatment programs were financed—only prevention programs. The right to health did not touch or mobilize anyone in power.

During DREAM's first years, its rapid expansion in several African countries was only possible thanks to the support of private donors. Thousands of people in European civil societies formed partnerships with DREAM, some donating a lot, some a little. Both young people and the elderly carried out fundraising activities. Artists sold their works and gave the proceeds to DREAM. Families looked after African HIV-positive children through long-distance adoptions.

Schools and parishes collected donations. All of these people coming together made it possible for DREAM to purchase the drugs for patients in the first years of the program. In 2004 DREAM was awarded the generous Balzan Prize, which called the DREAM program a "concrete model for African countries in difficulty."[30] Over time, large private donations were made, alongside the many small donations. The UniCredit banking group and the Unidea-UniCredit Foundation became DREAM's main sponsors in Mozambique, with long-term commitments, together with the Swiss FAI (Fondation Assistance Internationale) and funds from the Italian Catholic Church. The DREAM program in Malawi was made possible thanks to the long-term commitment of Banca Intesa and Fondazione Cariplo. Only later, after the 3 by 5 Initiative was approved for treating AIDS in Africa, were the partnerships with the World Bank and with the World Food Programme set up. Through the African governments, it was possible to receive more antiretroviral drugs from the Global Fund, while agreements were made with the European Union and with governments, regions, and towns in Belgium, Finland, France, Germany, Japan, Italy, Norway, Spain, and Switzerland, just to mention the most generous countries. In the meantime, the idea that treating was economically more advantageous than not treating was becoming more acceptable. The fact that the therapy itself was prevention because it inhibited contagion, and therefore represented a good investment, was slowly being understood. DREAM was aware of this, of course, but it was naturally not what motivated DREAM. Rather, it was humanitarian reasons, regardless of the economic analyses, which at the beginning of the program were admittedly very discouraging.

Today DREAM is still inevitably having to deal with the question of sustainability. There are some European volunteers, which reduces the financial needs, but the buildings and the local staff have to be paid for. The DREAM staff in Africa are all Africans, they have had training, both in theory and in the field, and they are highly motivated. This has made it less and less necessary to have European doctors present in Africa, although they are still very important for supporting the African doctors, especially during their professional apprenticeships. What is certain is that by now the African doctors and nurses, like the African activists and coordinators, are the people who run the centers. These local DREAM staff, just over five hundred people, are regularly paid according to the laws of each country, a cost that has to be taken into consideration. However, sustainability is not just a question of bookkeeping—it also concerns the stability of the health care personnel over time. In other words, it is necessary to guarantee that there will always be reliable personnel by motivating them professionally and with adequate salaries, which up to now DREAM has succeeded in doing.

Until 2010, DREAM's financial budget grew from year to year with the expansion of the treatment programs in new countries. Thanks to various agreements and synergies, it was then reduced, without compromising the further increase in the number of centers and of Africans treated. How did this happen? A growing number of private and public hospitals and health centers, often belonging to missionaries, joined DREAM and adopted its model of treatment with the costs involved, except for the training activities and the supervision of the centers. In the meantime, the costs for DREAM decreased because, according to a modus operandi carried out from the very beginning, costs of the antiretroviral drugs, laboratory reagents, nutritional supplementation, maintenance of diagnostic equipment, and sometimes individual members of staff were covered more and more by the individual African countries. This support came in the form of funds provided specifically for this purpose by the Global Fund, by Western governments, and by the vast American resources of PEPFAR. In 2010 DREAM's budget was over $11 million, and in 2018 it was around $7 million. Clearly the cost of treating hundreds of thousands of patients is far higher than a budget like this, but, as mentioned above, the drugs and laboratory reagents, as well as some services, are mainly guaranteed by international funds, whereas some health care centers that are affiliated with DREAM are financially supported by external organizations (missionaries, NGOs, etc.).

In any case, making ends meet is not easy. Resources are needed above all for the health centers and for the staff because these are the running costs that the international donors are usually reluctant to cover but are essential items on the list of costs involved in treating a chronic disease. The only way to balance such a budget is with very careful spending, a highly efficient use of resources, a large number of volunteers, scrupulous planning of stocks of drugs and reagents, and intense negotiations with suppliers in an economy of scale. The patients' adherence to the treatment also helps because it limits to under 5 percent the number of patients who need very expensive second- or third-line drugs.

One paradox is that in the context of international cooperation, where DREAM looks for sources of funds, its budget tends to be considered excessive. Furthermore, DREAM is constantly asked to explain its exit strategy, as though it were an ordinary development cooperation organization, operating on the basis of short-term projects. DREAM's decision was to have its own personnel and not to give them to the countries where they work because these countries do not always offer guarantees of long-lasting employment. As for the exit strategy, DREAM, as previously mentioned, is not an NGO that goes from one project to another but instead a Euro-African organization that, by treating chronically sick people and actually being a model for the African health care systems it collaborates with and has over time become a part of, does not correspond to the clichés of the Westerners who provide a fishing rod, teach people how to use it, and then leave. DREAM is European and African, white and Black, and everyone goes fishing together. This is precisely what the partnership is, instead of the ownership that the African governments like and also instead of the absence of responsibility of donors who are afraid of long-term programs that cannot be immediately translated into a series of successes.

It is therefore easy to understand why DREAM finds it hard to balance its budget. Like twenty years ago, whether DREAM is sustainable is a question that is asked every day, even though it is well stocked and has tested its ability to deal with temporary shortages of funds. People who are used to dealing with the precariousness of life in general in Africa can certainly face the precariousness of their funds without becoming discouraged. So far DREAM has never been short of generous small and large donors.

Moreover, as far as the availability of resources is concerned, there is reason to be optimistic due to the overall development of Africa. This is so both for DREAM and in general in the fight against AIDS in Africa: the economies of the sub-Saharan countries in the first two decades of the twenty-first century have grown. Africa is making economic progress despite social inequality and recurrent internal conflicts. The continent is fully involved in the process of globalization. In 2000 the UN set its ambitious Millennium Development Goals for 2015 and aimed for a dramatic reduction of poverty in all its forms, with Africa as the first beneficiary.[31] In the following years, many African countries made the transition to democracy, and their stability increased enough to consider "the decade of chaos," the 1990s, as something of the past.[32] These were the years when their usual partners (Europe and the United States) largely pulled out, leaving the continent in the hands of the international financial institutions. During the 1990s most of the countries in sub-Saharan Africa were governed by authoritarian regimes, whereas in 2004 this was the case for only a minority of five.[33]

When the Cold War ended, Africa was no longer divided between pro-West and pro-Soviet. The terrorist attacks of September 11, 2001, changed the international political climate, but Africa was not particularly involved. A book by Samuel Huntington, *The Clash of Civilizations*, which foresaw this historical phase, is significantly uncertain about attributing to Africa a role among the clashes. Throughout the world Africa is considered interesting, not from a point of view of strategic power but from an economic point of view, which is new. After the long season of reforms sponsored by the International Monetary Fund, many economic agreements were made within the free market, encouraged by the New Partnership for Africa's Development, which was set up by African presidents in order to introduce Africa to the world market. Following the example of China, which was then firmly in the lead in terms of business volume, the old and new strategic players—Europe and the United States but also Turkey, India, Brazil, South Korea, and others—started increasing their trade with African countries, which are rich in raw materials and also potential customers, each in their own way and with their own conditions. Over 320 new consulates and embassies were opened in Africa from 2010 to 2016, a phenomenon explained by the economic press:

> Africa is the last major emerging market. It is the continent that will have a massive increase in its population from now to 2050. It is the

region that has over 60 percent of all the unexploited arable land in the world. As well as vast deposits of hydrocarbons, raw materials and precious metals. It is a dynamic, growing continent. . . . Sub-Saharan economies are expected to increase by 20 percent between 2015 and 2020. . . . A new middle class is making its way in Africa. The per capital GDP in the sub-Saharan regions has increased by 40 percent compared to 2000.[34]

The rates of economic expansion in African countries since 2000 have been above the world average, especially since 2009, with annual percentages at 3 to 4 percent in sub-Saharan countries and peaks of nearly 10 percent in Angola, Ethiopia, Mozambique, Zambia, Nigeria, Rwanda, Kenya, and Tanzania.[35] The driving force came from the energy sector, but some countries are performing well economically even without oil or natural gas. In the twenty years from 1980 to 2000, the GDP of sub-Saharan Africa dropped by 20 percent, whereas from 2007 to 2017 it increased by around 30 percent.

Thanks to Africa's new social and economic dynamics, it is also no longer the continent with impossible communications. In just a few years, from 1999 to 2008, the percentage of Africans with a mobile phone increased from 10 to 60 percent.[36] It was the same for smartphones, with a six-fold increase from 2014 to 2019. The digital divide between sub-Saharan countries and the rest of the world, which was enormous in the 1990s, shrank year after year. In 2019, 526 million Africans used the Internet on the continent—39.3 percent of the population—compared with 53.6 percent in Asia and 87.2 percent in Europe, but from 2000 to 2019 telecommunications spread six times faster in Africa than in Asia and sixteen times faster than in Europe.[37] Having a mobile phone first, then a smartphone with access to Internet, transforms people's relationship with society and the whole world, acts as a driving force for the economy, and feeds the imagination of the young generations, who long to live in a consumer society. Technology makes up for the lack of other aspects of life and makes it possible for society to skip steps in its development. The smartphone, for example, compensates not only for the chronic inadequacy of the landline telephone networks but also for the difficulty in personal banking. By now in many African countries, payments are made with smartphones.

A whole continent is gradually moving into a new era, however with disparities, backlashes, neocolonial phenomena such as land grabbing,[38] and dramatic mass migration. There are also situations like those described by Alexis de Tocqueville: when resources, well-being, schooling, and culture increase fast in a society, what the public (and in particular young people) tolerated before in terms of poverty, injustice, and inequality suddenly becomes unbearable. Growing and acquiring a new geopolitical role, Africa wants a future, and its people are insisting on improvements in conditions in society and at work. A young middle class of Africans is emerging who want to study and become more aware of their potential. In 1990, 57 percent of all the people in Africa were poor; by 2012 the figure had fallen to 43 percent, according to the World Bank statistics.[39] This is encouraging, even though in many countries the gap between the small rich minority and the large majority of people who are by no means wealthy is increasing. In the larger countries the increasing number of nouveaux riche multimillionaires is not preventing the creation of a middle class. The spread of so-called nontransmissible diseases, such as obesity, diabetes, and heart conditions, indicates that Africa is less and less the continent of hunger and scarcity. In the meantime, the continent's leaders are again the proud protagonists, which leads them to constantly call for "African solutions to African problems," almost as though it were an official doctrine.

The challenge of sustainable development, with dignified health systems that are self-financed with national resources, more so than in the past involves the creation of efficient tax systems. The problem is that they are taking a very long time. DREAM has taken this into account, as have the many international development cooperation organizations, in the hope that African countries will become more autonomous and self-sufficient. In the specific case of DREAM, a sustainable balance will have to be found between the resources it can procure on its own and the amount provided by the countries that benefit from its naturally expanding programs. This is becoming more and more relevant because there are increasing interactions in DREAM's partnerships with African governments and their public health systems in the field of health care policy, in therapeutic practices, and in hiring and training personnel.

## GLOBAL HEALTH

The billions of dollars poured into the fight against HIV so far have produced more efficient infrastructures, better services, diagnostics that previously did not exist, and trained and motivated personnel. The history of AIDS in Africa is also the history of an opportunity offered and often taken. Stronger health care systems have been created and are easier to access thanks to decentralization processes, to a different extent from country to country. DREAM is a typical case of the effect of AIDS on the African health care system in that the fight against the pandemic made it possible to provide stronger and more widespread health care throughout the countries than there had ever been before.

DREAM built a system that is valid because of the therapies and diagnostics taken from Western medical practice and also because of its ability to make the patients aware of their clinical condition, which is essential for adherence. It makes sense to use this system to deal with other pathologies too. The day hospitals at the DREAM centers have the clinical data of hundreds of thousands of patients who arrived HIV-positive, immunodepressed, and vulnerable and who have to deal with countless infections and pathologies related to HIV. The acronym AIDS refers to a "syndrome," which means a "set of symptoms": people who are HIV-positive can get any disease because they no longer have effective barriers against viruses, bacteria, fungi, parasites, and all types of carcinogens. The HAART regimen reconstitutes their immune system within the limits indicated by the patients' condition at the beginning of the therapy, but the patients are not always able to fully recover their defenses, and they are more susceptible to infection than people who are HIV-negative. Anyone who has treated AIDS patients in Africa knows that several pathologies often have to be treated at the same time. This is true in the initial phases of the treatment but also, to a lesser extent, when the disease becomes chronic. So, having fought AIDS now makes it possible to do much more with the same infrastructures and with the same know-how acquired to fight AIDS. In particular, the molecular biology laboratories that DREAM has set up in many countries and then entrusted to ad hoc trained African biologists and technicians are useful not only for AIDS but for all infectious diseases and for cancer.

This is how, in 2015, DREAM 2.0 was set up,[40] which meant that DREAM no longer represented only a model for fighting HIV/AIDS and malnutrition. It was now also a multipurpose platform, a model for the treatment of other infectious diseases and chronic pathologies common in Africa. The same software that tracks every contact of every DREAM patient and makes it possible to check on them at a distance has over time become useful for telemedicine, asking for second opinions and specialists' opinions, remote diagnostics, and prescriptions for patients with different needs.[41] DREAM personnel were first trained to treat AIDS patients and then to prevent and treat other pathologies too. For example, there is cervical cancer, which affects African women more than women elsewhere. HIV-positive women are particularly vulnerable to cervical cancer, and many die from it. While treating AIDS, DREAM often ended up treating this pathology too. Screening had been taboo because it was carried out with a vaginal smear, but DREAM was able to overcome this. African women are not used to going to a gynecologist, they do not generally have medical examinations, and they often give birth without the assistance of an obstetrician. Cervical cancer can be prevented and can be cured if dealt with in time, but it thrives in conditions of ignorance and concealment. The familiarity and trust created in the DREAM centers among the activists, personnel, and patients make it possible to overcome this ancestral reserve and therefore to prevent and treat this cancer.

Cervical cancer is an example of how facilities and services created to treat HIV/AIDS can be used for many other pathologies too, from TB, which is increasing and has become very resistant and difficult to treat, to epilepsy, which is neglected in African societies, to COVID-19 and new noncommunicable diseases. In fact, there is a considerable increase by now in Africa in risk factors for chronic diseases such as obesity. There is the need to address what is called the double burden of malnutrition due to excess, which is new for the continent and therefore also for its public health systems. High blood pressure, heart diseases, and diabetes are increasing in Africa, along with the number of adults and elderly people, thanks to their longer life expectancy. For the DREAM centers with clinics and laboratories that specialize in treating HIV-positive patients' nutritional issues, it is not difficult to start paying attention to these pathologies, with blood tests, electrocardiograms, specialist teleconsultations, and so on.

The concept of global health is therefore also involving Africa, and for this reason HIV/AIDS may finally be eradicated. It may be through a perfectly optimized 90-90-90 Initiative, perhaps in the perspective of eradicating the virus progressively, district by district, thanks to widespread coverage, as proposed by DREAM.[42] The spread of the HAART regimen has already produced a considerable reduction of the virus. But it is also reasonable to hope for the continuous progress of medical research. There may not be a vaccine, which everyone has been expecting for decades, but maybe, just maybe, it will be possible to eliminate HIV from the sanctuary cells where it hides and where the triple therapy, despite making it harmless, is unable to eradicate it. This would change AIDS from a chronic disease needing constant therapy to one that people can fully recover from, with no further need for treatment.

In any case, the Afro-pessimism that dominated the history of AIDS in Africa is by now groundless, and this book proves how wrong it was. There is still the challenge of the economic sustainability of the treatment, which has marked the history of AIDS in Africa from the very beginning. However, this financial distress, which has never diminished, does not prevent Africa from seeing that it can be free of HIV.

However, the hope of overcoming the HIV emergency must not mean forgetting that AIDS killed tens of thousands of people in Africa, produced countless orphans, destroyed entire generations, and reduced life expectancy. Since 1996 the triple antiretroviral therapy has made it possible for many people to survive AIDS, but for years only the West had been able to benefit from it. Yet most of the AIDS patients throughout the world lived south of the Sahara. The development cooperation agencies talked about the right to treatment, but they denied Africa this right. They said that the antiretroviral drugs were for everyone, but it was not considered possible to use them in Africa, and there was a list of logical reasons to justify this standpoint. The same politicians, senior officials, academics, and scientists who advocated the universal right to treatment were also trying to convince public opinion worldwide that Africans could not be treated, for both economic and anthropologic reasons, and that they just had to be taught to be sexually responsible and be provided with condoms. This was happening while in Europe, North America, and elsewhere there were wealthy people, AIDS was being treated. What prevailed was a blanket of indifference, not reasoning. The leaders of the international multilateral organizations, as well as the "most important" countries, all followed their own interests and decided who would live and who would die.

An overall picture the history of AIDS in Africa cannot be formed unless it starts from single, decisive elements. This commonsense rule, which is well known in every branch of science, was applied here, starting with the experience of DREAM. The way DREAM evolved is symbolic of the way AIDS was stemmed in Africa: not mainly thanks to plans and announcements from illustrious international institutions but by virtue of the sensitivity of civil society, of the secular or religious piety of many people, of the patients' refusal to give in when they were close to dying.

AIDS was finally dealt with in Africa the right way (how else if not with therapy and a sense of humanity?), thanks to the unconventional initiatives of compassionate men and women, idealistic development cooperation organizations, African patriots, HIV-positive activists, nonconformist intellectuals, and doctors determined to carry out their profession fully, all of whom refused to accept the prevailing Afro-pessimism and who dared go beyond the idea of prevention alone. Then, of course, there were international officers, large multilateral agencies, wealthy countries with their development cooperation organizations, presidents, and famous philanthropists who contributed to fighting AIDS effectively in sub-Saharan Africa and who to some extent made up for the previous attitudes of indifference and inertia. However, they did so after all the volunteers on the front line against therapeutic denial were already active in the fight against AIDS. It is to the latter that this unconventional book on AIDS is dedicated.

## NOTES

1. Elisa Manacorda, "Peter Piot: "Per battere Hiv, i farmaci non bastano," *La Repubblica*, December 1, 2016, https://www.repubblica.it/salute/prevenzi

one/2016/11/29/news/world_aids_day_hiv_virus_epidemia_novartis-153089754/.

2. Sachs, "End of AIDS."
3. Denis, "Pour une histoire sociale du sida," 26.
4. Marseille, Hofmann, and Kahn, "HIV Prevention before HAART," 1851.
5. See UNAIDS, "HIV Treatment in Africa: A Looming Crisis," June 15, 2015, http://www.unaids.org/sites/default/files/media_asset/HIVtreatmentinAfrica_en.pdf.
6. The U=U campaign was launched internationally by anti-AIDS activists in 2016 in order to show that the antiretroviral therapy taken properly made it possible to avoid transmitting HIV to one's partner(s) through sexual intercourse.
7. The mathematical result of an initial baseline of 90 out of 100, which at the second stage became 81 and at the third stage became 72.9.
8. UNAIDS, *UNAIDS Data 2018*.
9. UNAIDS, *UNAIDS Data 2019*.
10. UNAIDS, *UNAIDS Data 2018*, 2.
11. See Médecins Sans Frontières, "Despite Better Access to Treatment, Many AIDS Patients in African Hospitals Still Die," press release, November 27, 2015, https://www.msf.org/hivaids-despite-better-access-treatment-many-aids-patients-african-hospitals-still-die.
12. Jean-Baptiste Sagno, a doctor at the Blantyre DREAM center, interview by the author, May 22, 2018.
13. See Palombi et al., "Predicting Trends in HIV-1 Sexual Transmission."
14. Lewis, *Race against Time*, 201. The French edition, *Contre la montre*, is even harsher.
15. See Kates, Wexler, and Lief, *Financing the Response to HIV*.
16. Because of waste and scandals, many national commissions set up to fight AIDS were subject to sanctions by the international aid community, including interruptions of funds. Above all, it was the single development cooperation organizations from Western countries that stopped providing funds or suspended them (but there were also some multilateral organizations, such as the Global Fund).
17. "'For God's Sake, Please Stop the Aid!,'" *Spiegel*, July 4, 2005, https://www.spiegel.de/international/spiegel/spiegel-interview-with-african-economics-expert-for-god-s-sake-please-stop-the-aid-a-363663.html.
18. See Moyo, *Dead Aid*.
19. "The Wit and Wisdom of Dambisa Moyo, Her Supporters and Critics," *Telegraph*, January 8, 2011, https://www.telegraph.co.uk/finance/economics/8247831/The-wit-and-wisdom-of-Dambisa-Moyo-her-supporters-and-critics.html.
20. "Wit and Wisdom."
21. Afewerki has supported these theories in various interviews. This is one of the best known: "Anyone who takes aid is crippled. Aid is meant to cripple people." YouTube, April 5, 2015, https://www.youtube.com/watch?v=khFTrp7AygQ.

See also "Interview with Eritrea's Isaias Afewerki," *Financial Times*, September 18, 2009, in which Afewerki refers to Moyo's book, which had just been published.

22. "Aid Is Political, Markets Are Neutral," speech to the Capital Markets East Africa International Conference in Kigali, February 12, 2015, YouTube video, https://www.youtube.com/watch?v=Qh26sXNj7eY.

23. Paul Kagame, "Africa Has to Find Its Own Road to Prosperity," *Financial Times*, May 7, 2009.

24. *The Paris Declaration on Aid Effectiveness and the Accra Agenda for Action*, OECD (Organisation for Economic Co-operation and Development), 3, https://www.oecd.org/dac/effectiveness/34428351.pdf.

25. Knight, *UNAIDS*, 38.

26. See UNAIDS, "'Three Ones' Key Principles," conference paper, April 25, 2004, http://data.unaids.org/una-docs/three-ones_keyprinciples_en.pdf. On the origins of "Three Ones," see Piot, *No Time to Lose*, 335–36.

27. Katherine Marshall, "Opening Remarks" (3rd International DREAM Conference, "A Dream for Africa: Children without AIDS," Rome, May 27, 2005), text in DAR.

28. Mario Giro (handwritten notes), DREAM meeting with the Ghanaian, Nigerian, DRC, and Kenyan ministries of health, Rome, May 28, 2005, in DAR.

29. Instructions sent by mail from Massimo Magnano to Mario Giro regarding Accordo Congo, July 5, 2005, copy in DAR.

30. "The Community of Sant'Egidio – DREAM. 2004 Balzan Prize for Humanity, Peace and Fraternity among Peoples," https://www.balzan.org/en/prizewinners/comunita-di-sant-egidio-dream.

31. For more about the Millenium Development Goals adopted in September 2000 through the *United Nations Millennium Declaration*, and about the reached targets, see See http://www.un.org/fr/millenniumgoals/bkgd.shtml.

32. Brunel, *L'Afrique*, 79.

33. Marshall, *Conflict Trends in Africa*, 3.

34. Roberto Bongiorni, "Economia e demografia, crescita doppia dell'Africa," *Il Sole 24 Ore*, June 16, 2019.

35. See the reports on sub-Saharan Africa published by the International Monetary Fund in 2010, *Regional Economic Outlook: Sub–Saharan Africa, Back to High Growth* (https://www.imf.org/en/Publications/REO/SSA/Issues/2017/01/07/Regional-Economic-Outlook-Sub-Saharan-Africa6), and in 2020, *Regional Economic Outlook: Sub–Saharan Africa, A Difficult Road to Recovery* (https://www.imf.org/en/Publications/REO/Issues/2020/10/20/Regional-Economic-Outlook-October-2020-Sub-Saharan-Africa-A-Difficult-Road-to-Recovery-49787)..

36. Aker and Mbiti, "Mobile Phones and Economic Development," 208.

37. See the data provided by the Internet World Stats and Peroni and Bartolo, "Digital Divide," 101–9, 105.

38. This involves taking land and selling it to foreign governments or multinational companies without the consent of the communities that live on and cultivate it.

39. See Beegle et al., *Poverty in a Rising Africa.*
40. The acronym is the same, but what it stands for today is different: no longer "Drug Resource Enhancement against AIDS and Malnutrition" but rather "Disease Relief through Excellent and Advanced Means."
41. See Bartolo and Ferrari, *Multidisciplinary Teleconsultation.*
42. See Palombi et al., "Predicting Trends in HIV-1 Sexual Transmission."

# 5

# Access for All

The history of AIDS in Africa has two main phases, the first of which was a tragedy in terms of the cost of human lives, and goes from the years of prevention alone to the start of the antiretroviral treatment in 2002 and 2003. Until 1996 prevention alone was fully justified because there was no therapy for AIDS, whereas from 1996 to 2002 it was more of an ideological approach because the therapy now existed. The second phase goes from 2002 and 2003, when the treatment became legal, up to today and consists of a gradual transition from an initially minimalistic approach to a commitment to universal access to treatment.

The economic aspect of the history of AIDS in Africa is crucial from a cost-effectiveness perspective. This perspective was often conditioned by the intention to spend and fund as little as possible. Actually, saving the lives of people with AIDS in sub-Saharan countries was economically advantageous. Moreover, it became more and more obvious, on the basis of what had been done in the West, that universal access to treatment could bring the epidemic under control. This was the main way to eradicate or at least stem HIV/AIDS. Nonetheless, the large development cooperation agencies and politicians generally persisted in establishing restrictive criteria and limiting access to the therapies in Africa. It was as though they were compelled to limit themselves, not to dare—even the health experts who were aware that it was possible to attack the pandemic more effectively.

What was behind this attitude? There are several possible explanations: fear of wasting resources, reluctance to fall out of line with the generally acknowledged Afro-pessimism, the tendency to act according to short-term economic calculations, the idea that the Africans did not deserve to receive investments, acceptance of unequal standards in different regions in the world, and so on. It was a sort of mental dissociation: the experts knew what had to be done but were afraid of violating the restrictions that they themselves had enforced.

The first phase, from prevention alone to the start of therapy, has been discussed at length in this book. The second phase is described in detail here: overcoming therapeutic minimalism, in which the story of DREAM is an example in the history of AIDS in Africa.

In 2002 people who wanted to take HAART to Africa could refer to the new guidelines for treating AIDS in resource-limited settings, which the WHO had finally drawn up.[1] These guidelines were necessary for the governments to be able to authorize the therapies, but at the same time they were too restrictive. The therapeutic protocols that DREAM wanted to adopt in Africa were perfectly acceptable because they followed what was already being done in the West.[2] However, what DREAM wanted was radically different from the WHO's guidelines, which involved procedures, therapies, and diagnostics that aimed to save money and were therefore second-rate and frequently produced poor results. Neither were there any alternatives for limiting the mother-to-child transmission of HIV, such as caesarean section and formula milk, which could only be carried out safely in developed countries. In Africa they were out of the question because of the poor hygiene in the hospitals where the procedure could be performed and the lack of clean water available for formula milk, which in any case was far too expensive for most mothers.

Given the difference between DREAM's protocols, taken from its experience in the West, and those prescribed by the WHO for countries with limited resources, there was no alternative for DREAM but to invest as much as possible in scientific research. Western medical excellence not only had to be made acceptable in the African context but improved, based on the empirical observation of what was being done for all the people with AIDS, of whom there were far more than in the United States and Europe. Once the protocols used in rich countries had been brought to sub-Saharan Africa, they had to be studied and their effectiveness checked, also in terms of their practicability. The advantage of DREAM lay in the vast number of patients who would be reached year after year and whose clinical data could be entered and stored in a unique database and used for research. These were not clinical trials carried out in vitro, in a specifically equipped environment and with limited timing. DREAM's researchers carried out studies in real situations, with large numbers of patients and over long periods of time.

The first obstacle to overcome was when to start the therapy. This was a critical point on which the expansion of the treatment to millions of HIV-positive people and also universal access to treatment depended. HAART was prescribed in the West to patients with fewer than 350 CD4s, whereas in the 2002 WHO guidelines for starting the treatment in poor countries, the threshold was under 200 CD4s. When it was impossible to measure this immunological threshold, which was often the case, only symptomatic patients in a severe condition could receive the antiretroviral therapies because they definitely had very few CD4s.[3] The WHO classified HIV/AIDS patients according to four clinical stages: (1) asymptomatic, (2) mild symptoms, (3) advanced symptoms, and (4) severe symptoms. Stage 4 patients were to be treated regardless of their CD4 count, and stage 3 patients were to be monitored and put on therapy before their CD4s fell below 200, whereas stage 2 and stage 1 patients were not to be treated unless their CD4 count was extremely low.

When the treatment was carried out on patients whose bodies were very weak, it was not always able to help the immune system recover from HIV. The consequences were dramatic mortality in the short term and decreased chances of long-term survival because the immune defense system only recovered partially and the patients were highly exposed to infection and disease. How was it possible to start treating African patients without waiting for the often fatal fall in their CD4 count to below 200 or for the devastation wrought by acute opportunistic diseases? It was a question of reaching as many HIV-positive people as possible, which was the opposite approach to that taken by experts who, as mentioned above, gave the go-ahead to the antiretroviral treatment in Africa but at the same time, for economic reasons, tried to limit the number of HIV-positive people to treat. In fact, the legal threshold of 200 CD4s was established in order to create a *numerus clausus* (a limit on the number) of patients. The slogan was "cost and feasibility." This was epidemiologically counterproductive: the fewer patients treated, the longer HIV stayed infectious because the HIV-positive people who were not treated were carriers of the virus, unlike those who were treated, whose viral load decreased until they were no longer infectious.

DREAM could only operate in every country with authorizations from local governments that followed the international guidelines to the letter. Moreover, its ability to receive financial and logistic resources also mainly depended on its staying within these guidelines. For example, the Global Fund provided the antiretroviral drugs only if the organizations using them followed the internationally approved therapeutic schemes. It was therefore impossible to elude the WHO protocols, even though the WHO did have a double standard in order to take into account the different spending capacities of rich and poor countries and the resistance in funding of the various donor countries. In order to counter these strict guidelines, DREAM qualified its initiatives, where the governments allowed it, as operative research through pilot projects—that is, experimental activities aimed at innovation, which as such could be carried out despite the guidelines. This way the HIV-positive people monitored by DREAM were able to start treatment without waiting for their CD4s to fall below 200, when their immune system had already been affected but was not compromised, which was the approach generally taken in the West.

The comparison between the therapeutic protocols adopted by DREAM experimentally in sub-Saharan Africa and the therapeutic protocols established by the WHO shows that the former were constantly ahead of the latter in terms of results. There was absolutely nothing wrong with that because the WHO provides indications for the whole world; it has to study and compare scientific progress very carefully before accepting any new proposals and cannot afford to jump the gun. The WHO is neutral, and its school of thought does not rule out anything. It brings together and legitimizes advances in knowledge, treatments, and health policies that are presented and then studied impartially by its experts. What counts is the experimental data, not ethical prejudice. The WHO is the mirror of, and is guided by, the scientific community. If the scientific community is held back by economic scruples, as in the case of AIDS in countries with limited resources, this conditions the WHO. Besides, the WHO guidelines for countries with limited resources have changed continuously from the first ones issued in 2002 to today's, in a constant search for what is best. Year by year the guidelines extended the criteria for administering the triple antiretroviral therapy in countries with limited resources. The first guidelines, whether out of skepticism regarding the resources available or in order to endorse the very cautious scientific opinions of the time, adopted minimal criteria, which at least guaranteed that the standard would not be too low, whereas high-quality therapy could be administered in certain circumstances. It was believed that because of the economic and social conditions of many countries, only limited action was possible, and in the meantime the scientific community, the large development cooperation agencies, and the organizations working in these countries would propose new and better solutions. If they were convincing, they would be approved.

From 2002, DREAM researchers worked to make it possible for the WHO to approve the operative findings of the DREAM program to treat AIDS in Africa in terms of its feasibility, safety, and the efficacy of Western therapeutic solutions as well as to be adopted in countries with limited resources. The aim was to bring the standards accepted in the Global North and Global South in line with each other. For this purpose, essays and scientific papers were produced, and researchers also looked for allies among the organizations working in the field, in the research centers, in the universities, and in the institutions.[4] DREAM's philosophy was shared by prominent figures in the fight against AIDS, including Kevin De Cock, Karin Nielsen-Saines, Jeffrey Sachs, Stefano Vella, and others and also by institutions such as the prestigious CDC and the Italian National Institute of Health.

As far as the threshold for starting therapy was concerned, in 2002, depending on the geographical area, it was either 350 CD4s or 200 CD4s, or else it just depended on the clinical symptomatology. DREAM immediately took an antiminimalist position. It is worth mentioning the first results of the observation carried out on thousands of DREAM patients, presented in 2004 on various occasions.[5] It was summed up by three academic scholars connected with DREAM (Leonardo Palombi, Carlo Federico Perno, and Cristina Marazzi) in an article in *AIDS*, the International AIDS Society's journal. The authors questioned the effectiveness of limiting the treatment to severe cases of full-blown AIDS. The better the condition of the immune system to start with, the better the patient's response to the therapy—that is, the outcome of the interaction between the drugs and the patient's immune system. By contrast, patients whose immune system was severely compromised and who started treatment with only a few CD4s and a high viral load responded poorly to the treatment. Mortality in the subgroup of patients who started treatment with less than 50 or between 51 and 200 CD4s was 6.6 and 3.4 times greater, respectively, than in patients who started treatment when they had more than 200 CD4s. Likewise, the risk of dying was higher in patients who started treatment with a high viral load (above 100,000 HIV-RNA copies/milliliter).[6]

After studying the effectiveness of the therapy in relation to the condition of the immune system, Palombi, Perno, and Marazzi wanted to stop treating only the weakest HIV-positive people and instead involve as many patients as possible. They also reported that the therapy itself made a decisive contribution to prevention because it reduced the viral load, so with a larger number of HIV-positive patients on therapy, fewer HIV-positive people were infectious.[7] This concept was not accepted at all internationally. Only in 2012 did the WHO formally end the prevention or treatment dichotomy with the publication of its report *Antiretroviral Treatment as Prevention (TasP) of HIV and TB*.[8] In 2004 this was a long way off. For years the condom had been turned into an ideal, and the antiretroviral drugs had been completely ignored, as though one approach excluded the other. So, the lesson from the experience of HIV in the West from 1996 onward had not been learned: treatment also meant prevention, and prevention did not exclude the use of the condom but was much more than that.

According to Palombi, Perno, and Marazzi, the only way to understand that treatment was the best form of prevention was by treating vast numbers of HIV-positive people, including the asymptomatic patients, who were the majority. If a decision was taken to treat only the symptomatic patients, the benefits in terms of prevention were very limited. It was, in fact, mainly apparently healthy people who transmitted the virus, through sexual intercourse.[9]

The approach these scholars recommended, then, involved

treating as many patients as possible and as well as possible, not only for ethical reasons but also in order to get the disease under control, which in the medium term would compensate the high short-term costs of offering valid treatment to many people, if not everyone. There was not yet even any talk about universal access to treatment for all HIV-positive people in 2004. It was unthinkable, would have sounded utopian, and was very different from the idea of relaxing the tight limits of the official guidelines.

Palombi, Perno, and Marazzi's request for extended access to treatment went together with their request for excellent treatment, with particular reference to diagnostics. After the question of the eligibility thresholds for treatment, this was another way that DREAM challenged the minimalist approach to treatment. At the beginning, the international guidelines limited diagnostics to just the CD4 count and ignored the measurement of the viral load, which, despite being far more complex and expensive, was standard practice in the West. The widespread opinion was that the lack of adequate health facilities in the poor countries justified the distribution of antiretroviral drugs, with no virological studies carried out on the patients—just immunological or clinical findings, which were easier and cheaper to obtain. In the case of severely symptomatic patients, these diagnostic procedures were considered superfluous for starting treatment. These minimalistic criteria were also accepted by the 3 by 5 Initiative launched by the WHO in 2002 (three million AIDS patients to be treated in Africa by 2005), which estimated that there were three million Africans with fewer than 200 CD4s or who had severe symptoms. However, without good diagnostics, the treatment was necessarily carried out badly because HAART required constant and precise monitoring.

DREAM constantly clashed with the double clinical and diagnostic standard between poor countries and rich countries. In 2005 the WHO acknowledged the validity of DREAM's accomplishments by publishing a case study summarizing DREAM's work and scientific progress called *DREAM: An Integrated Faith-Based Initiative to Treat HIV/AIDS in Mozambique; Case Study*. This was official recognition, although with some reservations. A WHO official added the following significant note to the description of the molecular biology laboratories that DREAM considered necessary for the measurement of the patients' viral load and for monitoring the results of the therapy as well as possible:

> Viral load testing is not currently considered essential under World Health Organization (WHO) antiretroviral treatment guidelines for resource-poor settings as a mean of guiding decision-making on initiating treatment or the regular monitoring of ART response. . . . These [viral load] tests are undertaken for patients by the DREAM project on an exceptional basis through the availability of specially dedicated laboratory resources.[10]

In fact, in the first guidelines in 2002 and the next ones in 2004, it was not considered necessary to measure the viral load in countries with limited resources because of the high costs and technical complexity of the test.[11]

DREAM argued that measuring the viral load was decisive both for starting therapy and in the clinical follow-up because referring to the CD4 count alone led to treating the patients at an advanced stage, when their immunological system was already compromised and they had severe opportunistic diseases. Moreover, with the CD4 count alone, it was not possible to diagnose a therapeutic failure in time to be able to save the patients. The advantage of measuring the viral load was that it provided an early and precise indication of the patient's condition so the treatment could be decided quickly and carried out properly, thus saving many more people's lives. DREAM's experience on the field had shown that a high viral load, and then also a certain level of anemia and a significant reduction in the body mass index were powerful predictors of mortality. In other words, they warned of the danger better than the condition of the immune system—that is, the number of CD4s left. Above all, when the treatment had started, measuring the viral load was the best way of monitoring the therapy: it made it possible to prevent resistances and consequent early abandonment of the first lines of therapy, to verify the effectiveness of the therapy and avoid failure, to highlight side effects, and to see when the patients were not adhering to the therapy.[12]

Naturally there were great differences in costs between counting CD4 lymphocytes and measuring the viral load. The CD4 count was cheaper and faster, but it offered less precise and less immediate information. Measuring the viral load indicated earlier than by counting the CD4s whether the therapy was working. One could say that the viral load represented the actual situation, whereas the CD4 count was just an indication. However, looking at the real situation instead of an indication of it is more expensive because of the complexity of the laboratories, the need for specialized personnel, and the cost of the reagents. The CD4 count was also useful, though. Because it could be performed easily and often, it could be carried out as one of the ordinary monitoring activities and could indicate if there was a need to measure the viral load urgently and more often than twice a year, which was the frequency generally indicated in the Western protocols.

This approach is similar to how all patients in hospitals have their temperature and blood pressure measured every day regardless of the various diagnostic tests or complex operations they may have to undergo. Another example is how patients with diabetes have their blood sugar level checked every day, regardless of how complex their therapy may be. The same applies to AIDS patients, whose CD4s are checked frequently so that if there is a problem with the therapy, it can be caught in time. The viral load, however, is measured less often or when the therapy is not working, which is be indicated by the CD4 count. Checking the number of CD4s is also useful because low levels of these lymphocytes correspond to a high risk of opportunistic infectious diseases (tuberculosis, cryptococcosis, pneumocystis carinii pneumonia, and more). It was therefore good for both the immunological and the virological aspects to be taken into consideration. The DREAM protocols used the two diagnostic procedures, following the example of what was done in the West.

The international guidelines for countries with limited resources, which were initially against measuring the viral load, gradually started to include this test. In 2006 the WHO confirmed: "Because resources are limited, laboratory testing should generally be directed by signs and symptoms and should be done only when the results can be used to guide management decisions. . . . Routine monitoring of CD4 cell counts (if available) is recommended every six months, or more frequently if clinically indicated."[13] As for the viral load, "HIV viral load measurement is currently not recommended for monitoring patients on ART in resource-limited settings."[14] Also: "Viral load measurements . . . are unlikely to be widely available in low-resource settings at present and are an expensive way to monitor adherence."[15] There did, however, seem to be an initial acknowledgment of its value: "In adults and adolescents, viral load testing may contribute to the diagnosis of ART failure earlier than would happen if only clinical and CD4 monitoring were in place."[16] In the meantime, many advocates of very simple treatments in Africa were changing their mind. This may have been the consequence of the very different results of therapy between the rich countries and the poor countries, which by now was well known,[17] or else it was because of new parameters in assessing cost-effectiveness.

An article published in January 2007 was a typical example of this approach: "HIV Viral Load Monitoring in Resource-Limited Regions: Optional or Necessary?" Its many authors came from MSF, the Harvard Medical School, the Clinton Foundation, and Swiss, Belgian, Australian, and Ugandan scientific and health institutions. Just a few years earlier these organizations had differing views on the matter: some were in favor of prevention and some of treatment. The beginning of the article seemed to confirm the minimalist mainstream approach: "Scaling up antiretroviral therapy in resource-limited regions requires a simplified approach."[18] However, a few lines on, the tone changed completely: "As the need for viral load testing increases, technologies to determine the viral load are becoming simpler, and costs are decreasing. Given the $8.3 billion annual investment in HIV treatment in resource-limited settings, the question of whether high-quality, effective HIV care can be provided without viral load monitoring needs to be revisited." One aspect was essential: "The prices of second-line regimen drugs are currently 10-fold higher than the prices of first-line regimen drugs."[19] Switches to second-line therapies had to be avoided as much as possible. This is where the measurement of the viral load helped with first-line therapies, with suggestions of different cocktails of drugs or that the patients might not be adhering to the treatment properly. The conclusion emphasized that despite the high cost of measuring the viral load, it was useful for preventing expensive and unnecessary switches to second-line therapies.

Moreover, the article criticized the fact that in countries with limited resources, HIV-positive people could only be treated according to their CD4 count or clinical symptoms, which was considered delayed action, produced poor results, and caused resistance to the drugs. It said that instead of concentrating on providing access to the drugs to a large number of people, it would be better to offer excellent treatments and limit the costs connected to second-line therapies.

The economic aspect prevailed, of course. However, this time it aimed for an increase in the standard of the treatment offered rather than minimalism. The WHO gradually accepted this point of view, and in 2010 it updated the 2006 guidelines, recommending measuring the viral load at the first signs of immunological alarm provided by the CD4 count. Therefore, if the lymphocytes, which indicate the strength of the immune system, were decreasing instead of increasing during the treatment, this clear and worrying clinical condition would justify measuring the viral load. Countries with limited resources, above all in Africa, could finally use advanced diagnostics. Over the years the WHO's approach had changed completely. In 2013 the viral load became the first form of diagnosis of treatment failure for all populations: "Viral load is recommended as the preferred monitoring approach to diagnose and confirm ARV treatment failure."[20] In 2015 the indication was not to perform the CD4 count when it was possible to measure the viral load, which was described as routine for therapies, instead of the CD4 count.[21] In 2017 the CD4 count was no longer even necessary for eligibility for treating HIV-positive people because by then there was universal access to treatment according to the so-called test-and-treat approach.[22]

The timeline of the WHO guidelines may look unremarkable, but it highlights two important points. The first is in regard to what development cooperation agencies euphemistically call a "lesson learned"—that is, correcting a wrong approach, in this case the minimalistic and simplistic approach to AIDS in poor countries—when so many patients' lives could have been saved if higher diagnostic and therapeutic standards had been applied. There was a gradual understanding that treatments carried out well are more advantageous than treatments that aim to save money: they are economically valid because they allow people to live, become healthy again, and go back to work. They are also worthwhile because they constitute prevention: overcoming the dichotomy between treatment and prevention was essential for understanding that excellence in treatment, in particular in terms of universal access, is a profitable investment rather than a waste. It is a decisive way of blocking the pandemic.

The second point concerns the transition from one extreme to the other, from the absolutism of the CD4 count to the absolute control of the viral load. Actually, as explained above, both diagnostic procedures have a part to play in the treatment. It is worth mentioning that the world of health care is a combination of science and business. Setting up a molecular biology laboratory to measure the viral load is very expensive, and the reagents used for the tests are also very expensive. When Siemens stopped manufacturing the equipment for measuring the viral load and supplying the necessary reagents, the market became a monopoly of the United States. With millions of viral load measurements to be performed every year and no competition, a large profit was guaranteed.

## UNIVERSAL ACCESS

Overcoming the minimalistic approach to the fight against AIDS in Africa was a gradual process that started with the 3 by 5 Initiative and ended with universal access to treatment. In Africa this meant that from eight hundred thousand people with AIDS who were being treated in 2005,[23] there are now millions of people in treatment because the therapy has been extended to everyone who is HIV-positive.[24]

The WHO guidelines for resource-limited settings gradually relaxed the eligibility requirements for therapy. After years of the threshold of 200 CD4s, in 2010 it was possible to treat people with 350 CD4s regardless of their clinical condition. Moreover, it was recommended that all patients with WHO stages 3 or 4 be treated regardless of their CD4 count.[25] In 2013 the threshold was raised to 500 CD4s for starting treatment, and a series of exceptions were indicated: HIV-positive patients who have tuberculosis or hepatitis B, have HIV-positive partners, are pregnant, or are breast-feeding.[26] These HIV-positive patients could start the antiretroviral treatment regardless of any immunological or clinical observation. In September 2015 the WHO finally removed all limitations to therapy: "ART should be initiated among all adults living with HIV regardless of WHO clinical stage and at any CD4 cell count."[27] An additional "good practice statement" advocated testing and treating: "Efforts should be made to reduce the time between HIV diagnosis and ART initiation based on an assessment of a person's readiness."[28] This was universal access, and it had two goals, the first of which was for the year 2020: "90% of people living with HIV being aware of their HIV infection, 90% of those receiving antiretroviral treatment, and 90% of people on ART having no detectable virus in their blood." The second goal was to be reached in 2030, and it consisted of simply putting an end to the AIDS epidemic.[29] By then the economic aspect encouraged mass treatment: "The increased cost of earlier ART would be partly offset by subsequent reduced costs (such as decreased hospitalization and increased productivity) and preventing people from acquiring HIV infection."[30]

DREAM had always wanted to extend access to treatment, and it overcame all the thresholds one after the other. Apart from ethics, it seemed right from a medical and epidemiological point of view. For years, the way to win against minimalism was through the programs for the prevention of mother-to-child transmission (PMTCT) of HIV.[31] In the case of pregnant women, it was easier to get around the threshold for starting treatment established by the international guidelines because it was a question of prevention, more so than for other patients. Basically, progress could be made within a specific sector. The success rates were extraordinarily high because if pregnant women were put onto HAART quickly, over 98 percent of their babies were born free of HIV. This supported the decision to offer the triple antiretroviral therapy also to women who were asymptomatic and apparently in good health. Thanks to the results achieved with PMTCT, DREAM could spread the awareness that limiting, if not ending, the scourge of AIDS would take place through universal access to treatment.

In May 2011 DREAM dedicated one of its international conferences held regularly with African ministers of health to the topic of "universal access to treatment: the decisive step toward eliminating AIDS."

The following is from an article prepared by DREAM in December 2010 in preparation for the conference:

> In the past few years, over five million people in the countries in the Global South have had access to the antiretroviral treatment. This is a major success that has resulted in the decrease in new HIV infections. Many people are in therapy thanks to the efforts made by various international development coordination agencies, NGOs, and by several countries. There is hope. The antiretroviral treatment itself represents real and effective prevention with its potential to eliminate the virus from the plasma and from all the body fluids, which makes people with the virus almost not infectious at all. Practically completely eliminating the virus from the infected person's body means reducing the possibility of this person infecting other people to the same extent. In recent years this theory has often been confirmed directly and indirectly. The number of new cases in the United States and in Western Europe decreased almost five times when over 95 percent of infected people needing treatment were treated.[32]

It did look as though the scientific community was becoming familiar with the concept of universal access to treatment. Some articles that had been published over the previous two years talked about it, and in September 2010 the WHO published a progress report, *Towards Universal Access: Scaling Up Priority HIV/AIDS Interventions in the Health Sector*, authored with UNAIDS and UNICEF, which predicted that if universal access to treatment were achieved, there would be a drastic reduction in the number of HIV infections. Universal access, however, meant "universal access to treatment by 2010 for all those who need it." This concept had been formulated years before, on December 23, 2005, in UNGASS Resolution 60/224,[33] in preparation for a follow-up meeting from May 31 to June 2, 2006, when UN member states formally committed to extending the fight against AIDS in order to achieve "universal access to HIV prevention, treatment, care and support by 2010." This time, universal access meant for "at least 80% of the population in need."[34] Based on this definition, the 2010 WHO report stated that after four years, eight out of

144 countries with low or medium incomes that were supervised had reached that goal (two of these countries were African: Botswana and Rwanda). The problem was the definition of "universal access" and, in particular, the definition of "all those who need it"—that is, who the "population in need" referred to. First mentioned were the 2010 WHO guidelines, which established a threshold of 350 CD4s (raised from 200 CD4s in the 2006 WHO guidelines) or clinical stage 3 or 4 for starting treatment. The universal access they were talking about did not apply to all HIV-positive people but only the minority who presented a certain immunological or clinical condition. In fact, the 2010 report stated that administration of antiretroviral drugs had increased from 28 percent at the end of 2008 to 36 percent at the end of 2009, but it was clearly specified that this figure only concerned HIV-positive people with not more than 350 CD4s.[35]

The universal access discussed in the 2010 WHO report was not exactly universal. It would have been if it had been addressed to everyone who tested positive for HIV, but it was still a long way from the test-and-treat approach. The latter was only established by the WHO in 2015, together with the 90-90-90 goal for 2020. At the time, in 2010, putting a greater number of HIV-positive people on therapy in order to limit and control the pandemic went against the WHO's restrictions and classifications. A rough estimate of universal access according to the 2010 WHO report was around six million HIV-positive people and, according to the guidelines for starting treatment, this figure could have reached eleven million infected people throughout the world, out of a total of thirty-three million HIV-positive people.[36] Instead of universal access, this meant access to treatment for only one third of all the people who were HIV-positive.

On the other hand, the May 2011 DREAM conference was about access to treatment for all HIV-positive people. DREAM tried to motivate this option from both an economic and an epidemiological point of view in order to overcome the main objections to access that would be truly universal, concentrating on cost and feasibility.

As far as cost was concerned, Stefano Orlando, an economist, took a district of three hundred thousand people in Malawi as a model. He compared two scenarios: one of partial therapeutic coverage, which corresponded with the current system, costing $11 million a year, added to which was the cost of health care and social costs for HIV-positive people who were not treated, and a scenario of universal access to treatment, which would have cost $23 million. It turned out that the second scenario would have cost more at the beginning, but within four years the costs would have been equal. From the fifth year onward, true universal access would have been more convenient from an economic point of view because there would have been net savings for the health care system due to the reduction in both the incidence and the prevalence of the disease—that is, the number of HIV-positive people needing treatment. Orlando added a further fact: after a few months on the HAART regimen, the patients recovered their strength, increased the number of hours they worked, and their individual income increased (therefore the national revenue increased too). According to Orlando, this model would have only been valid if all the adults in the area were tested and treated immediately if they were HIV-positive because this would have radically prevented the spread of HIV. With a little imagination, Orlando hypothesized a program of test and treat for all the HIV-positive people among the 770 million inhabitants of sub-Saharan Africa, which according to a necessarily approximate calculation would cost $29 billion. This figure looks huge, but it would be a good investment considering the inversion in the trend of the economies of many African countries caused by a quarter of a century of AIDS, which lost a third of their potential GDP.[37]

The extent of the study on the area taken into consideration was less theoretical than Orlando's algorithms suggested. This was demonstrated by the epidemiological contributions to the conference. In fact, after discussing the cost of true universal access, the conference concentrated on the objection regarding feasibility. Two doctors from DREAM, Noorjehan Abdul Majid and Leonardo Palombi, presented the results of research carried out on 26,563 patients treated in Mozambique and Malawi from 2002 to 2010.[38]

Abdul Majid and Palombi were impressed by an article by Reuben M. Granich, De Cock, and other WHO researchers who were in favor of true universal access to treatment, "Universal Voluntary HIV Testing with Immediate Antiretroviral Therapy as a Strategy for Elimination of HIV Transmission: A Mathematical Model."[39] This study, which was published in 2009, took into consideration existing studies, but it was very innovative and sparked a bitter debate within the WHO. In fact, years later Margaret Chan, the director general of the WHO, said jokingly, "When the article by Granich and De Cock came out, they wanted to kill them."[40] The study proposed that therapy for everyone, after they took the test, was the best chance for eradicating HIV/AIDS. A mathematical model, in which everyone had access to the test and to the treatment, was developed in order to simulate epidemic trends over time. The result was a drastic reduction of the epidemic, with a decrease in both the incidence rate, which fell to less than 0.3 percent in three years, and in mortality. In the long run, there were no more infected people at all. Abdul Majid and Palombi supported the results of this study, with the difference that they reported the results, not of a theoretical simulation, but of research carried out on a cohort of more than twenty-six thousand real patients who had been treated for eight years. This was, therefore, not a mathematical model but one based on clinical cases, thanks to the constant computerized collection of the data on DREAM's patients.

The fact that the viral load had been measured in patients since 2002, when the international guidelines still considered it an unnecessary luxury for Africa, provided a significant scientific advantage. Moreover, the patients did not have to wait for their CD4s to fall below 200 to be treated. They started the treatment when they were near 350 CD4s, bypassing the international guidelines with the previously mentioned pilot projects. This therapeutic threshold led to a decrease not only of mortality but also of the number of contagious people. Going against the tide, both in measuring the viral load and in terms of the CD4 threshold, was now paying off. It was possible to retrospectively study patients who had been treated in the past, not following the minimalistic regulations but with far more generous criteria, similar to the ones that became part of the 2010 WHO guidelines that then led to universal access.

The study carried out by Abdul Majid and Palombi highlighted a remarkable progressive reduction of the viral load in the population—that is, of the average quantity of the virus in circulation: "A dramatic 5-fold decrease in infectivity from 1,6% to 0,3% was observed, reflecting the reduction of individual viral load with a collective reduction in infectivity after the use of triple ART in the community."[41] The annual incidence of the infection in the areas involved decreased from 7 percent to 2 percent in two years and then to 1 percent over the following years. The prevalence decreased from 12 percent to 6 percent from 2000 to 2010. Mortality decreased by 50 percent in five years. The number of HIV-positive pregnant women also decreased by 50 percent in the first five years and continued to decrease over time. An analysis of the costs indicated that this approach was economically valid after four years. Finally, there was the prospect of eradicating HIV, with the reduction to practically zero new infections in a range of 5–10 years and zero HIV-positive people within a few decades. It was not difficult for Abdul Majid and Palombi to emphasize universal access as the right policy for controlling and eradicating HIV/AIDS, by supporting the conclusions of the theoretical study by Granich et al. with real-life data. As they later stated in the journal *Clinical Infectious Diseases*, "treatment of all infected individuals translates into a drastic reduction in incident HIV infections and leads to the 'sterilization' of the epidemic."[42]

The study by Abdul Majid and Palombi was in line with the main scientific contributions to the international epidemiological debate at the time that supported truly universal access to treatment: the mathematical model of the eradication of HIV by Granich et al. of 2009; the US national HIV Prevention Trials Network research called HPTN-52, carried out on 1,763 serodiscordant couples, which ended in 2011[43]; and the studies presented by DREAM from 2007 to 2010 on mother-to-child transmission, which demonstrated how the almost total elimination of the viral load with HAART made it possible for almost 100 percent of babies to be born healthy.[44]

Abdul Majid and Palombi considered that the best way to fight AIDS in Africa was district by district, area by area:

> The DREAM model offers the advantage of gradual implementation at a district level that is chosen as a priority area. The main obstacle to universal voluntary counseling, testing, and treatment is the dimension of the ordeal, which poses enormous and unsolvable challenges from the economic and human resources perspective, and

therefore, a focused approach is preferable. Sustainability cannot be attained in a short period of time, because these changes would profoundly affect the entire health system and require a complex organizational process. . . . The focus on districts would facilitate policy choices, because areas of high prevalence or incidence could be targeted initially, or districts could be chosen if they possess adequate communication facilities and infrastructure. . . . Sterilization of the HIV epidemic, district by district, would offer the opportunity for furthering a strategy that could be scaled up, with substantial benefits to health care systems in sub-Saharan Africa.[45]

The large development cooperation agencies had a different approach. In order to provide universal access for everyone who was HIV-positive, their idea was to cover vast areas and just distribute the antiretroviral therapy, even in the absence of the necessary health care facilities. In other words: simplify matters in order to save money, offer a little but to everyone, and concentrate on distributing the drugs rather than on the more expensive diagnostic monitoring of the therapy. DREAM's model for eradicating HIV involved treating people in limited areas because this made it easier for the patients to adhere to the therapy and was more feasible for the health care facilities and less expensive in the medium term. The idea was to start from one point and gradually reach everyone through a process that would lose only very few patients and would expand to cover more and more patients.

It is worth mentioning the ideology that DREAM had to deal with at the beginning of the treatment in Africa: everybody or nobody. Something similar occurred for universal access. The hypothesis described by Abdul Majid and Palombi received scientific consensus.[46] Nonetheless, it was not accepted as a model by the international health care policies because they were conditioned by the relationships with the local governments and their political needs, which implied equality with consequential low standards if it was not possible to provide everyone with high standards all at the same time. Above all there was the question of cost—not in terms of a calculation of the costs and benefits over time but just how much had to be spent immediately. If the large development cooperation agencies and international donors had taken into greater consideration the benefits as well as the costs, they might not have acted with the aim of simplifying everything but might have acted in order to provide high standards and in a few years also to enable the African countries to benefit from an economic point of view.

## PEDIATRIC AIDS

From a historical point of view, for several reasons, children with AIDS started to receive treatment in large numbers only recently. Until a few years ago there was a significant gap in access to the antiretroviral treatment between adults (defined as older than fifteen) and children. In 2007 an HIV-positive adult had three times the possibility of receiving HAART than a child did.[47] By 2012 the gap had been halved: 58 percent of HIV-positive adults were on HAART, compared to 25 percent of the children (26 percent in Africa).[48] When there was universal access to treatment with no eligibility thresholds for treatment, the difference was far less dramatic: in 2017 it was 59 percent for HIV-positive adults and 52 percent for HIV-positive children.[49] This progress, however, must not let one forget that for years the weakest HIV-positive subjects, the children, were not treated at all. Around 2000 the infected, sick children were not even counted, as though they did not exist. The sentinel sites did not investigate them. In 2003 almost half the countries with a widespread HIV epidemic still did not have a specific health care policy for infected children. Later the disparity gradually started to decrease.

Africa is full of orphans due to AIDS. In 2006, when the antiretroviral drugs started to be administered, there were 11.5 million children who had been orphaned due to AIDS according to UNICEF.[50] However, this figure does not represent the phenomenon properly: over time AIDS produced far more orphans but with very high mortality. In any case, 2 million of these 11.5 million orphans were HIV-positive.

African HIV-positive children were much more fragile than other children, and they had to deal with a social and health care context that was in itself inhospitable. In 2010 in sub-Saharan Africa, child mortality at the fifth year of life was 10.3 percent, around fifteen times the percentage at the time in developed Western countries, where it was 0.7 percent.[51] Before universal access to treatment vastly increased the number of children in triple therapy, only 40 percent of African HIV-positive children lived until they were five years old. Death comes sooner in young infected children than in adults because the disease evolves faster. Children's immune systems are not yet fully developed, so when HIV attacks, they are immediately susceptible to serious infections, and the time of survival from infection to the full-blown stage and then death is shorter than in adults. HIV-positive children are weak, they have severe respiratory and intestinal pathologies, they are unable to absorb their food and they look undernourished, they suffer from neurological deficits, their growth is slow, and they are often so exhausted that they cannot speak or even cry.

DREAM has been looking after children since the beginning because otherwise they would have been left to a certain and early death. As the DREAM centers were being set up, they specialized in pediatric AIDS, with space provided for treating the children every week. As mentioned, very few children received treatment for AIDS in Africa at the beginning of the 2000s. Adults with AIDS were at least included in the 3 by 5 Initiative, which indicated that the administration of HAART would increase, whereas from a pharmacological point of view children were practically not catered to at all. Treating HIV-positive children involved more problems than treating adults.

First of all, there was the question of diagnosis for children under eighteen months old. Babies have their mothers' antibodies because they shared their blood flow until they were born. HIV tests are based on the search for antibodies to the virus developed by the body, so at birth all the children born from HIV-positive mothers are HIV-positive even if they are not infected themselves.

Then there was the question of administering the treatment and everything that implied. Children have to be accompanied and looked after, but there was not always anyone available to do this, given the vast numbers of orphans in the country. (Most of the HIV-positive children that DREAM looked after came from families that had been destroyed by AIDS, and 80 percent of them were left without one or both their parents.) So, there were the practical problems of adherence to the treatment and retention since the children depended on adults who were often absent or unreliable as well as the fact that the children themselves did not always even know they had AIDS.

Another crucial problem was that the antiretroviral drugs were not available with a pediatric formula. Until 2010 the pediatric antiretroviral drugs were administered as syrup, but the dosage changed continuously as the children grew, both in terms of height and weight.[52] In Europe and North America, people just about managed to use these syrups. In Africa it was different. One can imagine what it was like for these children's mothers, or more often their grandmothers, to measure the exact amount of the drug with a syringe and administer it three times a day, in a context of widespread illiteracy. HAART had become simple for adults thanks to the fixed dose of the three drugs in a single pill. This solution did not exist for children. The multinational pharmaceutical companies that produced branded antiretroviral drugs were not interested in investing in new drugs for pediatric AIDS because there was no market for them. In 2005 there were seven hundred new HIV infections in children under fifteen years old in industrialized countries, whereas there were 630,000 in children in sub-Saharan Africa. There was also a huge gap between the prevalence data on children under fifteen years old: fourteen thousand and two million, respectively.[53]

In 2006 a DREAM doctor explained the situation as follows:

> The generic first line [pediatric] drugs are formulated as syrups, three syrups, to take three times a day. Let's imagine what it means to administer the drug nine times a day and to adapt it in three cases to the square meters of the body surface, and in the other cases to the children's weight in kilogrammes. Everything to be measured in milliliters and that's not all: if the children are anemic, and this often happens, also because malaria is everywhere, if they need a second line, at least one of the syrups has to be replaced by a drug that is only available in pills. There are no pediatric formulations for these pills. So the pill has to be broken up, with the risk that the active principle is over or under dosed. The result is that taking the

therapy is extremely complex, far more so than taking the two pills a day that are necessary to control HIV in adult patients.[54]

What could be done? The DREAM activists went to the children's homes if they did not have any relatives who could look after them. In most cases, the children were orphans and lived with their grandparents, who were illiterate and had to be helped. They were given a graduated syringe with the amount they had to give marked on it with a felt-tip pen. Centiliters and milliliters are not part of their culture. Every day the activists went to check that the syrup was being administered properly. This was a sort of home-assisted therapy. It was difficult and not always satisfactory, but the alternative was the even greater risk of breaking up the pills produced for adults to take whole.

Going to the children's homes made it possible to assess their context and to identify any other primary needs that would condition the effectiveness of the therapy and to provide essential all-round health education. The children had to be guaranteed a balanced diet, clean water, basic hygiene, and mosquito nets to prevent malaria. They also had to be registered so they would not stay "invisible," and finally they had to go to school. If they were left to themselves, not supported in their health and in their social life as well, they would not be able to adhere to the treatment and would easily fall prey to opportunistic diseases brought on by AIDS. In the context of poverty in Africa, HIV and malnutrition constitute a vicious circle that can lead to death even when the children are taking antiretroviral drugs. Every HIV-positive child in need is provided with basic food (oil, flour, sugar, etc.) as well as food fortified with micronutrients until their nutritional indexes stabilize at standard values.

What is depressing, a similar topic that is always lurking, is that children who are saved from AIDS, born healthy of HIV-positive mothers, often die early anyway because, like so many other African children, they are malnourished.[55] Such children are monitored and supported by DREAM until they are two years old in order to protect their health while their mothers receive HAART so they can breast-feed safely.[56] Weaning is a crucial moment and requires nutritional education for the mothers. This is a high-risk time. When the children are around two years old, after they have been breast-fed for a long time, which is normal in Africa, their mother's milk is more water than nutrients and antibodies. The children suddenly start eating the same food as their parents (beans, meat, fried food, spices). This type of weaning often causes malnutrition, which plays a significant role in African child mortality. The DREAM staff teach the mothers how to properly wean their children who have been saved from AIDS, in order to avoid enteritis, infections, growth failure, and even death. The mothers are shown how to cook vegetable broth with fresh vegetables and are encouraged to give their children fruit such as mango, bananas, avocado, and papaya, which are easily found in the wild or at the small local markets. They are shown the nourishing food that is suitable for toddlers, which is easy to make and is cheap. If necessary, they are given food supplements with flour that is enriched with minerals and vitamins, to add to the food. What is important is that the children who have been saved from AIDS do not die because of nutrition illiteracy.

Although in Africa having children means happiness for the mothers in particular, in general whatever happens to the children does not upset society very much. Children are often not even given a name during their first year of life because of the high possibility that they might die. In many sub-Saharan countries, fewer than half the children's births are registered, so if they die or are kidnapped or sold or abused, the situation goes unnoticed by the local authorities. Their mothers have to be helped to protect their children

Another aspect of pediatric AIDS concerns adolescents. Until 2006 there were only a few adolescents who had been infected at birth by their mothers for the simple reason that their life expectancy was very short, so only a few of them had even reached puberty. Nonetheless, there were a number of African HIV-positive adolescents who did not have HIV at birth but were infected later in various ways, such as being raped on the street, sexual abuse at home, early sexual experiences, abuse carried out in religious sects, incisions performed by traditional healers, sexual blackmail from teachers in exchange for good marks, unsterilized instruments used in hospitals, and circumcision performed with blades that were not disinfected. In the following years there were many long-term adolescent patients because they were born HIV-positive but survived in a good condition, thanks to the availability of the antiretroviral drugs.

Young children usually trust adults and take their medicine without asking too many questions, but when they become teenagers they often start wondering why they have to take so much medicine. If they are not orphans, it is up to their parents to explain it to them. However, their parents are often embarrassed. Parents of adolescents often come to the DREAM centers to ask for help. They do not want to be the ones to tell their children how things stand, so they ask the DREAM staff to talk to their children. They feel guilty. On the other hand, when the teenagers find out they have AIDS, they panic and often accuse their parents of infecting them. It is easier for DREAM activists to deal with the teenagers' inner turmoil than for the parents. When teenagers find out they are HIV-positive, they are filled with distressing questions. Am I going to die soon? Will I be able to find a partner? Will I be able to love someone? Will I be able to have children? Will I have a normal life? Then there is the problem of stigma. Their peers do not know, and as they themselves did not know until shortly before, there is the fear of talking about the disease. It is not easy to hide it if they have to take all those pills at fixed times, and they are with the others at school. HIV-positive teenagers tend to be short, and adolescents are always measuring each other. A DREAM coordinator pointed out the following:

> Teenagers are in the prime of life—they have the right to smell every smell and get dirty with every color. Their life should be light and intense at the same time. When they discover that they are sick, they feel their world collapse around them. They suddenly feel fragile and alone. They look at their peers and think that their life will never be like theirs. They are envious and ashamed. The most common reaction is to close up. You take a step toward them, and they take two steps back. Then, when they accept and start the therapy, they feel naked compared to the others. The treatment does not allow for distractions. The adolescents have to follow it regularly and take their dose, and they have to do it with the fear of being discovered and isolated. . . . In general, when they start their secondary school, they go through a deep crisis and are tempted to stop the

treatment. It is not easy to deal with them. You have to listen to them and be firm, show the importance of the medicine and of a regular life, offer positive models and hope for the future, explain that science is making enormous progress.[57]

## PMTCT

In the message for the World AIDS Day of December 1, 2005, Stephen Lewis, the UN special envoy for HIV/AIDS in Africa, talked about the mother-to-child transmission of the HIV virus and of the double standard between African children, who were deprived of effective protection, and Western children, who were guaranteed the triple therapy that their mothers also benefited from:

> Why do we tolerate one regimen for Africa (second-rate) and another for the rich nations (first rate)? Why do we tolerate the carnage of African children, and save the life of every Western child? Is it possible to do full therapy in Africa rather than single dose nevirapine? Of course it is. . . . It leaves the mind reeling to think of the millions of children who should be alive and aren't alive, simply because the world imposes such an obscene division between rich and poor. That's about to change, but why does it always come after a horrific toll is taken?[58]

The path toward overcoming therapeutic minimalism in the fight against AIDS in Africa owes much to the work carried out on PMTCT of HIV. Preventing transmission of the virus depends on various factors regarding the condition of the mother from clinical, immunological, and virological points of view, the method of delivery, and the way the baby is fed. Around the year 2000 in sub-Saharan Africa, hundreds of thousands of babies were born with HIV, and they all probably died very early on. Depending on the different places and circumstances, between 35 percent and 45 percent of the children born from HIV-positive African women were infected by their mother in the uterus, during delivery, or while breast-feeding.

PMTCT was classified as prevention, so paradoxically it escaped the antitherapeutic approach of the late 1990s. Since the purpose was prevention, the use of antiretroviral drugs was permitted, although not as a triple combination but in a one-off single dose with a negligible cost, and that was easily administered. The mother was given a Nevirapine pill during labor and two similar doses were given to the newborn baby in a syrup, within the third day of life. In 1999 two similar doses of Nevirapine, at a cost of $4, were presented as a miraculous novelty that would dramatically reduce the infection rate in newborns in the poorest countries. At that time in Western countries, most pregnant women were already receiving the triple therapy, with guaranteed success in almost all cases. But the triple therapy in pregnancy cost around $900 and was considered impossible to implement in countries with limited resources. So, Nevirapine was immediately successful. Actually, its efficacy was no greater than that of another antiretroviral drug used in pregnancy in Western countries, AZT,[59] which cost around $250, and which it was also thought might be used in some way in countries with limited resources before Nevirapine was proposed in 1996. Neither Nevirapine nor AZT, administered in a single dose or together with another antiretroviral drug, was able to reduce the viral replication enough and keep it stable enough to prevent it from integrating with the DNA of the cells like the triple therapy did. Nonetheless, both Nevirapine and AZT lowered the viral load for a period, with an ephemeral semblance of efficacy.

The same illusory shortcut as AZT was adopted with Nevirapine, with additional enthusiasm due to the extremely low cost of the drug. Nevirapine was immediately sponsored as the perfect regimen for PMTCT outside the Western world. For years, many reports on AIDS produced by the most important international newspapers and the most prestigious scientific journals praised Nevirapine. The figures regarding its results varied over time, but it was generally believed that Nevirapine reduced the risk of infection by half.

Nevirapine was launched as a preventative for mother-to-child transmission by a laborious trial funded by the US National Institutes of Health. The study was carried out in Uganda from November 1997 to April 1999 on 618 women at their ninth month of pregnancy. It concluded that "Nevirapine lowered the risk of HIV-1 transmission during the first 14–16 weeks of life by nearly 50% in a breastfeeding population. This simple and inexpensive regimen could decrease mother-to-child HIV-1 transmission in less-developed countries."[60] Everyone was influenced by the concept of "simple and inexpensive" and took it for granted, as it was written in the *New York Times* in July 1999, that HAART was "impractical and too costly for third world countries."[61] The idea of a shortcut in view of saving money and of a simple procedure, was very attractive: "The low cost of Nevirapine makes it feasible for wide-scale use in many developing countries."[62] It was very good that Nevirapine was inexpensive, but unfortunately the drug was not very effective. It worked to a certain extent in the clinical trials far away from the dust of an African village or from the poverty of a rural health care center. In the field, PMTCT carried out with Nevirapine struggled to make an impact, for a variety of reasons.

Roughly speaking, half of HIV-positive pregnant women refused to be identified as such, so only half of them took the test, especially if there was no offer of treatment. Only half of the women who took the test came back for the result because the others were terrified that they were HIV-positive. Half of this remaining 25 percent were lost in desperation and stigma and did not take the Nevirapine pill, which would not have given them any guarantee of survival. So, in the end, just one-eighth of the initial number of pregnant women would have taken the single dose of Nevirapine, and an even smaller number of mothers would have completed the process by going for the subsequent checkups with their child. It was difficult to accept being condemned to a disease with an inevitable destiny and at the same time bring a child into the world who would soon become an orphan.

In any case, then, there was the breast-feeding, without the mothers receiving the therapy to bring the viral load in the milk down. Moreover, if there had been the idea of putting them on HAART, it would have been necessary to take into consideration the fact that in most cases, Nevirapine used as a single therapy develops resistance to the group to which the drug belongs (nonnucleosides; at the time, the other two groups of the triple therapy used most were nucleosides and protease inhibitors). Consequently, any therapy containing drugs of the Nevirapine group—that is, all the first line therapies used in Africa until 2010—would be compromised at least for a year. The same drawback penalized the children who were briefly exposed to Nevirapine.[63] This was known but ignored. The 2004 WHO guidelines state that "viral resistance has also been detected in HIV-infected infants exposed to short-course ARV regimens. Resistance to NVP develops rapidly and has been noted following single doses of NVP. . . . The clinical consequences of viral resistance following short-course MTCT 3 prophylaxis are unclear. The concern about resistance should be balanced with the programmatic simplicity and practicality of the single-dose NVP regimen compared with other regimens and the urgent need to expand programs to prevent MTCT."[64] The advocates of Nevirapine reaffirmed that the percentage of infected children would decrease from 35–45 percent to 15–20 percent. As already mentioned, the effects of an antiretroviral drug taken alone are only short-lived or even nonexistent. In the various trials performed on Nevirapine, a greater number of babies were observed to have been born HIV-positive. This, however, was a misleading outcome that disappeared after the perinatal period. The transmission of the virus occurs during both pregnancy and delivery and also while breast-feeding. Nevirapine had no effect at all on what happened during pregnancy. During delivery the drug appeared to be able to considerably limit the percentage of infected newborn babies, reducing the transmission of the virus since for a few days, or for a few hours, it lowered the mothers' viral load. Breast-feeding then exposed the babies to the risk of contracting HIV because they had no form of protection. The solution of formula milk was in fact impractical in Africa, not only because of the costs but also because of inadequate hygiene, which would result in high infant mortality from gastroenteritis and other infections.

Breast milk is a plasma filtrate, a yellow serum that may contain the virus, which can also be transmitted through minimal lesions of the nipple or skin. The longer the breast-feeding lasts, the greater the risk of transmission. In the 1990s the WHO, UNICEF, and UNAIDS recommended formula milk for all the babies born from HIV-positive women, but it was commonly accepted that this was not practical in

Africa because of the costs and the lack of clean water. Moreover, an African woman who used formula milk would immediately be identified as HIV-positive and therefore stigmatized. It looked like an impossible choice. Breast milk could transmit HIV, but even if the mothers could afford formula milk, it would cause death by various events induced by the lack of clean water. Also, even if breast milk could carry HIV, it had its well-known advantages in terms of antibodies and essential nutrients. It was difficult to decide between these two options because either way the consequences could well be dramatic. PMTCT, as indicated by the WHO, prescribed formula milk, but the WHO knew perfectly well that outside the West this practice went against culture and traditions. It stated the following, in a Solomon-like way: "HIV-infected women should avoid all breastfeeding when replacement feeding is acceptable, feasible, affordable, sustainable and safe. Otherwise, exclusive breastfeeding is recommended during the first months of life."[65]

Regardless of what was decided about breast-feeding, the world health systems welcomed Nevirapine in PMTCT with enthusiasm. Mother-to-child prevention was carried out throughout sub-Saharan Africa with this monotherapy for many years, in some places until 2015, like in Cameroon, which was the last country to drop it. In South Africa, on December 14, 2001, a judge of the High Court of Pretoria ordered the government, whose position was of HIV denial as requested by President Thabo Mbeki, to make Nevirapine available for women who were about to give birth, on the grounds that failure to distribute the drug violated the South Africans' constitutional right to health care. In the international press, this was called the *affaire Nevirapine*. For the occasion, the *Economist* defined the administration of Nevirapine as "this cheap and simple life-saver" because it was so easy and inexpensive:

> Judges do not normally prescribe drugs, but these are not normal times in South Africa. . . . Nevirapine is what most health economists would agree is a "no- brainer." Between 70,000 and 100,000 babies are born each year in South Africa with HIV, the virus that leads to AIDS. A couple of doses of Nevirapine have been shown to reduce by half the proportion of infected mothers who pass the virus on to

their babies around the time of birth. At its full retail price, the drug is cheap.[66]

In 2004 the WHO stated, "The simplest regimen consisted of single-dose NVP at the onset of labour plus a single dose for the infant soon after birth. Programmes to prevent MTCT (mother-to-child transmission) based on this regimen have been shown to be feasible and acceptable. There have been several years of experience in implementing such programmes."[67]

DREAM began its activities in February 2002 convinced that therapy was the decisive element of prevention. PMTCT was the ideal area in which to demonstrate this hypothesis. So, the triple therapy, or HAART, was to be administered to all the HIV-positive pregnant women from the twenty-fifth week and continued until the sixth month after delivery for those who were not eligible for treatment (those with more than 200 CD4s at the beginning of therapy that DREAM took, up to 350 CD4s, with the justification of the pilot projects), obviously to be continued indefinitely for those who were already eligible. This was the maximum allowed in an experimental context, considering that in Africa there was no HAART in PMTCT. The triple therapy, administered from the beginning of pregnancy and including the period after delivery, brings HIV infection down to practically zero during pregnancy, during delivery, and while breast-feeding (for as long as the treatment is continued). This is how 98 percent of the children born to HIV-positive mothers treated by DREAM were born and stayed HIV-negative through their first year. Without the triple therapy, it should be remembered, around 40 percent of these children would have tested HIV-positive by then. Another important aspect is that these HIV-positive women received the triple therapy because they were pregnant, without having to wait to be at an advanced stage.[68]

So, there are then two fundamental points: although the only stated intention of PMTCT was to protect babies from HIV, there was the additional aim to protect their mothers' lives too. In Africa, being an orphan is a sort of death sentence if the children are not fortunate enough to have relatives to look after them. The idea of saving babies with Nevirapine at birth did not deal with the question of maternal survival, which was as necessary for these babies as being born free of HIV.

## BREAST MILK

In the history of PMTCT, the breast milk / formula milk dilemma indicated a stark difference between the developed West and sub-Saharan Africa. For the latter, both choices were "wrong." There were serious contraindications for breast-feeding and for giving formula milk: in the first case there was the risk of a sharp increase in the number of HIV infections in children with consequent early death, and in the second case excessive mortality from gastroenteritis and other infectious diseases and related conditions.

Some scientific advances made by DREAM in the area of PMTCT concern breast-feeding for babies born from HIV-positive mothers who had been previously put on HAART. This practice was not even included in the international guidelines for Western countries, where the limited number of cases and easy replacement of breast milk with formula milk distracted researchers from investigating the possibility of breast-feeding for mothers on the HAART regimen. During the first three years of activity, the DREAM staff found it difficult to give the new mothers the specific kits with water filters, formula milk, and bottles because bottle feeding was such an unusual challenge for African women. This is what had to be done to comply with the international guidelines because it had not yet been scientifically proven that the breast milk of HIV-positive women treated with HAART was healthy. In fact, before DREAM became operative, its founders were already convinced, as they said in 2001, that the triple therapy would "allow mothers to breastfeed safely, both because of the significant reduction of the viral load in their milk and because the antiretroviral drugs were present in the mothers' milk."[69] It was now a question of translating a belief into scientific proof on the field. A series of measurements of the viral load in the milk of mothers on HAART offered reassuring data. When the triple therapy was continued after delivery it brought the transmission of HIV during breast-feeding down to zero because it significantly reduced the viral load present in the breast milk. Of course, deciding to let the mothers breast-feed involved regularly monitoring the mothers because if they did not adhere to the treatment, the viral load could increase in their milk and infect it. If, on the other hand, the mothers did adhere to the treatment, they could breast-feed their children with no risk of them becoming infected.

The scientific community became aware of this evidence through articles published by DREAM researchers in 2007.[70] One article in particular, *Treatment Acceleration Program and the Experience of of Mother-to-Child Transmission of HIV*, was based on the comparison between two cohorts of 879 and 341 children, the first given formula milk (hygiene standards respected) and the second breast-fed by their mothers. The results showed that the HIV rate of transmission was extremely low in both groups. The mortality rate at one year was 2.7 percent in the children given formula milk and 2.8 percent in those breast-fed, which are significantly lower than the general infant mortality rates of around 10 percent in their countries of origin (Mozambique, Tanzania, and Malawi).[71]

The experts were astonished with the results for breast-feeding in mothers with HIV/AIDS, but in fact DREAM was simply filling a gap in the studies. In the West, as already mentioned, there was no apparent need to investigate the matter. At the end of 2009 the WHO incorporated this scientific approach in its new recommendations on feeding infants in the context of HIV.[72] If the HAART regimen had not been so totally neglected in PMTCT in Africa, perhaps the harmlessness of breast-feeding while on the triple therapy would not have been explored only by DREAM. The fact is that DREAM did not accept therapeutic minimalism: HAART had to be administered on a wide scale in order to study the right way to feed these children. Already in 2005 DREAM had stopped giving mothers the impractical formula milk kits and was letting them breast-feed. So, in May of that year DREAM started working with young African mothers:

> We always believed that prevention should be integrated with therapy. This is how the idea of introducing the triple combination

of antiretroviral drugs, together with nutritional support, during pregnancy came about, even though it was strongly opposed in 2002, when we started putting it into practice. The aim was both to prevent mother-to-child transmission and to protect the mothers' health. One point should be underlined: the women's ability to follow an apparently complex therapeutic protocol is one of the highest in the world. . . . The transmission rate is less than 2%. What is the reason for this success? We will never get tired of repeating that the prospect of being treated and of surviving is the key element of their adhesion. This [happens] unlike with other experiences that only contemplate the preventive phase of treatment, with the administration of Nevirapine in a single dose, or similar protocols that often stop at 40–50% precisely because these approaches dramatically leave the question of maternal survival unanswered. Until now we have also assisted our women by giving them formula milk in order to avoid the transmission of the virus during breastfeeding. [Our] study, carried out in collaboration with the Italian National Institute of Health, offers precious indications regarding the safety of the breast milk of women treated with antiretroviral drugs, which removes our last reservation, so the mothers can breastfeed again.[73]

The following is a clarification regarding the above-mentioned "opposition" to the triple therapy for pregnant women. In its 2004 guidelines for countries with limited resources, the WHO recommended various regimens with one or two drugs for PMTCT, in which Nevirapine always stood out as "the simplest regimen to deliver." It also expressed some reserves regarding the triple therapy:

Although triple-combination regimens are widely used in industrialized countries for preventing MTCT in women who do not yet require ARV treatment for their own health, their safety and effectiveness have not been assessed in resource-limited settings. There is serious concern about risk to the woman if possible toxicity cannot be carefully monitored. Information on the safety of various ARV regimens shows that short-course regimens are, in general, well tolerated, with few mild and transient side-effects for the woman and her infant. There is more concern about the safety of ARV drugs taken by pregnant women for extended periods, especially those who do not yet require ARV treatment.[74]

Similar claims were obviously based on scientific findings. A series of studies performed in the early 2000s raised concern about the toxicity of Nevirapine used in HAART outside the Western countries during pregnancy.[75] Nonetheless, these studies were not consistent with each other, in particular regarding the relationship between toxicity and CD4 levels. According to some of the studies, HAART was toxic for pregnant women with a high number of CD4s, and these were the women who, according to the WHO criteria, were not supposed to be given the antiretroviral therapy. It was therefore argued that it was necessary to greatly reduce the number of pregnant women to be given HAART. According to other studies, however, this was not the case. The results were probably contradictory because the number of patients included in each study was too small. In any case, the alarm regarding the toxicity of Nevirapine, as well as the opposition to including pregnant women who had high CD4 levels or were asymptomatic, corresponded to the still strong international mistrust of adopting HAART regimens in countries with limited resources.

What is certain is that for years DREAM had to defend itself from accusations of toxicity connected above all to the presence of Nevirapine in the triple therapy administered to pregnant women. Even in 2009, the Institute of Tropical Medicine and International Health in Berlin accused DREAM of putting the lives of pregnant women and their babies at risk, which led to the German public funds for DREAM being suspended. Basically, DREAM was criticized for operative recklessness because there was no certainty that administering HAART in pregnancy did not have toxic effects on the mothers and their children or lead to subsequent tragic resistances to the antiretroviral drugs. In particular, the fetuses risked even lethal consequences from prolonged exposure to drugs that were too strong for them. The institute claimed that DREAM should not administer HAART to pregnant women or encourage breast-feeding without having previously carried out convincing studies.

DREAM replied that the therapeutic protocols applied in PMTCT in Africa corresponded to those of Western countries. The institute answered that the compliance of the Africans in HAART must not "in any case be accepted as problem-free" because of "the notoriously more difficult conditions for adherence in African countries."[76] Furthermore, the evidence found by DREAM was considered dubious because it was proven by observational studies of real situations and not by randomized clinical studies.

The opinions of the Institute of Tropical Medicine and International Health were soon proved wrong at the highest level. Within a year the WHO guidelines for countries with limited resources legitimized the so-called Option B for health care throughout the world, which had exactly the same therapeutic criteria for PMTCT that DREAM followed with the triple therapy. In any case, in 2005 the WHO had already expressed consent for the PMTCT that DREAM administered by publishing the previously mentioned *DREAM: An Integrated Faith-Based Initiative to Treat HIV/AIDS in Mozambique*, which included the scientific protocols followed in PMTCT.

In July 2006 the DREAM researchers published the results of a long study on the safety of Nevirapine, as much an excellent drug in a triple combination as it was useless and detrimental to subsequent therapies if taken alone. This article was called "Safety of Nevirapine-Containing Antiretroviral Triple Therapy Regimens to Prevent Vertical Transmission in an African Cohort of HIV-1-Infected Pregnant Women."[77] The long academic title took into account the first scientific article on Nevirapine used in the field, not in the laboratory, where it was seen that only one out of 703 women treated by DREAM and monitored from 2002 to 2004 suffered from severe toxicity that was probably caused by Nevirapine used in the HAART regimen (not the single dose in mother-to-child prevention). The article reported levels of typical Nevirapine toxicity (hepatotoxicity, skin rashes and Stevens-Johnson syndrome) that were no higher than those observed with the same therapeutic protocols in Western countries. This type of toxicity was mainly relatively insignificant: the conditions were treated without even having to interrupt the triple antiretroviral therapy, obviously while constantly monitoring the liver functions and the general clinical status.

One criticism of DREAM concerned the fact that all the pregnant women received the triple therapy, even the ones who in normal conditions would not have been eligible for the treatment because they were in good health or because they still had plenty of CD4s. In particular, it was said that the HAART regimen was toxic in subjects with high numbers of CD4s. "Safety of Nevirapine-Containing Antiretroviral Triple Therapy" produced data that proved there was no association between a high number of CD4s and any toxicity. This was very important for PMTCT. If a link between a good immunological condition (a high number of CD4s) and toxicity had been proved, only immunologically depressed women would have been administered the therapy, whereas mother-to-child transmission was mainly a question of the mother's viral load, not her immunological status. More precisely, if a low CD4 count had been the parameter for putting pregnant women on the therapy, according to the therapeutic eligibility criteria adopted for any other HIV-positive person, only 10 percent of the African pregnant women would have been put on HAART. PMTCT would have lost its raison d'être, with tragic consequences for many newborns. Why was the figure 10 percent? The fact is that in order to get pregnant, the women usually had to be in fairly good health. Only a few of the pregnant women with low CD4 levels would have carried out a cytofluorimetric test certifying that they had 200 or fewer CD4s.

It should be added that the success rate of PMTCT achieved by DREAM—that is, in the specific treatment protocol that motivated access to treatment for all HIV-positive pregnant women regardless of their clinical, immunological, and virological data—was over 98 percent, which was not less than that observed in the West. "Safety of Nevirapine-Containing Antiretroviral Triple Therapy" therefore concluded by praising the triple therapy:

> The results obtained here, showing a high rate of prevention of mother-to-child transmission, suggest that the use of triple therapy is effective in greatly reducing the number of HIV-infected new born infants. The use of formula milk to avoid transmission after delivery could be limited by social and economic difficulties. Triple therapy after delivery could therefore be an effective means of preventing HIV transmission after delivery in resource-limited settings. In

conclusion, the low frequency and mainly minor consequences of adverse reactions to a NVP-based regimen in poor women in this resource-limited environment suggest that such a regimen should be considered by policy makers and those involved in HIV programmes as the preferred treatment regimen for HIV-positive pregnant women.[78]

Three years after this article was published, the Institute of Tropical Medicine and International Health considered DREAM's scientific activity to be a series of unreliable *deskriptive Kohortenstudien*—merely "descriptive cohort studies." And yet it was through "Safety of Nevirapine-Containing Antiretroviral Triple Therapy" that Gianni Guidotti and Leonardo Palombi were invited to collaborate with the WHO on drawing up the new guidelines on AIDS in resource-limited settings.

## THE TRIPLE THERAPY

In Geneva, Guidotti and Palombi were able to certify the safety of the HAART regimen in pregnancy, its efficacy in PMTCT, and the advantages of allowing access to all pregnant women, with no eligibility thresholds. These therapeutic guidelines were gradually adopted, amid recurrent attempts to limit eligibility for treatment and to continue administering single or double therapies, since they were simpler and less expensive.[79]

The single and double therapies were encouraged by the large international development cooperation agencies. The hypothesized economic advantages were decisive. The two doses of Nevirapine for the mother and baby, as previously mentioned, cost $4. On the other hand, in 2010, putting a five-months-pregnant woman on HAART until six months after delivery cost around $400 in sub-Saharan Africa.[80] According to DREAM, it was a question of demonstrating that it was economically worthwhile to carry out PMTCT with HAART, like in the West—that is, to invest more in the short term in order to have a profitable return in the medium and long terms. The economist Stefano Orlando presented this financial sustainability:

Over the last years the situation has changed considerably: the cost of antiretroviral drugs has been reduced and the single dose of Nevirapine has proved less efficient than was hoped. The economic analyses claiming that the most effective approach was not sustainable, should be reviewed. We have tried to analyse the cost/efficacy ratio of DREAM's mother-to-child prevention programme, which gives all the mothers the triple therapy until their children are weaned. The results are very reassuring: the cost per avoided infection is US$998 and the cost per recovered DALY[81] is US$35 (for those who are not familiar with this indicator, DALY stands for a year of life in good health, so that figure tells us how much it costs with this therapy to add a year of life in good health to a patient. It is commonly accepted that it can be considered efficient if a year of life gained costs under US$50, so I would say it is). However, up to now we have only been talking about direct costs. In reality, a sick child is also a cost to the state, so one less sick child is a saving for the whole society, as well as good news for the country's future.[82]

In addition, according to Orlando, there were the economic advantages provided by the reduction of the number of orphans, thanks to the fact that the mothers lived longer, and the long-term investment in human capital: a child saved would become a worker years later. Training qualified staff and setting up health facilities would have positive effects on the whole public health system and counter the transmission of AIDS not only in terms of mother-to-child prevention but also by reducing the viral load in the mothers. So, PMTCT based on the HAART regimen was shown to be cost-effective in Africa.

The WHO approved the HAART regimen for pregnant women in its guidelines for countries with limited resources in 2010 and provided two possibilities for PMTCT, Option A, which had been adopted up to then (single or double therapy), and Option B (triple therapy). The guidelines did not indicate a clear preference between the two options, but they supplied percentages of transmission of the virus that revealed the greater efficacy of Option B. Option B was exactly what DREAM had been implementing since 2002.

In the following years another option appeared, Option B+, which recommended not interrupting the therapy at six months after delivery, whatever the clinical stage, CD4 count, and viral load. According to the previous options, only the mothers who were eligible according to the international guidelines—basically those in bad health—could continue the therapy from six months after delivery. In 2013 the WHO dropped Option A and kept Option B, together with Option B+, stating, "Key new clinical recommendations include . . . immediate ART for all pregnant and breastfeeding women (prevention of mother-to-child transmission [PMTCT] options); ART for all pregnant and breastfeeding women with the option to discontinue treatment after the MTCT risk period has ceased for women who do not meet the eligibility criteria (Option B); or lifelong ART in all pregnant and breastfeeding women (Option B+)."[83] This was what DREAM had been waiting for too, since it considered interrupting HAART at six months after delivery for the mothers in good health as a disastrous limit. Apart from putting the women's lives in danger, interrupting the therapy six months after delivery also meant that if breast-feeding was continued, it would no longer be safe, or else that the children would have to be weaned early, with all the risks this involved in Africa. The continuation of the therapy was justified, when possible, because of a need to breast-feed up to twelve months. Sometimes the mothers had one pregnancy so soon after the previous one that they were always able to stay on the triple therapy.

Supporting the HAART regimen in PMTCT gave DREAM its excellent results: high adherence to the therapies, rare switches to second-line therapies, survival of mothers, healthy babies who were not orphans. Administering HAART during pregnancy meant reducing maternal mortality, which was usually much higher in HIV-positive women, who were particularly physically stressed by their pregnancy. This reduction in mortality was not limited to bringing the mortality of pregnant HIV-positive women in line with the national averages but reduced it to under the average because their health was monitored. In the same way, PMTCT with HAART decreased premature births, miscarriages, and stillbirths, as well as low birth weight, statistically bringing these events to a level that was equal to or below the national averages.[84] And the mortality of the babies born in DREAM's PMTCT program was lower than that of healthy babies born from healthy mothers.

Furthermore, the DREAM patients have always enjoyed an even better physical condition than their HIV-negative fellow citizens. According to Cristina Marazzi,

> the paradox, so to say, is that AIDS patients treated by DREAM live longer than people who do not have AIDS because they look after themselves, they are health-conscious, they have a healthy lifestyle, they know the value of health for themselves, they are strong enough to work, they have enough to eat, they go to the doctor, and above all they have a doctor to go to. . . . Who goes to the doctor in Africa? In DREAM there have been paradoxical cases of people wanting to be HIV-positive because they consider this condition as fortunate.[85]

To summarize: the fight against AIDS in sub-Saharan countries did not require extraordinary skills—it required the serious application of the triple therapy. The HAART regimen, at first excluded for Africa, was introduced later on but with no ambitions of excellence because it was considered expensive and tiresome. In PMTCT in particular, the triple therapy was considered a luxury for the poorest and most underdeveloped continent in the world. Many of DREAM's scientific contributions are to be understood as an attempt, from various points of view, to motivate a HAART regimen carried out well for Africans, explaining its positive clinical effects, suggesting less narrow eligibility margins, disproving excessive fears of toxicity, showing the good adherence of the patients, indicating the need for careful diagnostic monitoring, describing the completeness of the treatment that includes nutritional support, ascertaining the economic advantages, and so on.

Since HAART worked and saved lives in Europe and in North America, why would it not work and save lives in Africa too? Nonetheless, this simple assumption went against two principles, the first concerning prevention and the second minimalism. The work carried out by DREAM, and by many other health care professionals, consisted in overcoming these two principles. These beliefs were based on similar convictions: that HAART was economically impractical and unsustainable. This is why DREAM argued that the HAART regimen carried out with the best Western standards with the test-and-treat approach was also advantageous in Africa. In fact, it was not only cost-effective but even cost-saving because it generated net savings for the finances of the countries in which it was administered. The more people were treated, the more hospitalizations, complications, infections, opportunistic infections, work disabilities, and deaths would be avoided. In other words, it was not a question of stopping an epidemic disaster in the best possible way but of conceiving the fight against AIDS in Africa as an investment that would provide advantageous returns.

The principle of prevention, made unsustainable by the millions of deaths in countries with limited resources, was gradually overcome at the beginning of the 2000s. The minimalist principle was more resilient. From 2010 onward in particular, various medical-economic studies,[86] in perfect agreement with UNAIDS (which at the time was run by Michel Sidibé) and with the WHO (while Margaret Chan was the director general) encouraged investments in universal access to treatment and high-level therapy. Nonetheless, the tendency to save on salaries and resources in African countries has not completely disappeared and slows down the fight against AIDS. Despite this, the fight continues, and it is being won.

## NOTES

1. WHO, *Scaling Up Antiretroviral Therapy.*
2. In particular, DREAM followed the protocols drawn up by the CDC, which were used in the United States.
3. WHO, *Scaling Up Antiretroviral Therapy.*
4. The invitations to the eight international conferences organized by DREAM in Rome from 2004 to 2012 are examples of this strategy. The speakers included academic scholars, representatives of the large development cooperation agencies, and African politicians.
5. Such as the AIDS conference in San Francisco in February 2004.
6. Palombi, Perno, and Marazzi, "HIV/AIDS in Africa."
7. "The probability of developing viral resistance in this subgroup is higher and, ipso facto, the need for close virological monitoring is highly recommended. On the basis of these considerations, one must highlight the substantially greater benefits associated with an initiation of therapy in accordance with international guidelines for the greatest possible number of patients." Palombi, Perno, and Marazzi, 536.

8. WHO, *Antiretroviral Treatment as Prevention (TasP)*.
9. WHO.
10. Marazzi et al., *DREAM*, 13.
11. "Because of its high cost and poor availability in resource-constrained settings, however, [viral load testing] is not recommended as an assessment tool for managing ARV treatment in the present guidelines. The lack of availability of viral load monitoring implies that treatment failure has to be assessed immunologically and clinically rather than virologically." WHO, *Scaling Up Antiretroviral Therapy*, 84. See also the 2003 revision of this volume (Geneva: WHO, 2004), which states the following on pages 9–10, 25: "An assessment of viral load (e.g. using plasma HIV-1 RNA levels) is not considered necessary before starting therapy. Because of the cost and complexity of viral load testing, WHO does not currently recommend its routine use in order to assist with decisions on when to start therapy in severely resource-constrained settings. . . . Because of the cost and technical issues associated with viral load testing, this test is not currently recommended as part of the present treatment guidelines".
12. Besides, in developed countries, the viral load had been measured as part of the treatment of AIDS from the beginning of the triple therapy and was considered the most effective parameter for monitoring the patients. See van Praag, Fernyak, and Katz, *Implications of Antiretroviral Treatments*. See also Hammer, "Advances in Antiretroviral Therapy"; Shearer et al., "Viral Load and Disease Progression"; and Hughes et al., "Monitoring Plasma HIV-1 RNA Levels."
13. WHO, *Antiretroviral Therapy for HIV Infection in Adults and Adolescents: 2006 Revision*, 65.
14. WHO, 68.
15. WHO, *Antiretroviral Therapy of HIV Infection in Infants and Children* (2006), 60.
16. WHO, *Antiretroviral Therapy for HIV Infection in Adults and Adolescents* (2006) 68.
17. Braitstein et al., "Mortality of HIV-1-Infected Patients."
18. Calmy et al., "HIV Viral Load Monitoring," 128.
19. Calmy et al., 129.
20. WHO, *Consolidated Guidelines on the Use of Antiretroviral Drugs: Summary of New Recommendations*, 32
21. "Clinical assessment and laboratory tests play a key role in assessing individuals following a positive diagnosis of HIV. Viral load is the preferred monitoring approach to diagnose and confirm treatment failure. New recommendations encourage routine viral load testing to be carried out at six and 12 months after initiating ART and, if the patient is stable on ART, every 12 months thereafter. . . . WHO supports stopping routine CD4 count testing where viral load testing is available and can be used instead." WHO, *Consolidated Guidelines on the Use of Antiretroviral Drugs: What's New*, 8.
22. "HIV Treatment and Care: What's New in Treatment Monitoring; Viral

Load and CD4 Testing," WHO, July 2017, http://apps.who.int/iris/bitstream/handle/10665/255891/WHO-HIV-2017.22-eng.pdf?sequence=1.

23. UNAIDS, *2006 Report.*
24. UNAIDS, *Global AIDS Update 2016.*
25. WHO, *Antiretroviral Therapy for HIV Infection in Adults and Adolescents: 2010 Revision*, 24.
26. WHO, *Summary of New Recommendations*, when to start ART in people living with HIV (part 1).
27. WHO, *Guideline on When to Start Antiretroviral Therapy*, 24.
28. WHO, *Consolidated Guidelines on the Use of Antiretroviral Drugs: What's New*, 6.
29. WHO, "Treat All People."
30. WHO, *Guideline on When to Start Antiretroviral Therapy*, 29.
31. As indicated in Gabriella Bortolot's master's thesis "The DREAM Model" (Faculty of Medicine, University of Genoa, 2005), DREAM's strategy was the opposite of the ideology of "everybody or nobody," which until 2002 contributed to blocking the antiretroviral treatment in Africa: "In fact it is not possible to offer everything to everyone at the same time. Decisions in terms of priorities have to be made. During the first phase of DREAM priority was given to pregnant women, to the mother and child couple," 20.
32. Memoria per Conferenza DREAM: Maggio 2011, documento preparatorio della Conferenza Internazionale del 13 maggio 2011, non datato, senza indicazione d'autore, in DAR.
33. "Resolution Adopted by the General Assembly on 23 December 2005," UN, https://undocs.org/en/A/RES/60/224.
34. WHO, UNAIDS, and UNICEF, *Towards Universal Access.*
35. "Based on the new criterion for treatment initiation (CD4 cell count of or below 350 cells/mm$^3$), antiretroviral therapy coverage increased from 28% [26–31 percent] in December 2008 to 36% [33–39 percent] at the end of 2009. Under the previous criterion for treatment initiation (CD4 count of or below 200 cells/mm$^3$), global coverage would have reached 52% [47–58 percent] in 2009." WHO, UNAIDS, and UNICEF, *Towards Universal Access*, 6.
36. The figure of eleven million corresponds to the estimated number of HIV-positive people eligible for treatment according to the 2010 guidelines, reduced by 20 percent in that universal access at the time aimed to treat 80 percent of the people who were acknowledged as needing treatment.
37. Report by Stefano Orlando, 7th International Dream Conference, Accesso universale al trattamento: Il passo decisivo per sconfiggere l'AIDS, May 13, 2011, text in DAR.
38. Report by Noorjehan Abdul Majid and Leonardo Palombi, 7th International DREAM Conference, "Universal Access to Treatment: The Crucial Step for Defeating AIDS," May 13, 2011, text in DAR. Part of the research was presented in San Francisco at the Conference on Retrovirus and Opportunistic Infections

held on February 16–19, 2010. On the basis of this material, Palombi and Abdul Majid then published "Predicting Trends in HIV-1 Sexual Transmission."

39. Published in *Lancet* 373, 9657 (January 3, 2009).

40. During a conference on the Global Fund at the Italian National Institute of Health in Rome, June 27, 2016 (related to the author by Leonardo Palombi, February 3, 2018).

41. Palombi et al., "Predicting Trends in HIV-1 Sexual Transmission," 271.

42. "Our findings . . . support the main conclusions of the Granich study, that is, treatment of all infected individuals translates into a drastic reduction in incident HIV infections and leads to the 'sterilization' of the epidemic. Both modeling approaches demonstrate a clear reduction of new cases well below the substitution threshold. Randomized controlled studies such as HPTN 052, which evaluated HIV sexual transmission in serodiscordant couples, effectively demonstrated a 96% reduction in HIV transmission when the index partner was treated with triple ART at a relatively higher CD4 cell count threshold (350–550 cells/mm$^3$). Data from mother-to-child transmission studies have extensively demonstrated that a marked reduction in HIV transmission is achievable with viral load suppression. The model from our study, based on real-life parameters, confirms this assumption." Palombi et al., "Predicting Trends in HIV-1 Sexual Transmission," 5

43. Cohen et al., "Prevention of HIV-1 Infection."

44. Marina Giuliano et al., "Triple Antiretroviral Prophylaxis"; Palombi et al., "Treatment Acceleration Program"; Marazzi et al., "Increased Infant Human Immunodeficiency"; Marazzi et al., "Extended Antenatal Antiretroviral Use."

45. Palombi et al., "Predicting Trends in HIV-1 Sexual Transmission."

46. Starting with the Harvard School of Public Health. See Goyal, Wang, and DeGruttola, "Editorial Commentary."

47. Prendergast et al., "International Perspectives."

48. UNAIDS, *UNAIDS Report*, 51.

49. UNAIDS, "Global HIV and AIDS Statistics."

50. UNICEF, UNAIDS, and WHO, *Children and AIDS*, 23.

51. UNICEF, WHO, World Bank, and United Nations, *Levels and Trends in Child Mortality*, 10.

52. In 2005 the WHO approved the pediatric formulations for antiretroviral drugs, but in fact these drugs could not be used in most African countries until 2009. See Brenda Waning et al., "Global Pediatric Antiretroviral Market." Only in 2010 did simplified pediatric formulations start to become available in Africa. See also WHO, *Antiretroviral Therapy for HIV Infection in Infants and Children* (2010).

53. Presentation by Francesca Moneti in DREAM, *We Want to Live Too!*, 90–108, 101.

54. Presentation by Maria C. Marazzi, in DREAM, *We Want to Live Too!*, 32–55, 40–41.

55. Maria C. Marazzi and Leonardo Palombi, presentation at the fifth international conference organized by DREAM, "Long Life for Africa! Fighting AIDS and Malnutrition," Rome, May 10, 2007, in DREAM, *Long Life for Africa!*

56. On breast-feeding by HIV-positive mothers, see later in this chapter.

57. Kawonga, *Un domani per i miei bambini*, 139–40. Around the DREAM centers, there are gatherings of adolescents who have overcome the stigma phase and are committed to talking about HIV with healthy peers in schools and meeting places. These adolescents, forced by the disease to become psychologically mature early on, thanks to the treatment and the inclusion in the group, find safety at the centers and contribute to break down the stigma of HIV among young people.

58. "Statement by Stephen Lewis, UN Special Envoy for HIV/AIDS in Africa, on World AIDS Day, December 1, 2005," http://data.unaids.org/media/speech es02/sp_lewis_wad_01dec2005_en.pdf.

59. In the West, even at the end of the 1990s, AZT was considered a possible alternative to the triple therapy but together with a caesarean section and formula milk.

60. Laura A. Guay et al., "Intrapartum and Neonatal Single Dose."

61. Lawrence K. Altman, "New Means Found for Reducing H. I. V. Passed to Child," *New York Times*, July 15, 1999.

62. Anthony Fauci, quoted in Altman. Fauci was the head of the National Institute of Allergy and Infectious Diseases at the time.

63. Lockman et al., "Response to Antiretroviral Therapy."

64. WHO, *Antiretroviral Drugs for Treating Pregnant Women*, 2–3.

65. WHO, 30.

66. "One Battle Won, Still Losing the War," *Economist*, December 14, 2001.

67. WHO, *Antiretroviral Drugs for Treating Pregnant Women*, 2.

68. Marazzi et al., *DREAM*.

69. Presentation by Leonardo Palombi, "Sull'AIDS in Africa e in Mozambico," during a DREAM meeting, Rome, February 11, 2001, text in DAR.

70. See Giuliano et al., "Triple Antiretroviral Prophylaxis"; Palombi et al., "Treatment Acceleration Program."

71. Palombi et al. "Treatment Acceleration Program."

72. WHO, *HIV and Infant Feeding*. See also "Breast Is Always Best, Even for HIV-Positive Mothers," WHO, bulletin no. 88 (January 1, 2010), 9–10, and the review of 1,295 articles in Chikhungu et al., "HIV-Free Survival at 12–24 Months."

73. Maria C. Marazzi and Leonardo Palombi, presentation at the 3rd International DREAM Conference, "A Dream for Africa: Children without AIDS," Rome, May 2006, text.

74. WHO, *Antiretroviral Drugs for Treating Pregnant Women*, 2.

75. See Martínez et al., "Hepatotoxicity in HIV-1-Infected Patients"; de Maat et al., "Incidence and Risk Factors"; de Maat et al., "Case Series of Acute Hepatitis"; Ena et al., "Risk and Determinants"; Dieterich et al., "Drug-Induced Liver

Injury"; Hitti et al., "Maternal Toxicity"; and Martin et al., "Predisposition to Nevirapine Hypersensitivity."

76. Kommentierung der Stellungnahme zum PMTCT-Ansatz von DREAM, Gemeinschaft Sant'Egidio, von Frau Prof. Dr. Gundel Harms-Zwingenberger, July 8, 2009, in DAR. This is an answer to a note by DREAM (Anmerkungen zum Programm DREAM der Gemeinschaft Sant'Egidio) during a debate after a meeting at the Bundesministerium für wirtschaftliche Zusammenarbeit und Entwicklung on May 14, 2009 in Berlin. Text in DAR.

77. Marazzi et al., "Safety of Nevirapine-Containing Antiretroviral Triple Therapy."

78. Marazzi et al., 343.

79. The following is an example: Rapid advice on PMTCT published by the WHO in 2009 recommended previous CD4 count or at least a clinically advanced stage of the disease in order to decide whether to put the pregnant women on the triple antiretroviral therapy. Depending on the immunological results, prolonged monotherapy with AZT during pregnancy or, as an alternative, a triple therapy with massive doses of Efavirenz, was proposed again. Nevirapine was to be administered to breast-feeding babies every day. See WHO, "Rapid Advice." Palombi and Marazzi objected to the rapid advice, together with Karin Nielsen-Saines of the University of California, Los Angeles, and Marina Giuliano of the Italian National Health Institute, who had been working on PMTCT for a long time. These four researchers pointed out that it was almost impossible to measure CD4 levels in most African health centers, so connecting access to antiretroviral drugs to this immunological test meant delaying treatment with the triple therapy. They recalled that AZT had not been administered in monotherapy for a long time in developed countries and that Efavirenz, which is potentially teratogenic, was banned in developed countries in the first trimester of pregnancy. Moreover, there were no definitive tests on its contraindications with respect to hepatotoxicity. Regarding Nevirapine in monotherapy: "Results of clinical trials documenting the efficacy of this approach for extended periods of time are not yet available. Single dose nevirapine has been shown to compromise future treatment options in HIV-infected women and infants. In addition, the long-term safety profile of this agent in immune-competent infants has not been established." Palombi et al., "Easier Said than Done," 1.

80. Orlando et al., "Cost-effectiveness of Using HAART."

81. DALY is the acronym for "disability-adjusted life year."

82. Presentation by Stefano Orlando, 7th International DREAM Conference, "Universal Access to Treatment: The Crucial Step for Defeating AIDS," Rome, May 13, 2011, text in DAR. See Also Orlando et al., Cost-Effectiveness of Using HAART."

83. WHO, "Consolidated Guidelines on the Use of Antiretroviral Drugs."

84. Marazzi et al., "Favorable Pregnancy Outcomes"; Marazzi et al., "Extended Antenatal Use"; Marazzi et al., "Epidemia da HIV/AIDS."

85. Interview by the author with Cristina Marazzi, Rome, January 11, 2018.

86. The first of these were Robberstad and Evjen-Olsen, "Preventing Mother to Child Transmission"; Fleishman et al., "Economic Burden of Late Entry"; Shah et al., "Cost-effectiveness of New WHO Recommendations"; and Resch et al., "Economic Returns to Investment."

# Afterword

## Paul Elie

In the nearly sixty years since a group of young Italian Catholics came together in a nonviolent response to the upheavals in Europe in 1968, establishing a prayer group and then a social movement rooted in "the gospel and friendship," the Community of Sant'Egidio has become a fixture in Rome—to the life of the historic center and to Trastevere in particular as well as to the city's hardscrabble periphery, made familiar by the writer and filmmaker Pier Paolo Pasolini.

For a certain kind of visitor to Rome (Catholic, progressive, curious), Sant'Egidio represents qualities we identify with the city and find lacking in Catholicism where we come from. The nightly prayer service in the grand basilica of Santa Maria in Trastevere, held at the slack hour of 8 p.m., is mostly led by laypeople and draws a diverse congregation, all there out of desire rather than obligation—the crowd filling the great space and then spilling out at the conclusion onto the adjoining piazzas, conversations already in progress. Rather than in formal meetings, the Community's members strategize over coffee and during strolls through the neighborhood. Instead of a thickly layered bureaucracy, they maintain a pretty transparent web of relationships. Often Sant'Egidio's projects have the character of brainstorms rooted in common sense: Why not arrange for able-bodied young people to carry groceries upstairs to frail elderly ones who live on the upper stories of Trastevere's seventeenth-century apartment houses? Why not publish a little guidebook that indicates public buildings and monuments where homeless people can use washrooms, sleep, or get food at low cost or for free?

The Community's base of operations, in a restored convent on the small Piazza Sant'Egidio, a short walk from the basilica, is marked by a sculpture of a figure sleeping on a bench. If you look closely, you see he has holes—stigmata—on his feet; this is Jesus as a homeless person. But the entrance is so modest that you can pass it by on the way to the trattoria at the far end of the piazza (which the Community runs, employing people with intellectual disabilities as waiters and busboys). The tiny chapel alongside the old convent is decorated beautifully but simply, with a Franciscan crucifix, post–Vatican II Arte Povera, and icons from the Eastern churches. As far as I know, the Community maintains no exhibit spelling out its mission, no shop selling the many books its members have written over the years.

The Community of Sant'Egidio as most of us encounter it in Rome, then, embodies a set of distinctive qualities that seem to go to the heart of its undertaking: simplicity, informality, attention to the local (and the locale that is Trastevere), aliveness to the present, and a Christianity lightly worn—the gospel and friendship, as they put it.

And yet all the while, the Community, through its nearly seventy thousand members in Italy and seventy-one other countries, is pursuing projects that are daunting in their complexity—projects rooted in qualities often taken as opposites of those seen in Rome. The peacemaking efforts that brought an end to civil wars in Mozambique and Burundi in the 1990s demanded a global outlook; expertise in languages, governance, and international law; a commitment to problem-solving on a scale seemingly resistant to the personal coffee-and-a-stroll approach; and a long-term commitment to engaging in societies where Catholicism is itself on the margins. Its dealings involve cooperation, yes, but also hardheaded strategy and tactics because the problems it addresses—war, forced migration, state-sanctioned killing, religious strife—seem to have less to do with the gospel and friendship than with life and death. And yet—this is Sant'Egidio's essence—the Community manages to make the gospel and friendship seem synonymous with know-how and commitment and a way to heal from the solitude and fragmentation of postmodern life.

The DREAM Project (as this extraordinary book has made clear) is such a project. The simple and appealing acronym conceals plenty of conflict and complexity, as conveyed in the words it represented when the program was established in the late 1990s: Drug Resource Enhancement against AIDS and Malnutrition. Put simply, the program sought to address the AIDS crisis through the same means that had shown success in the developed world: a "triple therapy" of antiretroviral drugs, which enable people with HIV to live relatively healthy lives for decades. Sant'Egidio had grasped the evidence that

HIV, if treated, does not have to lead rapidly to AIDS and to death. Rather, the treatment gives hope: by allowing large numbers of people to live with a chronic disease, it offers a dream of a society surviving and even thriving in spite of HIV.

And the treatment has other consequences. When an effective treatment is present, people are willing to be tested. As people with HIV who live and thrive under treatment, the "silent slaughter" becomes the subject of public discussion. Those surviving with HIV share their knowledge of how the treatment works—and as Cristina Marazzi, one of the Italian epidemiologists associated with the Community who devised the program, puts it, "the patients themselves often become protagonists in the fight against AIDS." Through their work as volunteers, women who would have been stigmatized twice over—because they are women and because they have HIV—become the backbone of a newly healthy society. Throughout, the project does away with "il confine tra chi aiuta e chi è aiutato"—the divide between those helping and those who are helped.

It sounds commonsensical, and in many respects it is. But (as we learn, or are reminded, through Roberto Morozzo della Rocca's account) it ran against the conviction about AIDS, and AIDS "relief," that had emerged in the developed world and taken root, shaping the policies of governments and foundations. This was the notion that prevention is a preferable alternative to treatment because treatment, through a decades-long regimen of antiretrovirals, would be too expensive, too complex, and impossible to implement in Africa (which lacked adequate public health infrastructure and had strong folk-healing traditions) and for Africans (who could not be counted on to show up at clinics or to "take their meds"). There was the notion that treatment would introduce a new set of problems, bringing about a two-tier society across Africa in which the prosperous and the well-connected would gain access to treatment while the vast majority of Africans would not. Africa—the people atop many global aid organizations concluded—would have to make do with prevention only.

That the DREAM program has been a working refutation of those assumptions is the author's conviction, and the book itself is the supporting evidence. But what struck me, a layperson with no expertise in medicine or public policy, is how strongly the DREAM program also runs against conventional ideas of how social change comes about. Sant'Egidio's way of going about things with DREAM challenges the usual thinking about how people can join together to care for one another and so improve their lives and the society where they live—which in our time is at once a local and a global society.

Typically, international NGOs and humanitarian aid organizations are tightly focused on specific objectives: providing crisis health care, say, or resettling refugees or eliminating land mines or countering the practice of female genital mutilation. Over time, they develop expertise that is refined and then applied in different regions as a need emerges.

Sant'Egidio is different. It begins with the situation in which it finds itself and then figures out what to do and how to act, its leaders and members discerning what's needed to address the situation. This is what it did when its members created informal "schools for peace" on Rome's outskirts, giving basic education to poor people and immigrants who lacked access to the city's public schools. This is what it did when it set up programs enabling the Roma—people scorned even by other poor people in Italy—to live, work, and raise their families with health and dignity. And this is what it has done in addressing AIDS in Africa.

DREAM followed the October 1992 peace accords in Mozambique, in which Sant'Egidio took an unprecedented mediating role, bringing representatives of more than a dozen warring factions to Rome for eleven rounds of peace talks over twenty-six months. In important ways, the accord—a "Pax Romana," the French newspaper *Le Monde* called it—made DREAM possible. Due to its role in the efforts for peace, Sant'Egidio had relationships across Mozambique and friends among the parties, governors, tribes, and ethnic groups. The Community had credibility, for the peace efforts had actually brought about a long-sought accord. And it had a personal interest in the next stage of the country's history, through the lives of several thousand Mozambicans who had become members of the Community—laypeople leading prayer services and schooling and arranging aid to street children, elderly people, and those on the margins. Meanwhile, two Italian members—the movement's founder, Andrea Riccardi, and Fr. Matteo Zuppi, now the cardinal archbishop of Bologna—were intimately involved in the peace process, leading a group of four mediators that also included a young Mozambican bishop and an Italian parliamentarian.

Soon after a fragile peace had been achieved—following one million deaths, including, of course, the deaths of some members of the Community—the silent slaughter of AIDS began. Many mothers of the kids attending Sant'Egidio's schools of peace contracted the "slim disease," lost weight, grew weak, and died, leaving families grieving and bereft. That AIDS should strike the country at a moment of hope after years of strife is one of the cruel ironies of recent history.

And that Sant'Egidio had the energy and spirit—the audacity—to respond in the way it did is one of the marvels of recent history. Following the peace accords, the Community could have opted to focus its attention on mediation and peacemaking (and "building a brand" in the world of NGOs and philanthropy). It could have declared success in Mozambique and shifted its attention to other countries. Instead Sant'Egidio responded to the fresh challenge near at hand: a grim and unsparing pandemic that had already exhausted the attention span of much of the developed world and stymied the grand international aid organizations. And it did so in a way that prompted the Community to reinvent itself in midlife, so to speak.

Mozambique after the civil war was (as it remains) a religiously mixed country, its population half Christian (most of them Catholics), 20 percent Muslim, 10 percent animist, and 20 percent agnostic or unaffiliated. Given Sant'Egidio's profile—an informal movement of Catholic laypeople, ecumenically minded, with demanding jobs and families—the Community in Mozambique might have been expected to focus on prevention and care, say, by organizing its members to devote some (spare) time and effort to encouraging Mozambicans to make simple-seeming changes to their everyday behavior so as to help reduce the spread of HIV. That approach would have had the further advantages of keeping clear of controversy (which attended the Catholic Church's approach to AIDS in the United States when the disease was decimating gay men's communities there) and of aligning its efforts with Catholic teachings about monogamy and premarital sex that had been given fresh emphasis by Pope John Paul II, with whom the Community had worked through the annual World

Day of Prayer for Peace for nearly two decades, beginning in Assisi in 1986.

Sant'Egidio could have signed on to the prevention approach. But no. Instead the Community devised a new and different approach, rooted in medicine, epidemiology, and public health. It would be undertaken at scale throughout the country—in Maputo, in neighboring Matola, and step by step in other cities from south to north. It would require the mastery of highly specialized operations of blood testing, drug shipment, drug pricing, and the like and would involve the best practices that were sharply reducing deaths from AIDS in the developed world. It would mean erecting state-of-the-art laboratories in places where infrastructure was unreliable and power blackouts were common. It would involve standing aside from—if not actively opposing—the consensus around the prevention approach, one supported by vast philanthropic funding, strict government policies, and slick public relations. And it would be motivated—inspired—by voluntary human caring more than anything else.

"Excellence" is the word the Community uses, in retrospect, to capture the set of traits it sought to bring to the crisis of AIDS in Mozambique. The DREAM project would provide medical excellence to Mozambicans with HIV and AIDS, in the form of sustained drug-based treatment. It would provide treatment to seropositive mothers so that their babies were born without the virus, while also addressing the malnutrition that enables the virus to thrive in children born seropositive. The project would be rooted in the recognition that ordinary people are capable of excellence: the doctors and diplomats of Sant'Egidio who took coordinating roles and also the thousands of volunteers, many of them HIV-positive survivors, the preponderance of them women, who wished simply for themselves and their children and neighbors and friends to live, not to die. DREAM would strive for excellence as a form of friendship.

Twenty years on, DREAM has excelled in the treatment of people with HIV. In addition to Mozambique, the program is now present in ten countries: Malawi, Tanzania, Kenya, Nigeria, the Central African Republic, Cameroon, the Democratic Republic of Congo, Guinea, and Swaziland. It has treated more than half a million people, has seen patients in more than eight million visits to fifty clinics, and has performed more than four hundred thousand regular laboratory tests. It has involved about five hundred full-time staff—all of them Africans—and has trained some fifteen thousand people as health care volunteers. Through its treatment, about two hundred thousand babies born to HIV-positive mothers have emerged free of the virus. Over the past twenty years, the mortality of people with HIV in the countries where DREAM operates has decreased from 313 of every 100,000 inhabitants to 224. Average male life expectancy has increased from forty-seven to fifty-eight and that of females from fifty-two to sixty-four. Meanwhile, other activist groups have taken the treatment approach elsewhere and have seen similar outcomes.

Characteristically, Sant'Egidio hasn't sought to optimize its efforts by keeping a strict focus on HIV. Rather than specialize, the Community has adapted DREAM for the treatment of public health in Africa more broadly. A fresh iteration of the program, DREAM 2.0, adapted its acronym—which now stands for Disease Relief through Excellent and Advanced Means. The program still provides treatment for HIV and malnutrition, but it also provides a wide range of health care, involving both prevention and treatment. It uses prevention and education to help people to avoid opportunistic infections, such as the papillomavirus. It treats people with epilepsy and diabetes and offers them tests of their vision and hearing. It uses mammograms to screen women for breast cancer and colonoscopies to screen women and men for colon cancer. And in recent years it has tested people for COVID-19.

How does Sant'Egidio do all these things? Its Italian members work for DREAM on a volunteer basis—with doctors and nurses pledging to serve the project one month a year on-site and through telemedicine too. They seek donor funds that are then applied to the project's physical needs and to salaries for DREAM's full-time health care staff in Africa (some of them members of Sant'Egidio, some not). And it does all this with the aplomb that the Community brings to all its projects, whether its worldwide efforts to do away with capital punishment or its work (in a program called BRAVO! (Birth Registration for All Versus Oblivion) to register the personal identities of the several million "invisible children" in Africa who, lacking birth certificates and other state identification, cannot access basic services, are vulnerable to human trafficking, and can be said not to exist in the human population as the developed world reckons it. Through a combination of excellence and friendship—friendship being a way of life at which the members of Sant'Egidio truly excel—the Community has countered the complex global systems that (expressly or inadvertently) consider some lives more valuable than others, lead to silent slaughters, and render the lives of so many people inconsequential or invisible.

It's striking to me that Roberto Morozzo della Rocca has been able to tell the story of DREAM so persuasively while having little to say about religion as such. A key to Sant'Egidio's efforts, in my experience, is its lightness of touch—a Christian faith that is at once sophisticated and nimble, owing more to Rome's sunlight and soft earth colors than to its edifice-heavy Baroque architecture (and its equivalents in Catholic vocabulary and doctrine). Its end or objective is not direct evangelization or social transformation along Christian lines. (While some members are deeply rooted in prayer and the Bible, others are attracted, at first, by the everyday stress on love and justice.) Rather, the Community's end is more or less akin to the means it employs. The gospel and friendship are the main objectives of this people's movement as well as the means of bringing about its specific goals—whether the treatment of people with AIDS in Mozambique, the revival of a peace process in Guatemala after a third of a century of civil strife, a COVID-19 vaccination program in the Central African Republic (where it has helped to ease tribal conflict), or the creation of "humanitarian corridors" to enable refugees from wars in Syria and Ukraine to make their lives in Italy, Germany, France, Spain, Poland, and elsewhere. (The full range of the Community's projects can be read about—in thirteen languages—at www.santegidio.org.)

Pope Francis—whose pontificate has been rich in encounters and shared undertakings with Sant'Egidio—has spoken of the Community's "three Ps": prayer, peace, and the poor. It's impossible fully to know the role of prayer in the DREAM program. It's impossible to overstress the role of the poor—who, as much as anyone, have carried the program, sustained by their own human dignity and by

Sant'Egidio's respect for them as equal to the rich and for the neighborhoods deemed peripheral as the source of life for the so-called centers. And it's vital to recognize the role of peace. Without peace, it wouldn't have been possible for Sant'Egidio to join with the people of Mozambique to confront the silent slaughter of AIDS through co-ordinated long-term action.

More than that, the effort to achieve peace in Mozambique through dialogue and mediation schooled the Community in how to achieve the peace that is reflected in a healthy population, sustained at once by effective public health and by robust community—by friendship, that is. This is friendship in the deepest sense—a bond of feeling and solidarity that at its best joins youth and adults, healthy people, and those who are ill or infirm across borders of class, ethnic group, and nationality and through the pursuit of excellence for the common good. It's a people's movement worth emulating and an achievement the rest of us can learn from.

Paul Elie is a senior fellow in Georgetown's Berkley Center for Religion, Peace, and World Affairs and the author of *The Life You Save May Be Your Own: An American Pilgrimage* (2003) and *Reinventing Bach* (2012). He contributed an afterword to *13 Ways of Looking at the Death Penalty* by Mario Marazziti (2015), which spells out the Community of Sant'Egidio's efforts to eliminate the death penalty worldwide.

# Bibliography

Adler, Michael W. "Antiretrovirals for Developing World." *Lancet* 351, no. 9098 (January 24, 1998): 232.

Africa Region, World Bank. *Intensifying Action against HIV/AIDS in Africa: Responding to a Development Crisis.* Washington, DC: World Bank, 2000.

Ainsworth, Martha, and Waranya Teokul. "Breaking the Silence: Setting Realistic Priorities for AIDS Control in Less-Developed Countries." *Lancet* 356, no. 9223 (July 1, 2000): 55–60.

Aker, Jenny C., and Isaac M. Mbiti. "Mobile Phones and Economic Development in Africa." *Journal of Economic Perspectives* 24, no. 3 (Summer 2010): 207–32.

Aliou Diallo, Elhadj Mamadou. *Histoire politique et sociale de la Guinée : De 1958 à 2015.* Paris: L'Harmattan, 2017.

Alumando, Elard. "La prossimità nell'immensità dell'Africa." In DREAM, Comunità di Sant'Egidio, *Comunità e Salute*, 57–64.

Annan, Kofi A. "Address to the African Summit on HIV/AIDS, Tuberculosis and Other Infectious Diseases." Abuja, 2001. https://www.un.org/sg/en/content/sg/speeches/2001-04-26/address-kofi-annan-african-summit-hivaids-tuberculosis-and-other.

Attaran, Amir, and Jeffrey Sachs. "Defining and Refining International Donor Support for Combating the AIDS Pandemic." *Lancet* 357, no. 9249 (January 6, 2001): 57–61.

Barbaglia, Giorgio. "Plant for Africa and Renewable Energy." In Bartolo and Ferrari, *Multidisciplinary Teleconsultation in Developing Countries*, 111–34.

Barnett, Tony, and Alan Whiteside. *AIDS in the Twenty-First Century: Disease and Globalization.* Basingstoke, UK: Palgrave Macmillan, 2002.

Bartolo, Michelangelo, and Fabio Ferrari. *Multidisciplinary Teleconsultation in Developing Countries.* Berlin: Springer, 2018.

Becker, Charles. *La recherche sénégalaise et la prise en charge du sida: Leçons d'une revue de la littérature.* Dakar: Réser-Sida, 2000.

Becker, Charles, Jean-Pierre Dozon, Christine Obbo, and Moriba Touré. *Vivre et penser le sida en Afrique / Experiencing and Understanding AIDS in Africa.* Paris/Dakar: Karthala/CODESRIA, 1999.

Beegle, Kathleen, Luc Christiaensen, Andrew Dabalen, and Isis Gaddis. *Poverty in a Rising Africa.* Washington, DC: International Bank for Reconstruction and Development / World Bank, 2016.

Bibeau, Gilles. "L'Afrique, terre imaginaire du sida: La subversion du discours scientifique par le jeu des fantasmes." *Anthropologie et Sociétés* 15, nos. 2–3 (1991): 125–47.
Birdwell Wester, Kathryn. "Violated: Women's Human Rights in Sub-Saharan Africa." *Topical Review Digest: Human Rights in Sub-Saharan Africa.* https://www.du.edu/korbel/hrhw/researchdigest/africa/WomensRights.pdf.
Blixen, Karen. *Out of Africa.* London: Penguin, 1937.
Braitstein, Paula, Martin W. G. Brinkhof, François Dabis, Mauro Schechter, Andrew Boulle, Paolo Miotti, Robin Wood, et al. "Mortality of HIV-1-Infected Patients in the First Year of Antiretroviral Therapy: Comparison between Low-Income and High-Income Countries." *Lancet* 367, no. 9513 (March 11, 2006): 817–24.
Branswell, Helen. "History Credits This Man with Discovering Ebola on His Own: History Is Wrong." Stat, July 14, 2016. https://www.statnews.com/2016/07/14/history-ebola-peter-piot/.
Breman, Joel G., David L. Heymann, Graham Lloyd, Joseph B. McCormick, Malonga Miatudila, Frederick A. Murphy, Jean-Jacques Muyembé-Tamfun, et al. "Discovery and Description of Ebola Zaire Virus in 1976 and Relevance to the West African Epidemic during 2013–2016." *Journal of Infectious Diseases* 214, suppl. 3 (October 15, 2016): 93–101.
Brunel, Sylvie. *L'Afrique: Un continent en réserve de développement.* Rosny-sous-Bois: Bréal, 2004.
Butler, Anthony. "South Africa's HIV/AIDS Policy, 1994–2004: How Can It Be Explained?" *African Affairs* 104, no. 417 (October 2005): 591–614.
Buvé, Anne. "L'épidémie de VIH en Afrique subsaharienne: Pourquoi si grave, pourquoi si hétérogène? In Denis and Becker, *L'épidémie du Sida en Afrique subsaharienne,* 63–90.
Caldwell, John C., Pat Caldwell, and Pat Quiggin. *Disaster in an Alternative Civilization: The Social Dimension of AIDS in Sub-Saharan Africa.* Canberra: Health Transition Centre, National Centre for Epidemiology and Population Health, Australian National University, 1989.
Calmy, Alexandra, Nathan Ford, Bernard Hirschel, Steven J. Reynolds, Lut Lynen, Eric Goemaere, Felipe Garcia de la Vega, Luc Perrin, and William Rodriguez. "HIV Viral Load Monitoring in Resource-Limited Regions: Optional or Necessary?" *Clinical Infectious Diseases* 44, no. 1 (January 1, 2007): 128–34.
Caraël, Michel. "Face à la mondialisation du sida: Vingt ans d'interventions et de controverses." In Denis and Becker, *L'épidémie du sida en Afrique subsaharienne,* 43–61.
Chikhungu, Lana Clara, Stephanie Bispo, Nigel Rollins, Nandi Siegfried, and Marie-Louise Newell. "HIV-Free Survival at 12–24 Months in Breastfed Infants of HIV-Infected Women on Antiretroviral Treatment." *Tropical Medicine and International Health* 21, no. 7 (July 2016): 820–28.
Chirimuuta, Richard, and Rosalind Chirimuuta. *AIDS, Africa, and Racism.* London: Free Association Books, 1989.

Cohen, Jon. "A Call for Drugs." *Science Now*, April 6, 2001.
Cohen, Myron S., Ying Q. Chen, Marybeth McCauley, Theresa Gamble, Mina C. Hosseinipour, Nagalingeswaran Kumarasamy, James G. Hakim, et al. "Prevention of HIV-1 Infection with Early Antiretroviral Therapy." *New England Journal of Medicine* 365 (August 11, 2011): 493–505.
Colson, Elizabeth. "En quête de guérison: L'épidémie du sida dans la vallée Gwembe." In Denis and Becker, *L'épidémie du sida en Afrique subsaharienne*, 141–64.
Comunità di Sant'Egidio. *Como vai a saúde?* Milan: Guerini e Associati, 1999.
"Consensus Statement on Antiretroviral Treatment for AIDS in Poor Countries, by Individual Members of the Faculty of Harvard University." March 2001. https://www.coreysdigs.com/wp-content/uploads/2019/01/Harvard-AIDS-Consensus-Statement.pdf.
Creese, Andrew, Katherine Floyd, Anita Alban, and Lorna Guinness. "Cost-effectiveness of HIV/AIDS Interventions in Africa: A Systematic Review of the Evidence." *Lancet* 359, no. 9318 (May 11, 2002): 1635–42.
Delaunay, Karine. "Le Programme national de lutte contre le sida au Sénégal: Entre prévention et normalisation sociale." In Gruénais, *Organiser la lutte contre le sida*, 101–11.
de Maat, Monique M., Rob ter Heine, Eric C. M. van Gorp, Jan W. Mulder, Albert T. A. Mairuhu, and Jos H. Beijnen. "Case Series of Acute Hepatitis in a Non-selected Group of HIV-Infected Patients on Nevirapine-Containing Antiretroviral Treatment." *AIDS* 17, no. 15 (October 17, 2003): 2209–14.
de Maat, Monique M., Rob ter Heine, Jan W. Mulder, Pieter L. Meenhorst, Albert T. A. Mairuhu, Eric C. M. van Gorp, Alwin D. R. Huitema, and Jos H. Beijnen. "Incidence and Risk Factors for Nevirapine-Associated Rash." *European Journal of Clinical Pharmacology* 59, nos. 5–6 (October 2003): 457–62.
Denis, Philippe. "Pour une histoire sociale du sida en Afrique subsaharienne." In Denis and Becker, *L'épidémie du sida en Afrique subsaharienne*, 17–40.
Denis, Philippe, and Charles Becker, eds. *L'épidémie du sida en Afrique subsaharienne: Regards historiens*. Louvain-la-Neuve: Bruylant-Academia, 2006.
Desclaux, Alice, Isabelle Lanièce, Ibrahim Ndoye, and Bernard Taverne, eds. *L'Initiative sénégalaise d'accès aux médicaments antirétrovirales: Analyse économiques, sociales, comportementales et médicales; Octobre 2002*. Paris: Agence nationale de recherches sur le sida, 2002.
Devey Malu Malu, Muriel. *La Guinée*. Paris: Karthala, 2009.
Diallo, Boubacar Yacine. *Je m'appelle Conakry: Récits, mémoires et souvenirs*. Conakry: L'Harmattan Guinée, 2017.
Dieterich, Douglas T., Patrick Robinson, James Love, and Jerry O. Stern. "Drug-Induced Liver Injury Associated with the Use of Non-nucleoside Reverse-Transcriptase Inhibitors." *Clinical Infectious Diseases* 38, suppl. 2 (March 1, 2004): 80–89.
Dilger, Hansjörg. *Leben mit Aids: Krankheit, Tod und soziale Beziehungen in Afrika; Eine Ethnographie*. Frankfurt: Campus Verlag, 2005.
Dozon, Jean-Pierre. "Des appropriations sociales et culturelles du sida à sa

nécessaire appropriation politique: Quelques éléments de synthèse." In Becker, Dozon, Obbo, and Touré, *Vivre et penser le sida en Afrique*, 679–88.

DREAM, Comunità di Sant'Egidio. *Comunità e Salute: Un modello per l'Africa.* Rome: SAS, 2009.

———. *Curare l'AIDS in Africa*. Milan: Leonardo International, 2009.

———. *Long Life for Africa! Fighting AIDS and Malnutrition*. Milan: Leonardo International, 2007.

———. *Viva l'Africa viva! Vincere l'AIDS e la malnutrizione*. Milan: Leonardo International, 2008.

———. *We Want to Live, Too! Treating HIV+ Children in Africa: Proceedings of the 4th International DREAM Conference, Rome, May 19, 2007*. Rome: SAS 2007.

Duesberg, Peter H. *Inventing the AIDS Virus*. Washington, DC: Regnery, 1996.

Dybul, Mark, Tae-Wook Chun, Christian Yoder, Bertha Hidalgo, Michael Belson, Kurt Hertogs, Brendan Larder, et al. "Short-Cycle Structured Intermittent Treatment of Chronic HIV Infection with Highly Active Antiretroviral Therapy: Effects on Virologic, Immunologic, and Toxicity Parameters." *Proceedings of the National Academy of Sciences of the United States of America* 98, no. 26 (December 18, 2001): 15161–66.

"Editorial: The Economics of HIV in Africa." *Lancet* 360, no. 9326 (July 6, 2002): 1.

Elias, Norbert. *Über die Einsamkeit der Sterbenden*. Frankfurt am Main: Suhrkamp 1982.

Ena, Javier, Concepción Amador, Concepción Benito, Vicenta Fenoll, and Francisco Pasquau. "Risk and Determinants of Developing Severe Liver Toxicity during Therapy with Nevirapine- and Efavirenz-Containing Regimens in HIV-Infected Patients." *International Journal of STD and AIDS* 14, no. 11 (November 2003): 776–81.

Esparza, José G. "A Brief History of the Global Effort to Develop a Preventive HIV Vaccine." *Vaccine* 31, no. 35 (August 2, 2013): 3502–18.

European Commission. *HIV/AIDS and Population Related Operations in Developing Countries: Guidelines for Applicants 2000*. November 12, 1999.

Fleishman, John A., Baligh R. Yehia, Richard D. Moore, and Kelly A. Gebo. "The Economic Burden of Late Entry into Medical Care for Patients with HIV Infection." *Medical Care* 48, no. 12 (December 2010): 1071–79.

Freedberg, Kenneth A., Elena Losina, Milton C. Weinstein, A. David Paltiel, Calvin J. Cohen, George R. Seage, Donald E. Craven, Hong Zhang, April D. Kimmel, and Sue J. Goldie. "The Cost-effectiveness of Combination Anti-retroviral Therapy for HIV Disease." *New England Journal of Medicine* 344, no. 11 (March 15, 2001): 824–31.

Gehler, Monique. *Un continent se meurt: La tragédie du sida en Afrique*. Paris: Stock, 2000.

Germano, Paola, Ersilia Buonomo, and Giovanni Guidotti. *DREAM: An Integrated Public Health Programme to Fight HIV/AIDS and Malnutrition in Limited-Resource Settings*. Rome: World Food Programme / Community of Sant'Egidio, 2007.

"A Global Health Fund: Heeding Koch's Caution." *Lancet* 358, no. 9275 (July 7, 2001): 1.
Giuliano, Marina, Giovanni Guidotti, Mauro Andreotti, Maria F. Pirillo, Paola Villani, Giuseppe Liotta, Maria Cristina Marazzi, et al. "Triple Antiretroviral Prophylaxis Administered during Pregnancy and after Delivery Significantly Reduces Breast Milk Viral Load: A Study within the Drug Resource Enhancement against AIDS and Malnutrition Program." *Journal of Acquired Immune Deficiency Syndromes* 44, no. 3 (March 1, 2007): 286–291.
Goemaere, E., N. Ford, and S. R. Benatar. "HIV/AIDS Prevention and Treatment." *Lancet* 360, 9326 (July 6, 2002): 86.
Gonsalves, Gregg. "HIV/AIDS Prevention and Treatment." *Lancet* 360, 9326 (July 6, 2002): 87.
Goodman, Allen E., ed. *The Diplomatic Record, 1992–1993*. Boulder, CO: Westview, 1995.
Gostin, Larry O. *The AIDS Pandemic: Complacency, Injustice, and Unfulfilled Expectations*. Chapel Hill: University of North Carolina Press, 2004.
Gottlieb, Michael S. "Pneumocystis Pneumonia: Los Angeles." *Morbidity and Mortality Weekly Report* 30 (June 5, 1981): 250–52.
Government of Uganda, Uganda Aids Commission, UNAIDS. *The Draft National Strategic Framework for HIV/AIDS Activities in Uganda 2000/1–2005/6*. Kampala: Government of Uganda 1999.
Goyal, Ravi, Rui Wang, and Victor DeGruttola. "Editorial Commentary: Network Epidemic Models: Assumptions and Interpretations." *Clinical Infectious Diseases* 55, 2 (July 15, 2012): 276–78.
Granich, Reuben M., Charles F. Gilks, Christopher Dye, Kevin M. De Cock, and Brian G. Williams. "Universal Voluntary HIV Testing with Immediate Antiretroviral Therapy as a Strategy for Elimination of HIV Transmission: A Mathematical Model." *Lancet* 373, no. 9657 (January 3, 2009): 48–57.
Green, Edward C., Daniel T. Halperin, Vinand Nantulya, and Janice A. Hogle. "Uganda's HIV Prevention Success: The Role of Sexual Behavior Change and the National Response." *AIDS and Behavior* 10, no. 4 (July 2006): 335–46.
Grmek, Mirko. *Histoire du sida : Début et origine d'une pandémie actuelle*. Paris: Payot, 1989.
Gruénais, Marc-Éric, ed. *Organiser la lutte contre le sida: Une étude comparative sur les rapports états/société civile en Afrique (Cameroun, Congo, Côte-d'Ivoire, Kenya, Sénégal)*. Paris: ANRS, 1999.
Guay, Laura A., Philippa Musoke, Thomas Fleming, Danstan Bagenda, Melissa Allen, Clemensia Nakabiito, Joseph Sherman, et al. "Intrapartum and Neonatal Single Dose Nevirapine Compared with Zidovudine for Prevention of Mother-to-Child Transmission of HIV-1 in Kampala, Uganda: HIVNET 012 Randomised Trial." *Lancet* 354, no. 9181 (September 4, 1999): 795–802.
Hammer, Scott M. "Advances in Antiretroviral Therapy and Viral Load Monitoring." *AIDS* 10, suppl. 3 (December 1, 1996): 1–11.

Hitti, Jane, Lisa M. Frenkel, Alice M. Stek, Sharon A. Nachman, David Baker, Adolfo Gonzalez-Garcia, Arthur Provisor, et al. "Maternal Toxicity with Continuous Nevirapine in Pregnancy: Results from PACTG 1022." *Journal of Acquired Immune Deficiency Syndromes* 36, no. 3 (July 1, 2004): 772–76.

Hogg, Robert S., Amy E. Weber, Kevin J. P. Craib, Aslam H. Anis, Michael V. O'Shaughnessy, Martin T. Schecther, and Julio S. G. Montaner. "One World, One Hope: The Cost of Providing Antiretroviral Therapy to All Nations." *AIDS* 12, no. 16 (November 12, 1998): 2203–9.

Hogg, Robert. S., Aslam Anis, Amy E. Weber, Michael V. Schechter, and Martin T. Schechter. "Triple-Combination Antiretroviral Therapy in Sub-Saharan Africa." *Lancet* 350, no. 9088 (November 8, 1997): 1406.

Hogle, Janice Alene, ed. *What Happened in Uganda? Declining HIV Prevalence, Behavior Change and National Response*. Washington, DC: Office of HIV/AIDS, Bureau of Global Health, US Agency for International Development, 2000.

Hughes, Michael D., Victoria A. Johnson, Martin S. Hirsch, James W. Bremer, Tarek Elbeik, Alejo Erice, Daniel R. Kuritzkes, et al. "Monitoring Plasma HIV-1 RNA Levels in Addition to CD4+ Lymphocyte Count Improves Assessment of Antiretroviral Therapeutic Response." *Annals of Internal Medicine* 12, no. 126 (June 15, 1997): 929–38.

Hume, Cameron. *Ending Mozambique's War*. Washington, DC: United States Institute of Peace, 1994.

———. "The Mozambique Peace Process." In Goodman, *Diplomatic Record, 1992–1993*: 81–101.

Huntington, Samuel P. *The Clash of Civilizations and the Remaking of World Order*. New York: Simon & Schuster, 1996.

Iasilli, Gianna. "Malattia e resilienza: Una indagine sugli effetti dell'educazione sanitaria e di una rete di prossimità nei confronti dell'aderenza alla terapia antiretrovirale in un gruppo di persone HIV positive in Mozambico." PhD thesis in health education, University of Perugia, academic year 2010–11.

International Monetary Fund. *World Economic Outlook Database*. April 2018 edition. https://www.imf.org/en/Publications/WEO/weo-database/2018/April.

Jackson, Robin. "Presentation." In DREAM, Comunità di Sant'Egidio, *We Want to Live, Too!*, 110–27.

Johnson, Paul. "Abuse of HIV/AIDS-Relief Funds in Mozambique." *Lancet Infectious Diseases* 9, no. 9 (September 2009): 523–24.

Kalipeni, Ezekiel, Susan Craddock, Joseph R. Oppong, and Jayati Gosh. *HIV and AIDS in Africa beyond Epidemiology*. Malden, MA: Wiley-Blackwell, 2004.

Kates, Jennifer, Adam Wexler, and Eric Lief. *Financing the Response to HIV in Low- and Middle-Income Countries: International Assistance from Donor Governments in 2015*. Menlo Park, CA: Henry J. Kaiser Family Foundation, 2016.

Katona, Peter, and Judith Katona-Apte. "The Interaction between Nutrition and Infection." *Clinical Infectious Diseases* 46, no. 10 (May 15, 2008): 1582–88.

Katzenstein, David, Marie Laga, and Jean-Paul Moatti. "The Evaluation of the HIV/AIDS Drug Access Initiatives in Côte d'Ivoire, Senegal and Uganda: How

Access to Antiretroviral Treatment Can Become Feasible in Africa." *AIDS* 17 (July 2003): 1–4.

Kauffman, Kyle D., and David L. Lindauer. *AIDS and South Africa: The Social Expression of a Pandemic*. Basingstoke, UK: Palgrave Macmillan, 2004.

Kawonga, Pacem. *Un domani per i miei bambini*. Milano: Piemme, 2013.

Keusch, Gerald T. "The History of Nutrition: Malnutrition, Infection and Immunity." *Journal of Nutrition* 133, no. 1 (January 2003): 336–40.

Khonde, Nkuku. "L'histoire du sida au Congo selon les sources orales." In Denis and Becker, *L'épidémie du sida en Afrique subsaharienne*, 331–56.

Kirby, D. "Presentation on USAID's ABC Study." USAID. Washington, DC. October 23, 2003.

Knight, Lindsay. *UNAIDS: The First 10 Years, 1996–2006*. Geneva: UNAIDS 2008.

Kuyu, Camille. *Les Haïtiens au Congo*. Paris: L'Harmattan, 2006.

Lehideux-Vernimmen, Raymond. *La naissance de Conakry: Fille du vent et de l'Atlantique*. Paris: L'Harmattan, 2017.

Levy, Jay A. "Isolation of Lymphocytopathic Retroviruses from San Francisco Patients with AIDS." *Science* 225, no. 4664 (August 24, 1984): 840–42.

Lewis, Stephen. *Contre la montre*. Montréal: Leméac / Actes Sud, 2006.

———. *Race against Time: Searching for Hope in AIDS-Ravaged Africa*. Toronto: House of Anansi Press, 2005.

Liotta, Giuseppe, Sandro Mancinelli, Karin Nielsen-Saines, E. Gennaro, Paola Scarcella, Nurja Abdul Magid, Paola Germano, et al. "Reduction of Maternal Mortality with Highly Active Antiretroviral Therapy in a Large Cohort of HIV-Infected Pregnant Women in Malawi and Mozambique." *PLoS One* 8, no. 8 (August 19, 2013).

Lockman, Shahin, Roger L. Shapiro, Laura M. Smeaton, Carolyn Wester, Ibou Thior, Lisa Stevens, Fatima Chand, et al. "Response to Antiretroviral Therapy after a Single, Peripartum Dose of Nevirapine." *New England Journal of Medicine* 356 (January 11, 2007): 135–47.

Marazzi, Maria C. "DREAM: Le idee—guida." In DREAM, Comunità di Sant'Egidio, *Comunità e Salute*, 5–14.

———. "Presentation." In DREAM, Comunità di Sant'Egidio, *We Want to Live, Too!*, 110–27.

Marazzi, Maria C., G. Guidotti, Giuseppe Liotta, and Leonardo Palombi. *DREAM: An Integrated Faith-Based Initiative to Treat HIV/AIDS in Mozambique; Case Study*. Perspectives and Practice in Antiretroviral Treatment. Geneva: WHO, 2005.

Marazzi, Maria C., Giuseppe Liotta, Karin Nielsen-Saines, Jere Haswell, Nurja A. Magid, Ersilia Buonomo, Paola Scarcella, Anna M. Doro Altan, Sandro Mancinelli, and Leonardo Palombi. "Extended Antenatal Antiretroviral Use Correlates with Improved Infant Outcomes throughout the First Year of Life." *AIDS* 24, no. 18 (November 27, 2010): 2819–26.

Marazzi, Maria C., Karin Nielsen-Saines, Ersilia Buonomo, Paola Scarcella, Paola Germano, Nuria Abdul Majid, Ines Zimba, Susanna Ceffa, and Leonardo Palombi. "Increased Infant Human Immunodeficiency Virus-Type One Free

Survival at One Year of Age in Sub-Saharan Africa with Maternal Use of Highly Active Antiretroviral Therapy during Breastfeeding." *Pediatric Infectious Disease Journal* 28, no. 6 (July 2009): 483–87.

Marazzi, Maria C., Leonardo Palombi, E. Gennaro, Ersilia Buonomo, Paola Scarcella, Sandro Mancinelli, Anna M. Doro Altan, Susanna Ceffa, T. Staniscia, and Giuseppe Liotta. "Epidemia da HIV/AIDS: Il potenziale ruolo protettivo della HAART (Highly Active Antiretroviral Therapy) nel controllo della mortalità materna. Risultati del Programma DREAM." Proceedings of the 12th National Public Health Conference, Rome, October 12–15, 2011.

Marazzi, Maria C., Leonardo Palombi, and Karin Nielsen-Saines "Favorable Pregnancy Outcomes with Reduction of Abortion, Stillbirth, and Prematurity Rates in a Large Cohort of HIV+ Women in Southern Africa Receiving Highly Active Anti-retroviral Therapy (HAART) for Prevention of Mother-Child-Transmission (PMTCT)." Proceedings of the 5th IAS Conference on HIV Pathogenesis, Treatment and Prevention, Cape Town, July 19–22, 2009.

Marazzi, Maria C., Leonardo Palombi, Karin Nielsen-Saines, Jere Haswell, Ines Zimba, Nurja A. Magid, Ersilia Buonomo, et al. "Extended Antenatal Use of Triple Antiretroviral Therapy for Prevention of Mother-to-Child Transmission of HIV-1 Correlates with Favorable Pregnancy Outcomes." *AIDS* 25, no. 13 (August 24, 2011): 1611–18.

Marazzi, Maria C., M. Bartolo, Leonardo Emberti Gialloreti, Paola Germano, G. Guidotti, Giuseppe Liotta, Massimo Magnano San Lio, et al. "Improving Adherence to HAART in Africa: The DREAM Programme in Mozambique." *Health Education Research* 21, no. 1 (February 2006): 34–42.

Marazzi, Maria C., Paola Germano, Giuseppe Liotta, G. Guidotti, S. Loureiro, A. Da Cruz Gomes, M. C. Valls Blazquez, et al. "Safety of Nevirapine-Containing Antiretroviral Triple Therapy Regimens to Prevent Vertical Transmission in an African Cohort of HIV-1-Infected Pregnant Women." *HIV Medicine* 7, no. 5 (May 24, 2006): 338–44.

Marazziti, Mario. *Uno straordinario vivere: Storie di AIDS, solidarietà, speranze.* Casale Monferrato: Piemme 1993.

Marseille, Elliot, Paul B. Hofmann, and James G. Kahn. "HIV Prevention before HAART in Sub-Saharan Africa." *Lancet* 359, no. 9320 (May 25, 2002): 1851–56.

Marshall, Monty G. *Conflict Trends in Africa, 1946–2004: A Macro-Comparative Perspective.* London: Africa Conflict Prevention Pool, Government of the United Kingdom, October 14, 2005. http://www.systemicpeace.org/africa/AfricaCo nflictTrendsMGM2005us.pdf.

Martin, Annalise M., David Nolan, Ian James, Paul Cameron, Jean Keller, Corey Moore, Elizabeth Phillips, Frank T. Christiansen, and Simon Mallal. "Predisposition to Nevirapine Hypersensitivity Associated with HLA-DRB1*01 and Higher CD4+T Cell Counts." *AIDS* 19, no. 1 (February 2005): 97–99.

Martínez, Esteban, José L. Blanco, Juan A. Arnaiz, José B. Pérez-Cuevas, Amanda Mocroft, Anna Cruceta, Ma Angeles Marcos, et al. "Hepatotoxicity in

HIV-1-Infected Patients Receiving Nevirapine-Containing Antiretroviral Therapy." *AIDS* 15, no. 10 (July 6, 2001): 1261–68.

Martini, Carlo Maria. "Vivere e morire di AIDS oggi." In Marazziti, *Uno straordinario vivere*, 5–15.

Matsinhe, Cristiano. *Tábula Rasa: Dinâmica da Resposta Moçambicana ao HIV/SIDA*. Maputo: Texto Editores, 2006.

Mbali, Mandisa. "AIDS Discourses and the South African State: Government Denialism and Post-apartheid AIDS Policy-makers." *Transformation: Critical Perspectives on Southern Africa* 54 (2004): 104–19.

Mbonu, Ngozi C., Bart van den Borne, and Nanne K. De Vries. "Stigma of People with HIV/AIDS in Sub-Saharan Africa: A Literature Review." *Journal of Tropical Medicine* 2009 (August 16, 2009).

Minerva, Daniela, and Stefano Vella. *No AIDS: Globalizzare la salute*. Rome: Avverbi, 2002.

Ministério da Saúde, República de Moçambique. *Mozambique HIV/AIDS Care Initiative*. Maputo: MISAU, 2003.

Moneti, Francesca. "Presentation." In DREAM, Comunità di Sant'Egidio, *We Want to Live, Too!*, 90–108.

Morozzo della Rocca, Roberto. *Mozambique: Achieving Peace in Africa*. Washington, DC: Georgetown University, 2003.

Moyo, Dambisa. *Dead Aid: Why Aid Is Not Working and How There Is Another Way for Africa*. New York: Farrar, Straus & Giroux, 2009.

Mphande, Jane. "DREAM—dalla salute fisica alla 'vita piena': Le attiviste." In DREAM, Comunità di Sant'Egidio, *Comunità e Salute*, 47–56.

Msellati, Philippe, Laurent Vidal, and Jean-Paul Moatti. *L'accès aux traitements du VIH/sida en Côte d'Ivoire: Aspects économiques, sociaux et comportementaux*. Paris: ANS, 2000.

Müller, Olaf, Tumani Corrah, Elly Katabira, Frank Plummer, and David Mabey. "Antiretroviral Therapy in Sub-Saharan Africa." *Lancet* 351, no. 9095 (January 3, 1998): 68.

Mulwo, Abraham K., Keyan G. Tomaselli, and Michael D. Francis. "HIV/AIDS and Discourses of Denial in Sub-Saharan Africa: An Afro-Optimist Response?" *International Journal of Cultural Studies* 15, no. 6 (July 5, 2012): 567–82.

Ndoye, Ibrahim, Isabelle Lanièce, Alice Desclaux, Bernard Taverne, Éric Delaporte, Mounirou Ciss, Pape Salif Sow, and Omar Sylla. "Perspectives." In Desclaux, Lanièce, Ndoye, and Taverne, *L'Initiative sénégalaise d'accès aux médicaments antirétrovirales*, 243–49.

Ndoye, Ibrahim, Bernard Taverne, Alice Desclaux, Isabelle Lanièce, Marc Egrot, Éric Delaporte, Pape Salif Sow, Souleymane Mboup, Omar Sylla, and Mounirou Ciss. "Présentation de l'initiative sénégalaise d'accès aux antirétroviraux." In Desclaux, Lanièce, Ndoye, and Taverne, *L'Initiative sénégalaise d'accès aux médicaments antirétrovirales*, 5–19.

Newell, Marie Louise, Heena Brahmbhatt, and Peter D. Ghys. "Child Mortality

and HIV Infection in Africa: A Review." *AIDS* 18, suppl. 2 (June 1, 2004): 27–34.
Nucita, Andrea, Giuseppe M. Bernava, Michelangelo Bartolo, Fabio Di Pane Masi, Pietro Giglio, Marco Peroni, Giovanni Pizzimenti, and Leonardo Palombi. "A Global Approach to the Management of EMR (Electronic Medical Records) of Patients with HIV/AIDS in Sub-Saharan Africa: The Experience of DREAM Software." *BMC Medical Informatics and Decision Making* 9, no. 42 (September 11, 2009).
ONUSIDA/Sénégal. *Lutte contre le sida: Meilleures pratiques, l'expérience sénégalaise.* Geneva: ONUSIDA, 2001.
Oppenheimer, Gerald, and Ronald Bayer. "Choisir entre la vie et la mort : Le rationnement des soins de santé pendant l'épidémie du sida en Afrique du Sud." In Denis and Becker, *L'épidémie du SIDA en Afrique subsaharienne*, 167–92.
Oppong, Joseph R., and Ezekiel Kalipeni. "Perceptions and Misperceptions of AIDS in Africa." In Kalipeni, Craddock, Oppong, and Ghosh, *HIV and AIDS in Africa beyond Epidemiology*, 47–57.
Oransky, Ivan. "Annalena Tonelli." *Lancet* 362, no. 9399 (December 6, 2003): 1943.
Orlando, Stefano, Maria Cristina Marazzi, Sandro Mancinelli, Giuseppe Liotta, Susanna Ceffa, Pietro Giglio, Ellard Alumando, Isabelle Ziegler, Mary Shawa, and Leonardo Palombi,. "Cost-effectiveness of Using HAART in Prevention of Mother-to-Child Transmission in the DREAM-Project Malawi." *Journal of Acquired Immune Deficiency Syndromes* 55, no. 5 (December 15, 2010): 631–34.
Palombi, Leonardo. "Dove l'AIDS è un flagello incontenibile." *Limes* 5, no. 3 (1997): 121–30.
Palombi, Leonardo, Carlo Federico Perno, and Maria C. Marazzi. "HIV/AIDS in Africa: Treatment as a Right and Strategies for Fair Implementation: False Assumption on the Basis of a Minimalistic Approach." *AIDS* 5, no. 19 (March 25, 2005): 536–37.
Palombi, Leonardo, Giuseppe M. Bernava, Andrea Nucita, Pietro Giglio, Giuseppe Liotta, Karin Nielsen-Saines, Stefano Orlando, et al. "Predicting Trends in HIV-1 Sexual Transmission in Sub-Saharan Africa through the Drug Resource Enhancement against AIDS and Malnutrition Model: Antiretrovirals for Reduction of Population Infectivity, Incidence and Prevalence at the District Level." *Clinical Infectious Diseases* 55, no. 2 (May 21, 2012): 268–75.
Palombi, Leonardo, Karin Nielsen-Saines, Marina Giuliano, and Maria C. Marazzi. "Easier Said than Done: World Health Organization Recommendations for Prevention of Mother-to-Child Transmission of HIV; Areas of Concern." *AIDS Research and Human Retroviruses* 27, no. 8 (August 5, 2011): 807–8.
Palombi, Leonardo, Maria Cristina Marazzi, Albertus Voetberg, and N. Abdul Magid. "Treatment Acceleration Program and the Experience of the DREAM Program in Prevention of Mother-to-Child Transmission of HIV." *AIDS* 21, suppl. 4 (July 2007): 65–71.

Palombi, Leonardo, Maria Cristina Marazzi, Giovanni Guidotti, Paola Germano, Ersilia Buonomo, Paola Scarcella, Annamaria Doro Altan, Ines Da Vitoria M. Zimba, Massimo Magnano San Lio, and Andrea De Luca. "Incidence and Predictors of Death, Retention, and Switch to Second-Line Regimens in Antiretroviral-Treated Patients in Sub-Saharan African Sites with Comprehensive Monitoring Availability." *Clinical Infectious Diseases* 48, no. 1 (January 1, 2009): 115–22.

Parkhurst, Justin O. "The Ugandan Success Story? Evidence and Claims of HIV-1 Prevention." *Lancet* 360, no. 9326 (July 6, 2002): 78–80.

Pépin, Jacques. *The Origins of AIDS*. Cambridge: Cambridge University Press, 2011.

———. "The Origins of AIDS: From Patient Zero to Ground Zero." *Journal of Epidemiology and Community Health* 67, no. 6 (June 2013): 473–75.

Peroni, Marco, and Michelangelo Bartolo. "The Digital Divide." In Bartolo and Ferrari, *Multidisciplinary Teleconsultation in Developing Countries*, 101–9.

Piot, Peter. *No Time to Lose: A Life in Pursuit of Deadly Viruses*. New York: Norton, 2012.

Pitchenik, Arthur E., Margaret A. Fischl, Gordon M. Dickinson, Daniel M. Becker, Arthur M. Fournier, Mark T. O'Connell, Robert D. Colton, and Thomas J. Spira. "Opportunistic Infections and Kaposi's Syndrome among Haitians: Evidence of a New Acquired Immunodeficiency State." *Annals of Internal Medicine* 98, no. 3 (March 1983): 277–84.

Prendergast, Andrew J., Gareth Tudor-Williams, Prakash Jeena, Sandra Burchett, and Philip Goulder. "International Perspectives, Progress, and Future Challenges of Paediatric HIV Infection." *Lancet* 370, no. 9581 (July 7, 2007): 68–80.

Pridmore, Pat, and Roy Carr-Hill. *Addressing the Underlying and Basic Causes of Child Undernutrition in Developing Countries: What Works and Why?* Copenhagen: Ministry of Foreign Affairs of Denmark, 2009.

Putzel, James. "Histoire d'une action d'état: La lutte contre le sida en Ouganda et au Sénégal." In Denis and Becker, *L'épidémie du sida en Afrique subsaharienne*, 245–70.

———. "The Politics of Action on AIDS: A Case Study of Uganda." *Public Administration and Development* 24, no. 1 (February 2004): 19–30.

Quammen, David. *Spillover: Animal Infections and the Next Human Pandemic*. London: Vintage Books, 2013.

Ramsey, Sarah. "Global Fund Makes Historic First Round of Payments." *Lancet* 359, no. 9317 (May 4, 2002): 1581–82.

Rankin, William W., Sean Brennan, Ellen Schell, Jones Laviwa, and Sally H. Rankin. "The Stigma of Being HIV-Positive in Africa." *PLoS Medicine* 2, no. 8 (August 2005).

Resch, Stephen, Eline Korenromp, John Stover, Matthew Blakley, Carleigh Krubiner, Kira Thorien, Robert Hecht, and Rifat Atun. "Economic Returns to Investment in AIDS Treatment in Low and Middle Income Countries." *PLoS One* 6, no. 10 (October 5, 2011).

Robberstad, Bjarne, and Bjørg Evjen-Olsen. "Preventing Mother to Child

Transmission of HIV with Highly Active Antiretroviral Treatment in Tanzania: A Prospective Cost-effectiveness Study." *Journal of Acquired Immune Deficiency Syndromes* 55, no. 3 (November 2010): 397–403.

Robins, Steven. "From 'Rights' to 'Ritual': AIDS Activism in South Africa." *American Anthropologist* 2, no. 108 (June 2006): 312–23.

Rushing, William A. *The AIDS Epidemic: Social Dimension of an Infectious Disease.* Boulder: Westview, 1995.

Rushton, J. Philippe, and Anthony F. Bogaert. "Population Differences and Susceptibility to AIDS: An Evolutionary Analysis." *Social Science and Medicine* 28, no. 12 (1989): 1211–20.

Sachs, Jeffrey. "The End of AIDS." Project Syndicate, November 29, 2016. https://www.project-syndicate.org/commentary/end-of-aids-epidemic-by-jeffrey-d-sachs-2016-11.

———. "The Links of Public Health and Economic Development." Lecture, Office of Health Economics, London, 2001. https://www.ohe.org/publications/links-public-health-and-economic-development/.

Schwartländer, Bernhard, Ian Grubb, and Jos Perriëns. "The 10-Year Struggle to Provide Antiretroviral Treatment to People with HIV in the Developing World." *Lancet* 368, no. 9534 (August 5, 2006): 541–46.

Schwartländer, Bernhard, John Stover, Neff Walker, Lori Bollinger, Juan Pablo Gutierrez, William McGreevey, Margaret Opuni, et al. "Resource Needs for HIV/AIDS." *Science* 292, no. 5526 (June 29, 2001): 2434–36.

Scrimshaw, Nevin Stewart, Carl Ernest Taylor, John Everett Gordon, and World Health Organization. *Interactions of Nutrition and Infection.* Monograph Series no. 37. Geneva: WHO, 1968.

Selgelid, Michael J. "Ethics, Economics, and AIDS in Africa." *Developing World Bioethics* 4, no. 1 (April 8, 2004): 96–105.

Setel, Philip W., Milton Lewis, and Maryinez Lyons, eds. *Histories of Sexually Transmitted Diseases and HIV/AIDS in Sub-Saharan Africa.* Westport, CT: Greenwood, 1999.

Shah, Maunank, Benjamin Johns, Alash'Le Abimiku, and Damian Walker. "Cost-effectiveness of New WHO Recommendations for Prevention of Mother-to-Child Transmission of HIV in a Resource-Limited Setting." *AIDS* 25, no. 8 (May 2011): 1093–1102.

Shearer, William T., Thomas C. Quinn, Philip LaRussa, Judy F. Lew, Lynne Mofenson, Susan Almy, Kenneth Rich, et al. "Viral Load and Disease Progression in Infants Infected with Human Immunodeficiency Virus Type." *New England Journal of Medicine* 19, no. 336 (May 8, 1997): 1337–42.

Shelton, James D., and Beverly Johnston. "Condom Gap in Africa: Evidence from Donor Agencies and Key Informants." *British Medical Journal* 323, no. 7305 (July 21, 2001): 139.

Smith, Robert J. "Adherence to Antiretroviral HIV Drugs: How Many Doses Can You Miss before Resistance Emerges?" *Proceedings of the Royal Society B: Biological Sciences* 1586 (March 7, 2006): 617–24.

Sonntag, Diana. *AIDS and Aid: A Public Good Approach.* Berlin: Springer, 2010.

Spira, Rosemary, Philippe Lepage, Philippe Msellati, Philippe Van de Perre, Valeriane Leroy, Arlette Simonon, Etienne Karita, and François Dabis. "Natural History of Human Immunodeficiency Virus Type 1 Infection in Children: A Five-Year Prospective Study in Rwanda; Mother-to-Child HIV-1 Transmission Study Group." *Pediatrics* 104, no. 5 (November 1999).

Steenberg Olsen, Bent. "Structures of Stigma: Diagonal AIDS Care and Treatment Abandonment in Mozambique." PhD thesis in medical anthropology, Roskilde University, Denmark, 2013.

Stevens, Warren, Steve Kaye, and Tumani Corrah. "Antiretroviral Therapy in Africa." *British Medical Journal* 328, no. 7434 (January 31, 2004): 280–82.

Stillwaggon, Eileen. "Racial Metaphors: Interpreting Sex and AIDS in Africa." *Development and Change* 34, no. 5 (November 2003): 809–32.

Stover, John, Neff Walker, Geoff P. Garnett, Joshua A. Salomon, Karen A. Stanecki, Peter D. Ghys, Nicholas C. Grassly, Roy M. Anderson, and Bernhard Schwartländer. "Can We Reverse the HIV/AIDS Pandemic with an Expanded Response?" *Lancet* 360, no. 9326 (July 6, 2002): 73–77.

Swedish International Development Cooperation Agency, Department for Africa. *Country Analysis Mozambique. September 2001.* Stockholm: SIDCA, 2001.

Sweeney, Rosemary. "The U.S. Push for Worldwide Patent Protection for Drugs Meets the AIDS Crisis in Thailand: A Devastating Collision." *Pacific Rim Law and Policy Journal* 9, no. 2 (May 9, 2000): 445–71.

Thomas, Felicity. "'Our Families Are Killing Us': HIV/AIDS, Witchcraft and Social Tensions in the Caprivi Region, Namibia." *Anthropology and Medicine* 14, no. 3 (December 2007): 279–91.

Uganda Aids Commission. *Twenty Years of HIV in the World: Evolution of the Epidemic and Response in Uganda.* Kampala: Uganda Aids Commission, 2001.

Uganda Ministry of Health, UNAIDS, and CDC. *Preliminary Report: Uganda Ministry of Health–UNAIDS; HIV /AIDS Drug Access Initiative—August 1998–March 2000.* Geneva: UNAIDS, 2000. http://pdf.usaid.gov/pdf_docs/Pnacl448.pdf.

UNAIDS. *Accelerating Access to HIV Care, Support, and Treatment.* Geneva: UNAIDS, 2000.

———. *Collaboration with Traditional Healers in HIV/AIDS Prevention and Care in Sub-Saharan Africa.* Geneva: UNAIDS, 2000.

———. *Global AIDS Update 2016.* Geneva: UNAIDS, 2016.

———. "Global HIV and AIDS Statistics: 2018 Fact Sheet." Accessed June 23, 2019. http://www.unaids.org/en/resources/fact-sheet.

———. *The Global Strategy Framework on HIV/AIDS.* Geneva: UNAIDS, 2001.

———. *Report on the Global HIV/AIDS Epidemic: July 2002.* Geneva: UNAIDS, 2002.

———. *Report on the Global HIV/AIDS Epidemic: June 2000.* Geneva: UNAIDS, 2000.

———. *2004 Report on the Global AIDS Epidemic.* Geneva: UNAIDS, 2004.

———. *2006 Report on the Global AIDS Epidemic.* Geneva: UNAIDS, 2006.

———. *UNAIDS Data 2018.* Geneva: UNAIDS, 2018.

———. *UNAIDS Data 2019.* Geneva: UNAIDS, 2019.

———. *UNAIDS Report on the Global AIDS Epidemic 2012.* Geneva: UNAIDS 2012.
UNAIDS and WHO. *AIDS Epidemic Update: December 2000.* Geneva: UNAIDS/WHO, 2000. https://www.unaids.org/en/resources/fact-sheet.
———. *Report on the Global HIV/AIDS Epidemic: June 1998.* http://data.unaids.org/pub/report/1998/19981125_global_epidemic_report_en.pdf.
UNFPA and UNAIDS. "Report of the Planning Meeting on Strategic Options for HIV/AIDS Advocacy in Africa." 2001. Accessed July 22, 2019. https://www.unfpa.org/sites/default/files/pub-pdf/hiv_africa.pdf.
UNICEF, UNAIDS, and WHO. *Children and AIDS: Second Stocktaking Report; Actions and Progress.* New York: UNICEF, 2008.
UNICEF, WHO, World Bank, and United Nations. *Levels and Trends in Child Mortality: Report 2014.* New York: UNICEF, 2014.
United Nations, "Secretary-General Proposes Global Fund for Fight against HIV/AIDS and Other Infectious Diseases at African Leaders Summit." Press release, April 26, 2001. https://www.un.org/press/en/2001/SGSM7779R1.doc.htm.
United Nations Office for the Coordination of Humanitarian Affairs. "Overview: Focus on Mozambique." PlusNews, December 16, 2004. https://reliefweb.int/report/mozambique/africa-focus-mozambique-art-africa.
United Nations Office of the Special Adviser on Africa. *Community Realities and Responses to HIV/AIDS in Sub-Saharan Africa / La situation et l'action des communautés face au VIH/sida en Afrique subsaharienne.* New York: United Nations, 2003.
van der Vliet, Virginia. "South Africa Divided against AIDS: A Crisis of Leadership." In Kauffman and Lindauer, *AIDS and South Africa,* 48–96.
van Praag, Eric, Susan Fernyak, and Alison Martin Katz, eds. *The Implications of Antiretroviral Treatments: Informal Consultation, Geneva, 29–30 April 1997.* Geneva: WHO, 1997. https://apps.who.int/iris/handle/10665/63608.
Vogel, Gretchen. "Dollar and Cents vs. the AIDS Epidemic." *Science* 292, no. 5526 (June 29, 2001): 2420–22.
Waning, Brenda, Ellen Diedrichsen, Elodie Jambert, Till Bärnighausen, Yun Li, Mieke Pouw, and Suerie Moon. "The Global Pediatric Antiretroviral Market: Analyses of Product Availability and Utilization Reveal Challenges for Development of Pediatric Formulations and HIV/AIDS Treatment in Children." *BMC Pediatrics* 10, no. 74 (October 17, 2010).
Weidle, Paul J., Samuel Malamba, Raymond Mwebaze, Catherine Sozi, Gideon Rukundo, Robert Downing, Debra Hanson, et al. "Assessment of a Pilot Antiretroviral Drug Therapy Programme in Uganda: Patients' Response, Survival, and Drug Resistance." *Lancet* 360, no. 9326 (July 6, 2002): 34–40.
Whiteside, Alan. "Demography and Economics of HIV/AIDS." *British Medical Bulletin* 58, no. 1 (September 1, 2001): 73–88.
———. "Drugs: The Solutions?" *AIDS Analysis Africa.* April/May 2001.
WHO. *Antiretroviral Drugs for Treating Pregnant Women and Preventing HIV Infection in Infants: Guidelines on Care, Treatment and Support for Women Living with HIV/AIDS and Their Children in Resource-Constrained Settings.* Geneva: WHO, 2004.

———. *Antiretroviral Therapy for HIV Infection in Adults and Adolescents: Recommendations for a Public Health Approach; 2006 Revision.* Geneva: WHO, 2006.

———. *Antiretroviral Therapy for HIV Infection in Adults and Adolescents: Recommendations for a Public Health Approach; 2010 Revision.* Geneva: WHO, 2010.

———. *Antiretroviral Therapy of HIV Infection in Infants and Children: Recommendations for a Public Health Approach.* Geneva: WHO 2006.

———. *Antiretroviral Therapy for HIV Infection in Infants and Children: Towards Universal Access; Recommendations for a Public Health Approach—2010 Revision.* Geneva: WHO, 2010.

———. *Antiretroviral Treatment as Prevention (TasP) of HIV and TB: 2012 Update.* Geneva: WHO, June 2012.

———. "Consolidated Guidelines on the Use of Antiretroviral Drugs for Treating and Preventing HIV Infection: Questions and Answers." June 30, 2013. https://www.who.int/hiv/mediacentre/feature_story/hiv_arv2013/en/.

———. *Consolidated Guidelines on the Use of Antiretroviral Drugs for Treating and Preventing HIV Infection: Recommendations for a Public Health Approach, June 2013; Summary of New Recommendations.* Geneva: WHO, 2013.

———. *Consolidated Guidelines on the Use of Antiretroviral Drugs for Treating and Preventing HIV Infection: What's New; November 2015.* Geneva: WHO, 2015.

———. *Guidelines on When to Start Antiretroviral Therapy and on Pre-exposure Prophylaxis for HIV: September 2015.* Geneva: WHO, 2015.

———. *HIV and Infant Feeding. Revised Principles and Recommendations. Rapid Advice.* Geneva: WHO, 2009.

———. *Nutrient Requirement for People Living with HIV/AIDS: Report of a Technical Consultation.* Geneva: WHO, 2003.

———. "Rapid Advice: Use of Antiretroviral Drugs for Treating Pregnant Women and Preventing HIV Infection in Infants." November 2009. https://www.who.int/hiv/pub/mtct/rapid_advice_mtct.pdf.

———. *Scaling Up Antiretroviral Therapy in Resource-Limited Settings: Guidelines for a Public Health Approach.* Geneva: WHO, 2002.

———. *Summary of New Recommendations: Consolidated ARV Guidelines, June 2013; When to Start ART in People Living with HIV (part 1).* Geneva: WHO, 2013.

———. "Treat All People Living with HIV, Offer Antiretrovirals as Additional Prevention Choice for People at 'Substantial' Risk: New Policies Could Help Avert More than 21 Million Deaths and 28 Million New Infections by 2030." News release, September 30, 2015. https://www.who.int/mediacentre/news/releases/2015/hiv-treat-all-recommendation/en/.

———. "What's New in Treatment Monitoring: Viral Load and CD4 Testing." Update July 2017. http://apps.who.int/iris/bitstream/handle/10665/255891/WHO-HIV-2017.22-eng.pdf?sequence=1.

WHO and FAO. *Living Well with HIV/AIDS: A Manual of Nutritional Care and Support for People Living with HIV/AIDS.* Rome: FAO, 2002.

WHO, UNAIDS, and UNICEF. *Towards Universal Access: Scaling Up Priority HIV/AIDS Interventions in the Health Sector; Progress Report 2010.* https://www.afro

.who.int/publications/towards-universal-access-scaling-priority-hivaids-interventions-health-sector.

Williams, A. Olufemi. *AIDS: An African Perspective.* Boca Raton FL: CRC Press, 1992.

Worobey, Michael, Marlea Gemmel, Dirk E. Teuwen, Tamara Haselkorn, Kevin Kunstman, Michael Bunce, Jean-Jacques Muyembe, et al. "Direct Evidence of Extensive Diversity of HIV-1 in Kinshasa by 1960." *Nature* 455, no. 7213 (October 2, 2008): 661–64.

Zhu, Tuofu, B. T. Korber, A. J. Nahmias, E. Hooper, P. M. Sharp, and D. D. Ho. "An African HIV-1 Sequence from 1959 and Implications for the Origin of the Epidemic." *Nature* 391, no. 6667 (February 5, 1998): 594–97.

Zimba, Inês. "In Africa con gli strumenti migliori." In DREAM, Comunità di Sant'Egidio, *Comunità e Salute*, 29–38.

# Index

Accelerating Access Initiative, 58
access for all: breast milk, 243–49; overcoming therapeutic minimalism, 212–23; pediatric AIDS, 231–37; prevention of mother-to-child transmission, 237–43; triple therapy, 249–53; universal access, 223–31
Achmat, Zackie, 27, 176
acquired immunodeficiency syndrome (AIDS), 1; acknowledging as national emergency, 117–18; antitherapy obstinacy, 43–50; breast milk and, 243–49; case numbers, 2; characterizing as "gay plague," 2; collecting data on, 4–5; developments with respect to, 186–87; drug production for, 3; feasibility of treating, 23–24; getting from Léopoldville to United States, 7–9; global health and, 205–8; health care systems and, 60–63; highest rates of, 10–11; history in mind of Western individual, 1–4; investment in treating, 145; legitimizing treatment for, 170; limited resources for, 67–71; malnutrition and, 166–69; as multiplier of poverty, 15; multisectorial prevention, 71–88; 90-90-90 Initiative and, 184–87; ownership and, 187–97; partnership and, 187–97; pediatric AIDS, 231–37; prevention of mother-to-child transmission, 237–43; prevention *versus* treatment, 20–43; as priority concern, 3–4; reacting to lack of therapies for, 116–17; red herring regarding, 14–15; reporting cases in late 1970s, 10–11; resistances in treating, 157–61; sexual promiscuity and, 11–12; spread in sub-Saharan Africa, 11–12; sustainability and, 197–204; as sustainable chronic disease, 13; theories regarding origins of, 5–7; therapeutic management of, 63; traditional healers and, 78–79; and UNAIDS policy, 15–20; waste and scandals, 209n16
activism, 48, 85, 94, 98, 117, 151, 154
activists, 174–76; African, 27n 176n2, 199; becoming, 164–65; DREAM, 157–61; presence of, 80–81
Adler, Michael W., 21–22
*affaire Nevirapine*, 241–42
Africa: activists in, 157–61; and adherence to therapies, 63–67; "African solutions to African problems," 204; breast milk in, 243–49; "complex environment" of, 73; condom usage in, 83–85; fighting AIDS district by district, 229–31; following Cold War, 202–3; gender roles in, 85–88; having children in, 231–37; health care systems in, 60–63; new social and economic dynamics of, 203–4; 90-90-90 Initiative and, 184–87; pediatric AIDS and, 231–37; prevention of mother-to-child transmission in, 237–43; public health doctors, 152–54; reacting to lack of therapies, 116–17; sexual behavior in, 71–72; smartphones in, 203; thinking in scientific terms, 117–20; traditional healers, 77–79; triple therapy in, 249–53
African National Congress (ANC), 29
Afro-optimism, 110n13, 154
Afro-pessimism, 141–50, 207–8, 212
Afwerki, Isaias, 191

287

Agence nationale de recherches sur le sida (ANRS), 25
*AIDS* (journal), 216
*AIDS in the Twenty-First Century*, 46–47
AIDS. *See* acquired immunodeficiency syndrome
Alpha Condé, 161
*aménagement du territoire*, 162
Amin, Idi, 92
ANC. *See* African National Congress
Anderson, Roy, 14–15
Angola, 203
Annan, Kofi, 18, 29–30, 35, 60, 100, 188, 191
ANRS. *See* Agence nationale de recherches sur le sida
antiretroviral drugs, 3, 13, 15, 156, 233; activists and, 158, 162–63; antitherapy obstinacy, 43–44, 47–48; cocktails, 3, 58, 72, 95, 103, 158, 172, 221; condoms and, 83–86; DREAM and, 123–25, 130–32, 135, 137, 142–44, 153, 156; and failure of prevention, 64–70; intermittent therapy, 111n13; malnutrition and, 166–69; negotiating price reductions of, 52n37; prevention *versus* treatment, 20–29, 36, 39, 42; prevention-treatment inseparability and, 101, 104–6; second-line, 101, 156; in Uganda and Senegal, 88–97; unsustainable cost of, 58–60. *See also* highly active antiretroviral therapy (HAART)
*Antiretroviral Treatment as Prevention (TasP) of HIV and TB*, 170, 217
antitherapy obstinacy: controversial studies, 46–49; cost-effectiveness insistence, 47–48; economic analysis, 46–47; HIV as development crisis, 45–46; impossibility of treating AIDS, 43–44; Mozambique and, 126; radical change in perspective, 49–50; strengthening national health care systems, 44–45
*ars moriendi*, 2
Ashe, Arthur, 2
Australia, 221
azidothymidine (AZT), 72, 105, 238, 257n59, 258n79

Bactrim. *See* cotrimoxazole
Banca Intesa, 199
Barnett, Tony, 46–47
Barreto, Avertino, 124
Belgian Congo, 5
Belgium, 221
bilateralism, 188–90
Bill and Melinda Gates Foundation, 32
Blixen, Karen, 63
Blue Panther, 123
body mass index (BMI), 181n79, 181n82
Bortolot, Gabriella, 255n31
Botswana, 10, 15
Boutros-Ghali, Boutros, 18
Brazil, 27, 36, 59, 202
"Break the silence," slogan, 80
breast milk, 240–41, 243–49
British Columbia Centre for Excellence, 43
*British Medical Bulletin*, 46
*British Medical Journal*, 64
Brundtland, Gro Harlem, 30, 60, 100, 188
Burundi, 10, 58
Bush, George W., 38–39
Buvé, Anne, 16–17

Cairo Conference on Population, 37
Cameroon, 58, 196
Carr-Hill, Roy, 167–68
CD4s, 103, 135–36, 164–65, 187, 214, 216–17; identifying, 54n53, 74; universal access, 223–31; viral load measurement and, 219–23
CDC. *See* Centers for Disease Control and Prevention
Ceffa, Susanna, 179n45
Centers for Disease Control and Prevention (CDC), 1, 108
Central African Republic, 10, 196, 266
cervical cancer, 206–7
Chan, Margaret, 188, 228, 253
Chàuque, Luzete, 141
children, pediatric AIDS and, 231–37
Chile, 22
Chirac, Jacques, 21
Chissano, Joaquim, 120–21, 125, 129–33
Churchill, Winston, 1
*Clash of Civilizations, The* (Huntington), 202

INDEX                                                                 289

*Clinical Infectious Diseases*, 229
Clinton Foundation, 221
Clinton, Bill, 39, 60, 116
Clinton, Hillary, 133
cocktails, antiretroviral drugs, 3, 58, 72, 95, 103, 158, 172, 221
Cold War, 202
Combivir, 95
community engagement, 81
Community of Sant'Egidio, 121; base of operations, 261–62; excellence through DREAM, 266–69; first meetings, 125; as fixture in Rome, 261; mediating role in peace accords, 264–65; private meeting at, 130–31; projects of, 262–64; social roots in, 129–30
*Community Realities and Responses to HIV/AIDS in Sub-Saharan Africa*, 76–77
"Condom Gap in Africa," study, 83
condoms, 81–82, 83, 85, 142, 164; condom social marketing, 84. *See also* sexual behavior
Congo River, 6
Consensus Statement on Antiretroviral Treatment for AIDS in Poor Countries, 31–32
coordinators, DREAM, 150–52
corruption, 61, 75, 98–99, 146, 163–64; ownership/partnership and, 188–94
cotrimoxazole (Bactrim), 27, 74–75
COVID-19, 267
Creese, Andrew, 47

*Dead Aid* (Moyo), 191
decentralization, 174
de Cock, Kevin, 188, 216
Democratic Republic of the Congo (DRC), 5, 266; role in spread of HIV, 7–9
Denis, Philippe, 11–12
development cooperation agencies, 25, 28, 43, 63, 116, 118, 124, 127, 131–32, 186, 190, 198, 207, 212, 216, 222, 230, 249
Diogo, Luisa, 133
Diouf, Abdou, 24
directly observed therapy (DOT), 34, 158–59
disability-adjusted life year (DALY), 250, 258n81

DRC. *See* Democratic Republic of the Congo
DREAM. *See* Drug Resource Enhancement against AIDS and Malnutrition
DREAM 2.0, 206. *See also* Drug Resource Enhancement against AIDS and Malnutrition (DREAM)
*DREAM: An Integrated Faith-Based Initiative to Treat HIV/AIDS in Mozambique*, 218–19, 247
Drug Resource Enhancement against AIDS and Malnutrition (DREAM), 177n16; activists and, 157–61; adolescents and, 257n57; Afro-pessimism and, 141–50; Afro-pessimistic objection, 147–48; authorized patients, 131; beginning of, 120–33; breast milk and, 243–49; budget of, 200–202; centers in Africa, 150–51, 154; clashing with ownership, 195–97; coordinators of, 150–52; criticism of, 126–27; defining approach of, 146–47; diagnosis and, 170–71; doctors and, 152–54; dominant international trend before, 116–20; double standards and, 218–19; DREAM 2.0, 206; DREAM-WHO comparison, 215–19; Euro-African synergy, 150–57; European connection, 154–55; Fatoumata Sylla and, 161–66; first years of, 198–99; global health and, 205–8; health diplomacy, 173–74; health education manual produced by, 180n75; information technology, 149–50; laboratories, 122–24; lack of support, 129–30; long-term projects, 148; in Malawi, 199; malnutrition and, 166–69; medical excellence of, 125; minimalist approach and, 170–72; mission of, 142–43; model of good practices, 169–76; mother-to-child transmission, 171–73; Mozambique attitude, 120–22; as NGO, 155–56; nipping in bud, 127–28; operations of, 169–70; origins of, 141–42; overcoming therapeutic minimalism, 212–23; patients of, 146–47, 156–57; pediatric AIDS, 231–37; PMTCT and, 237–43; political and cultural movement, 174–76; presence of, 196; promoting, 127–28; question of treatment, 144–45;

Drug Resource Enhancement against AIDS and Malnutrition (DREAM) (*cont.*) stable interactions, 143–44; sustainability and, 197–204; system of, 148–50; treatment investment, 145–46; triple therapy, 249–53; universal access and, 223–31; viral load measurement and, 219–23; volunteers of, 128–29, 143; WHO protocols and, 174; women and, 155
Duesberg, Peter, 45, 57n104
Durban International AIDS Conference, 27–30
Duvalier, François "Papa Doc," 7
Dybul, Mark, 110n13

*Economist*, 30, 50, 84–85, 241–42
emergency cooperation, 194
Eswatini, 196
ethical principle, invoking, 69–71
Ethiopia, 49, 58, 203
Europe, 2, 12, 41, 47, 82, 105, 120–21, 154, 202–3, 208, 213, 225, 233, 252, 261
European Union, 26, 199
"everyone or no one," position, 69–71

family of the United Nations, 42
FAO. *See* Food and Agriculture Organization
*Financial Times*, 191
Fondazione Cariplo, 199
Food and Agriculture Organization (FAO), 117
food, receiving, 166–69
Francis, Pope, 268–69
FRELIMO. *See* Liberation Front of Mozambique
French Congo, 6
future, looking into, 183–86; global health, 205–8; ownership, 187–97; partnership, 187–97; sustainability, 197–204

Gallo, Robert, 45
Garrido, Ivo Paulo, 174
gay-related immune deficiency (GRID), 1
generic drugs, 59
Germano, Paola, 149–50, 154
Global Fund, 20, 28, 40, 47, 132, 163, 199, 200; applications for, 40–41; creation of, 29–32; financial question and, 101–2
Global Fund to Fight AIDS, Tuberculosis and Malaria, 35
global health, 205–8
Global HIV Prevention Working Group, 85
Global North, 27
Global Programme on AIDS (GPA), 51n31
Global South, 21
Gore, Al, 6
Gottlieb, Michael, 1, 8
GPA. *See* Global Programme on AIDS
grassroots, 75–77, 117, 176
GRID. *See* gay-related immune deficiency
Guidotti, Gianni, 249
Guinea, 61, 161–66, 196, 266

HAART. *See* highly active antiretroviral therapy
Hadja Djéné Condé Foundation, 162
Harvard Medical School, 221; statement from, 31–35
health care systems, inadequacy of, 60–63
Heckler, Margaret, 14
highly active antiretroviral therapy (HAART), 3, 47, 124, 126, 181n86; breast milk and, 243–49; global health and, 205; lowering viral load, 13–14; 90-90-90 Initiative, 184–87; pediatric AIDS and, 231–37; prevention of mother-to-child transmission, 237–43; regime of, 34–35; regimen of, 26; triple therapy, 249–53
HIV Prevention Trials Network (HPTN-52), 229
"HIV Viral Load Monitoring in Resource-Limited Regions: Optional or Necessary?," 221
HIV-2, 11, 89
HIV/AIDS. *See* acquired immunodeficiency syndrome (AIDS); human immunodeficiency virus (HIV)
Hogg, Robert, 43, 57n100
HPTN-52. *See* HIV Prevention Trials Network
Hudson, Rock, 2
human immunodeficiency virus (HIV), 1; 90-90-90 Initiative, 184–87; access for

all, 212–59; antitherapy obstinacy, 43–50; assessing individuals following diagnosis of, 254n21; average life expectancy, 139; babies infected with, 172–73; contesting thesis on origins of, 9–10; figures in 2000, 12–13; global health and, 205–8; highest rates of, 10–11; HIV-2, 11, 89; limited resources for, 67–71; malnutrition and, 166–69; mother-to-child transmission, 171–73; ownership and, 187–97; partnership and, 187–97; pediatric AIDS and, 231–37; predecessor of, 6; prevention of mother-to-child transmission, 237–43; progenitor of, 5; in rich countries, 13; spread in sub-Saharan Africa, 11; sustainability, 197–204; and UNAIDS policy, 15–20; universal access for treating, 223–31; women contracting, 140–41. *See also* acquired immunodeficiency syndrome (AIDS)
Huntington, Samuel, 202

India, 49, 59–60, 66, 202
Initiative sénégalaise d'accès aux antiretroviraux (ISAARV), 24–25
Institute of Tropical Medicine, 16–17
Institute of Tropical Medicine and International Health, 249
International AIDS Conference, 39
International AIDS Society, 216
international development agencies, 12, 22, 27, 61, 94, 124–29
ISAARV. *See* Initiative sénégalaise d'accès aux antiretroviraux
Italian National Institute of Health, 216

John Paul II, Pope, 82
Jong-wook, Lee, 100, 188

Kagame, Paul, 191–92
KAPB. *See* knowledge, attitudes, practices, behaviors
Kawonga, Pacem, 158
Kazatchkine, Michel, 40–41
Kenya, 15, 58, 196, 203, 266
Ki-moon, Ban, 18
Kinshasa, 6, 195

knowledge, attitudes, practices, behaviors (KAPB), 73–74
Kufuor, John, 191

*Lancet*, 21–22, 31, 44–45, 47–48, 49, 184
Lange, Joep, 39
Léopoldville, Belgium, 6
Lesotho, 10, 15
Lewis, Stephen, 37–38, 187–88, 237
Liberation Front of Mozambique (FRELIMO), 120–22, 175
lifelong, term, 40
Lilongwe, Malawi, 99
Limpopo River, 140

Machava-Maputo health center, 131–32
Machel, Samora, 120
Majid, Noorjehan Abdul, 147, 153, 227–30
Malawi, 196, 199, 226–27, 266
malnutrition, 166–69. *See also* Drug Resource Enhancement against AIDS and Malnutrition (DREAM)
Mandela, Nelson, 29, 176n2
Maputo, province, 123–24, 126, 128–32, 134, 141, 149, 153, 161, 266
Marazzi, Cristina, 141, 146–47, 216–18, 252, 263
Marseille, Elliot, 47–48
Marshall, Katherine, 195
Massango, Cacilda, 160–61
Mataka, Elizabeth, 167
Mbeki, Thabo, 29, 45, 111n15, 119, 153, 198
Médecins Sans Frontières (MSF), 104–5, 164
Mercury, Freddie, 2
Millennium Development Goals, UN, 36, 202, 169
Minerva, Daniela, 66
MISAU. *See* Mozambican Ministry of Health
Mocumbi, Pascoal, 125
model, DREAM, 169–76
*Monde diplomatique, Le,* 79–80
Montagnier, Luc, 45
mother-to-child transmission (MTCT), 171–73, 240, 242, 245, 256n42. *See also* prevention of mother-to-child transmission
Moyo, Dambisa, 191

Mozambican Civil War, 120
Mozambican Ministry of Health (MISAU), 123–24, 127–28, 131–33
Mozambican National Resistance (RENAMO), 121
Mozambique, 58, 175, 196, 203, 227; after civil war, 265–66; Ana Maria Muhai in, 133–41; attitude regarding AIDS, 120–22; beginning of DREAM in, 120–33; building molecular biology laboratories in, 131; civil war in, 140; DREAM negative atmosphere, 126–27; introducing HAART, 124; laboratories in, 123–24; obtaining consent from, 129–33; peace accords in, 264–65; prevalence rate in, 121–22; public health system, 128; reaching peace, 121; resources, 125–26; ruling class in, 122; skepticism, 124–25; stigma reigning in, 138–39; treating AIDS free of charge in, 122
Mphande, Jane, 175–76
MSF. *See* Médecins Sans Frontières
MTCT. *See* mother-to-child transmission
Muhai, Ana Maria, 161; AIDS diagnosis of, 134–35; confronting society stigma, 138–39; death of, 139; emotional resurrection of, 137–38; immune system of, 135–36; infection of, 139–41; starting therapy, 136–37; treating in Mozambique, 133–34; winning award, 133
Müller, Olaf, 44
multilateralism, 188–89
multisectorial prevention: activist presence, 80–81; advertising and entertainment, 81–82; civil society reliance, 75–76; community engagement, 81; condoms, 83–85; cotrimoxazole (Bactrim) administration, 74–75; gender roles, 85–88; grassroots action, 75–77; individual behavior, 73–74; outcome of, 71–88; religious institutions, 82–83; sexual behavior, 71–72, 79–80; traditional healer recruitment, 77–79; treating opportunistic infections, 72
Murphy, Eamonn, 36
Museveni, Yoweri, 92–94
Muzumbuka, 5–26

NACOSA. *See* National Conventional on AIDS
Nakajima, Hiroshi, 15–16
Namibia, 15
Narciso, Pasquale, 152
National Conventional on AIDS (NACOSA), 55n64
National Strategic Plan to Fight AIDS, 7
Ndoye, Ibrahim, 24
neocolonialism, 193
Nevirapine, 182n89, 258n79; breast milk and, 245–49; DREAM and, 171–73; and failure of prevention, 68, 105–6; PMTCT and, 238–43; triple therapy and, 249–50
*New England Journal of Medicine*, 58
New Partnership for Africa's Development, 202
*New York Times*, 39–40, 108
Ngangwa, Huberte Bashwa, 85
NGOs. *See* nongovernmental organizations
Nielsen-Saines, Karin, 216
Nigeria, 196, 203, 266
90-90-90 Initiative, 184–87, 207, 226
nongovernmental organizations (NGOs), 61–62, 74–75, 92, 100, 103–4, 113n66, 132, 150, 161, 175, 191, 194, 225, 264–65
nontransmissible diseases, 204
North America, 2, 8, 12, 82, 94, 108, 142, 208, 233, 252
Nureyev, Rudolf, 2

Obote, Milton, 92
Okello, Tito, 92
"One World, One Hope." *See* XI International AIDS Conference
Orlando, Stefano, 226–27, 249–50
*Out of Africa* (Blixen), 63
ownership: clashing with DREAM, 195–97; as criterion, 192; denouncing UN inaction, 187–89; meaning of, 193; in philosophy of international cooperation, 193; preference for, 194–95; UNAIDS and, 193–94; United Nations inaction, 187–92

Palombi, Leonardo, 216–18, 227–30, 249
parallel health care, 159, 196

Paris Declaration, 193
partnership, 147, 154, 187, 194–95, 201
Pasolini, Pier Paolo, 261
Paul VI, Pope, 82
pediatric AIDS, 231–37
PEPFAR. *See* President's Emergency Plan for AIDS Relief
Perno, Carlo Federico, 216–18
pills, 63–65, 108, 158, 166, 233–34, 236
Piot, Peter, 17–19, 28, 48, 52n37, 53n38, 60, 183–84
PMTCT. *See* prevention of mother-to-child transmission
pregnancy, therapy started during, 172–73
President's Emergency Plan for AIDS Relief (PEPFAR), 38–39, 89, 106–7, 200
prevention: Durban conference, 27–30; drug-access initiative results, 25–27; Global Fund creation, 29–32; Harvard statement, 31–35; ignoring lesson about, 37–42; as low-cost activity, 30; organizing UNGASS, 35–37; Senegalese initiative, 23–25; XI International AIDS Conference, 20–24. *See also* prevention of mother-to-child transmission (PMTCT); prevention, arguments in favor of
prevention of mother-to-child transmission (PMTCT), 237–43; Option A/B, 250–51; rapid advice on, 258n79; triple therapy and, 249–53
prevention, arguments in favor of: adherence to therapies, 63–67; antiretroviral drugs costs, 58–60; inadequate health care systems, 60–63; other health emergencies, 67–71. *See also* prevention
prevention, failure of: adherence to therapies, 63–67; inadequate health care systems, 60–63; other health emergencies, 67–71; outcomes, 71–88; success stories, 88–97; treatment and, 98–110; unsustainable cost of antiretroviral drugs, 58–60. *See also* prevention
Pridmore, Pat, 167–68
prophylaxis, 27, 35, 74–75, 142, 240

Qaddafi, Muammar, 94

Reagan, Ronald, 1
RENAMO. *See* Mozambican National Resistance
retroviruses, 3
Riccardi, Andrea, 129–30, 264
Rio Group, 36
Rockefeller Foundation, 32
Rome, Community of Sant'Egidio in, 261–62
Rwanda, 10, 203

Sachs, Jeffrey, 30–35, 79, 183–84, 188, 216
"Safety of Nevirapine-Containing Antiretroviral Triple Therapy," 247–49
sanctuary cells, 186
Sangaré, Hawa, 86–87
Sant'Egidio. *See* Community of Sant'Egidio
Schwartländer, Bernhard, 35, 102
*Science*, 102
Second Vatican Council, 121
Senegal, 23–25, 58; characteristics of, 89; epidemic breaking out in, 90–91; interpreting prevalence data, 91; multisectorial prevention in, 89–90; prevalence rates in, 89; prevention success story of, 88–97
sentinel sites, 50n7
sexual behavior, 71–72, 79–80; condom usage, 83–85; cultural stereotypes, 140–41. *See also* condoms
sexual promiscuity, 11–12
Shikwati, James, 190–91
Sidibé, Michel, 144, 185, 188, 253
Songane, Francisco, 125
South Africa, 10, 15, 198; annual per capita income in, 58; first human-to-human heart transplant in, 125–26; generic antiretroviral drug production, 59–60; responsibility for lack of action, 118–19
Spallanzani Hospital, 152
Steenberg Olsen, Bent, 87–88, 160
*Strategic Options for HIV/ AIDS Advocacy in Africa*, 36–37
sub-Saharan Africa, 4–5, 13, 26; AIDS in, 11–12, 76, 155, 173; antitherapy obstinacy, 43–44, 47–48; countries of, 43, 48,

sub-Saharan Africa (*cont.*)
202; funding in, 47; prevention *versus* treatment, 20–21; resources needed in, 35
sustainability, 197–204
Swaziland, 10, 15, 267
Switzerland, 221
Sylla, Fatoumata, 161–66

Tanzania, 10, 58, 78, 151, 159, 196, 203, 244, 266
test and treat, 170, 187, 222, 226–27, 252–53
Thailand, 26, 59
therapeutic minimalism: authorization from local governments, 215; classifying patients, 214–15; double clinical and diagnostic standard, 218–19; DREAM adopting therapeutic protocols, 213–14; DREAM-WHO comparison, 215–18; overcoming, 170, 212–13, 237, 244; viral load measurement, 219–23
therapy: absence of prospect of, 27–28, 81, 115n76; accepting idea of, 62; access to, 70, 149, 174; adherence to, 63–67; double, 23, 249–50; lines of, 185–86, 219; as prevention, 150, 183–84; responsibility for lack of action to, 116–20; single, 239, 249–50; triple antiretroviral, 3, 21, 31, 44, 53n38, 58, 65, 70, 74, 82, 92, 102, 118, 143, 170–73
3 by 5 Initiative, WHO, 38–42, 47, 65–66, 97, 100–101, 185, 199, 223; economic sustainability of, 106; interpreting, 104; time limit of, 103–4; treatment guaranteed by, 103. *See also* 90-90-90 Initiative; World Health Organization (WHO)
Three Ones, 193–95
Tocqueville, Alexis de, 204
Touré, Ahmed Sékou, 164
*Towards Universal Access: Scaling Up Priority HIV/AIDS Interventions in the Health Sector*, 225
traditional healers, recruiting, 77–79
transactional sex, 178n26
*Treatment Acceleration Program and the Experience of Mother-to-Child Transmission of HIV*, 244

Treatment Action Campaign, 27
treatment, inseparability of prevention and: advocating pragmatic shortcuts, 105–6; economic burden, 106–10; finances, 101–2; Medecins Sans Frontieres, 104–5; side effects, 101; therapy availability, 98–101; 3 by 5 Initiative, 103–4; universal treatment, 106–7
triple antiretroviral therapy, 3, 21, 31, 44, 53n38, 58, 65, 70, 74, 82, 92, 97, 102, 118, 143. *See also* highly active antiretroviral therapy (HAART)
triple therapy, 19–20, 24, 26–27, 35, 40, 43, 262; access for all and, 249–53, 258n79; breast milk and, 243–49; DREAM, 118, 172–74; and failure of prevention, 59, 68, 90, 95–96, 105–6; looking into future, 196. *See also* highly active antiretroviral therapy (HAART)
Turkey, 202

Uganda, 4, 10, 22, 58, 221, 238–39; *ad personam* regime in, 92–93; antiretroviral drugs, 95–97; controlling epidemic in, 97; current data in, 94; infections in, 92; prevention characteristics, 93–94; prevention success story of, 88–97; stopping epidemic in, 92
Ugandan Ministry of Health, 95–96
UNAIDS. *See* United Nations Programme on HIV and AIDS
UNFPA. *See* United Nations Population Fund
UNGASS. *See* United Nations General Assembly
UNICEF. *See* United Nations Children's Fund
Unidea-UniCredit Foundation, 199
United Nations, 7, 186; denouncing inaction of, 187–89; multilateralism of, 188–89; negotiations with, 59–60; representing overcoming nationalism, 188
United Nations Children's Fund (UNICEF), 18–19, 127, 173, 225, 231, 240
United Nations Foundation, 32
United Nations General Assembly

(UNGASS), 35–37, 108–10; UNGASS Resolution 60/224, 225
United Nations Population Fund (UNFPA), 16; lack of success of, 37; *Strategic Options for HIV/AIDS Advocacy in Africa*, 36–37
United Nations Programme on HIV and AIDS (UNAIDS), 15–20, 163; Accelerating Access Initiative, 58; AIDS national committees, 99; broad-ranging statistics, 85; community engagement, 81; cosponsoring agencies, 51–52n33; Dakar government and, 23; denouncing inaction of, 187–88; drug-access initiative of, 22–24; initiative results, 25–27; multisectorial prevention, 71–75; organizing UNGASS, 35–37; sexual behavior, 79–80; *Strategic Options for HIV/AIDS Advocacy in Africa*, 36–37; UNAIDS Board, 41
United States, 1, 7–8, 14; access for all, 213, 223, 225; DREAM and, 161; and failure of prevention, 58–60, 64, 71, 94, 106; looking into future, 189, 192, 202
United States Agency for International Development (USAID), 64
universal access, 223; concept of, 224–26; cost and feasibility of, 226–28; discussion of, 226–27; viral load, 228–29
"Universal Voluntary HIV Testing with Immediate Antiretroviral Therapy as a Strategy for Elimination of HIV Transmission," 227–28
University College London Medical School, 21
US National Institutes of Health, 56n87, 238–39
USAID. *See* United States Agency for International Development

Vancouver, XI International AIDS Conference in, 20–24
Vella, Stefano, 66, 216
Vietnam, 22
viral load, 50n5, 142; breast milk and, 243–44, 248; defined, 50n5; high viral load, 177n10, 217, 219; measurement of, 124, 128–29, 142, 171, 219–23; laboratory test, 177n10; lowering, 13–14, 33–34; PMTCT and, 239–40; prevention-treatment inseparability, 98, 102–3; sanctuary cells and, 186; testing, 219, 221, 254n11, 254n21, triple therapy and, 249–51; universal access and, 228–29

West Africa, 10, 164, 166
Whiteside, Alan, 45
WHO. *See* World Health Organization
Wolfensohn, James, 38–40
women: as activists, 157; DREAM centers run by, 155; mother-to-child transmission, 171–73. *See also* condoms; sexual behavior
World AIDS Day, 237
World Bank, 25, 38, 107, 195, 204; opposite of, 31
World Day of Prayer for Peace, 265–66
World Food Programme, 199
World Health Organization (WHO), 4; breast milk and, 243–49; classifying HIV/AIDS patients, 214; Commission on Macroeconomics and Health, 30; DREAM-WHO comparison, 215–19; Massive Attack on Diseases of Poverty, 30–31; 90-90-90 Initiative, 184–87; prevention of mother-to-child transmission, 237–43; promoting quality treatment, 197; taking brakes off of, 42–43; 3 by 5 Initiative, 38–42; triple therapy, 249–53; and UNAIDS policy, 15–20; universal access and, 223–31; viral load measurement, 220–23

XI International AIDS Conference, 20–24

Zaire, 5, 10, 52n37
Zambesi River, 140
Zambia, 4, 10, 15, 191, 203
Zimbabwe, 4, 10, 15
Zuma, Jacob, 119, 176n3
Zuppi, Matteo, 129–30, 264–65

## About the Author

Roberto Morozzo della Rocca is a professor of contemporary history at the Roma Tre University. For the last thirty years he has studied the theme of war and peace in contemporary Europe, Africa, and Latin America. He is the author of fifteen books in Italian, some of which have been translated into English and other languages.